Substance Abuse: Commonly Abused Substances and the Addiction Process

Second Edition

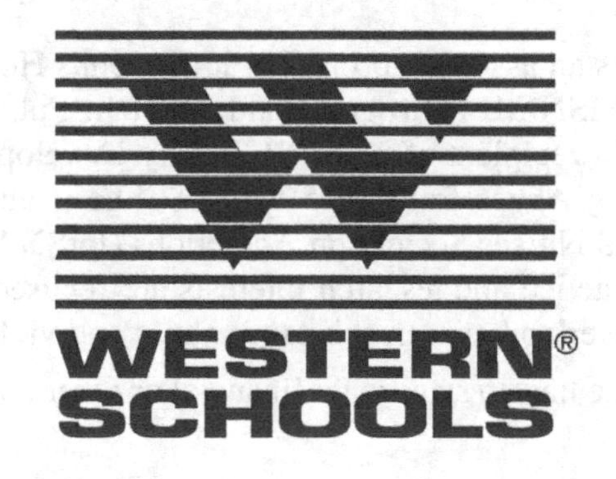

By

Benita Walton-Moss, DNS, APRN, BC
Kathleen Becker, MS, CRNP
Joan Kub, PhD, MA, APRN, BC
Kathleen Woodruff, MS, APRN, BC

Upon successful completion of this course, continuing education hours will be awarded as follows:

Social Workers, Counselors, Marriage and Family Therapists: 13 Clock Hours

Nurses: 32 Contact Hours*

*Western Schools is accredited as a provider of continuing nursing education by the American Nurses Credentialing Center's Commission on Accreditation.

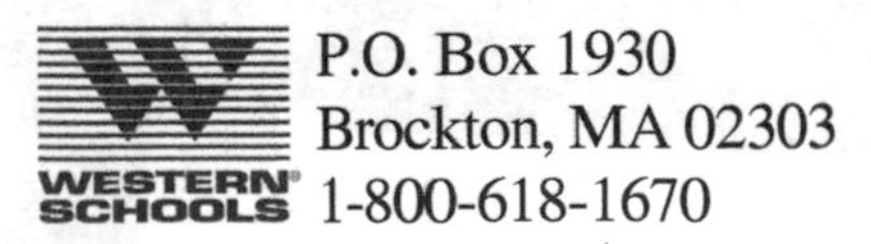
P.O. Box 1930
Brockton, MA 02303
1-800-618-1670

ABOUT THE AUTHORS

Benita Walton-Moss, DNS, APRN, BC, received her Bachelor's degree in Nursing from the Johns Hopkins University School of Health Services, Baltimore, in 1978. Her Master's in Nursing was obtained from the University of Rochester in 1982, during which time she was also prepared as a family nurse practitioner. She earned her Doctorate of Nursing Science from the University of California, San Francisco, in 1994. She is currently an assistant professor at the Johns Hopkins University School of Nursing. Dr. Walton-Moss delivers gynecologic care to women participating in a substance abuse clinic. Her area of research is women with substance abuse and intimate partner violence.

Dr. Benita Walton-Moss has disclosed that she has no significant financial or other conflicts of interest pertaining to this course book.

Kathleen Becker, MS, CRNP, is an assistant professor and an adult nurse practitioner (ANP) at the Johns Hopkins University School of Nursing in Baltimore. She is the coordinator of the Adult Nurse Practitioner Program and maintains a clinical practice at Health Care for the Homeless in Baltimore. She is currently a member of the Content Expert Panel for the Adult Nurse Practitioner Exam at The American Nurses Credentialing Center; a member of the review panel for *The Journal of Nursing Education;* and a member of the editorial board of the *Journal of Advanced Studies in Nursing,* Johns Hopkins Nursing. In 2006, she received the American Association of Colleges of Nursing Graduate End-of-Life Nursing Education Consortium (ELNEC) training for advance practice nurses award and, in 2004, received the American Academy of Nurse Practitioners State Award for Excellence in Maryland. Ms. Becker is actively involved in clinical practice with patients who have substance use disorders (SUDs) and lectures on the topics of screening and treating patients with SUDs.

Kathleen Becker has disclosed that she has no significant financial or other conflicts of interest pertaining to this course book.

Joan Kub, PhD, MA, APRN, BC, is an associate professor at the Johns Hopkins University School of Nursing, in Baltimore. She coordinates the MSN/MPH program and MSN in Public Health Nursing programs at the Johns Hopkins University. She was a recipient of a CSAP Faculty Development Fellowship for the Prevention of Alcohol, Tobacco, and Other Drug Abuse from 1995 to 1998. She is an active member of the research and policy committees of the International Nurses Society on Addictions (IntSNA) and is on the editorial board of the *Journal of Addictions Nursing.* Her practice and research interests are focused on the prevention of substance use in children and adolescents and the overlap between substance abuse and violence.

Dr. Joan Kub has disclosed that she has no significant financial or other conflicts of interest pertaining to this course book.

Kathleen Woodruff, MS, APRN, BC, received her Bachelor's degree in Nursing from the University of Maryland School of Nursing in 1981. Her Master's degree in Nursing was obtained from the University of Maryland School of Nursing in 1987. Her advanced degree prepared her as an adult nurse practitioner. She is currently an instructor at the Johns Hopkins University School of Nursing in Baltimore. She is currently working as a nurse practitioner, serving clients in the areas of substance abuse and HIV care.

Kathleen Woodruff has disclosed that she has no significant financial or other conflicts of interest pertaining to this course book.

ISBN: 978-1-57801-494-1

P.O. Box 1930
Brockton, MA 02303
1-800-618-1670 WESTERN SCHOOLS

ABOUT THE SUBJECT MATTER REVIEWERS

Lynette Jack, PhD, RN, CARN, has a Master's degree in Psychiatric/Mental Health Nursing and has been certified in addictions nursing. She has worked clinically in addictions treatment. She authored several texts in addictions nursing, and has served in elected office for the International Nurses Society on Addictions and the International Society of Psychiatric-Mental Health Nurses. Currently the Director of Accelerated Health Programs for Waynesburg College in Pennsylvania, which includes undergraduate, master's, and doctoral programs in nursing, Lynette has taught courses on addictions at undergraduate and graduate levels. She is an associate editor for the *Journal of Addictions Nursing* and a frequent presenter on topics related to addictions.

Dr. Lynette Jack has disclosed that she has no significant financial or other conflicts of interest pertaining to this course book.

Lori Holleran Steiker, PhD, CISW, ACSW, was an addictions therapist for more than 12 years. During her doctoral program at Arizona State University, Phoenix, she transitioned to research on adolescent substance abuse and prevention. She helped design and evaluate the model Drug Resistance Strategies Project's "Keepin' It REAL" curriculum and is presently working on a study of culturally grounded adaptations of that curriculum for high-risk youth in community settings. She is an associate professor at the University of Texas at Austin School of Social Work and was awarded a Mentored Research Scientist Development Award from the National Institute on Drug Abuse. She is the recent recipient of the Deborah K. Padgett Early Career Achievement Award given by the Society for Social Work and Research.

Dr. Lori Holleran Steiker has disclosed that she has no significant financial or other conflicts of interest pertaining to this course book.

Nurse Planner: Amy Bernard, MS, BSN, RN-BC

Behavioral Health Planners: Julie Guillemin, MSW, LICSW and Lys Hunt, MSW, LICSW

The planners have disclosed that they have no significant financial or other conflicts of interest pertaining to this course book.

Copy Editor: Tracy S. Diehl

Editor: Anne Manton, PhD, RN

Indexer: Sylvia Coates/Mary Kidd

IMPORTANT: PLEASE READ!

To begin this course, take the PRETEST on page xix of this book

Before starting Chapter 1:

Refer to the accompanying instruction booklet for instructions to assist you in completing this course and receiving your continuing education credits.

CONTENTS

FIGURES AND TABLES

Chapter 12

Chapter 13

Chapter 14

Chapter 15

Chapter 16

Chapter 17

PRETEST

1. Begin this course by taking the pretest. Circle the answers to the questions on this page, or write the answers on a separate sheet of paper. Do not log answers to the pretest questions on the FasTrax test sheet included with the course.
2. Compare your answers to the PRETEST KEY located at the end of the Pretest. The pretest key indicates the chapter where the content of that question is discussed. Make note of the questions you missed, so that you can focus on those areas as you complete the course.
3. Complete the course by reading the chapters and completing the exam questions at the end of each chapter. Answers to these exam questions should be logged on the FasTrax test sheet included with the course.

Note: Choose the one option that BEST answers each question.

1. A commonly used survey that provides data on recent trends in substance abuse among youth is the
   a. Monitoring the Future Survey.
   b. National Hospital Discharge Survey.
   c. National Survey of Children with Special Health Care Needs.
   d. National Survey on Health.

2. The group, *Adult Children of Alcoholics,* is an example of a prevention program that targets an at-risk subgroup within a larger population. This type of program is known as a(an)
   a. universal program.
   b. selective program.
   c. indicated program.
   d. primary prevention program.

3. A 10-item alcohol screening tool that can be used either by an interviewer or as a self-report is known as the
   a. CAGE-AID.
   b. DAST.
   c. MAST.
   d. AUDIT.

4. The initial phase of treatment where the client is withdrawn from substances is known as
   a. detoxification.
   b. treatment.
   c. continuing care.
   d. after care.

5. According to the Quadrants of Care model, the most appropriate setting for treating clients with a co-occurring substance abuse disorder and psychiatric condition that are both classified as less severe is
   a. the primary health care setting.
   b. the mental health system.
   c. the substance abuse system.
   d. a state hospital or prison.

6. The leading cause of preventable death and disability in the United States results from the use of
   a. cocaine.
   b. cannabis.
   c. nicotine.
   d. opioids.

7. The most common source of caffeine among children is
   a. chocolate.
   b. iced tea.
   c. coffee.
   d. soft drinks.

8. The National Institute on Alcohol Abuse and Alcoholism defines moderate drinking for healthy women as no more than a daily intake of
   a. one drink.
   b. two drinks.
   c. three drinks.
   d. four drinks.

9. Results of the Cannabis Youth Treatment study showed
   a. low rates of treatment completion and follow-up after therapy.
   b. improvements in days of abstinence and the percent of adolescents in recovery.
   c. motivational enhancement therapy is not an effective treatment for addiction.
   d. medications are effective in the treatment of marijuana abuse.

10. A street name for powder cocaine is
    a. fizzies.
    b. speed.
    c. snow.
    d. meth.

11. Methamphetamine differs from cocaine in that methamphetamine
    a. is derived from a plant.
    b. has medical use as a local anesthetic in many surgeries.
    c. is evacuated from the body within 1 hour.
    d. causes a high that lasts significantly longer than cocaine.

12. Codeine is classified as a(n)
    a. artificial opioid.
    b. natural opioid.
    c. semi-synthetic opioid.
    d. synthetic opioid.

13. A life threatening physical sign commonly associated with opioid overdose is
    a. heart failure.
    b. high fever and chills.
    c. decreased respirations.
    d. dilated pupils.

14. Alcohol is in the class of drugs known as a
    a. depressant.
    b. stimulant.
    c. designer drug.
    d. hallucinogen.

15. The inhalation of vapors from plastic bags containing a substance is called
    a. sniffing.
    b. snorting.
    c. huffing.
    d. bagging.

16. According to the National Survey on Drug Use and Health, new inhalant users are predominantly
    a. younger than 18 years old.
    b. 20 to 30 years old.
    c. 30 to 50 years old.
    d. older than 50 years old.

17. Which statement regarding the effects of LSD is correct?

    a. LSD does not produce tolerance so users generally stay with a set dose.
    b. LSD is not considered a physically or psychologically addictive drug.
    c. There are significant withdrawal symptoms when stopping LSD.
    d. Death related to an LSD overdose is common.

18. A date rape designer drug that renders its users incapacitated and later causes amnesia is

    a. LSD.
    b. PCP.
    c. rohypnol.
    d. Ecstasy.

19. A common steroid dosing technique where individuals use several different steroids to maximize the effect on muscle size is

    a. cycling.
    b. pyramiding.
    c. stacking the pyramid.
    d. stacking.

20. The prevalence of substance abuse among health care professionals

    a. is less than the general population.
    b. is equal to the general population.
    c. is greater than the general population.
    d. has never been studied.

PRETEST KEY

1.	a	Chapter 1
2.	b	Chapter 2
3.	d	Chapter 3
4.	a	Chapter 4
5.	a	Chapter 4
6.	c	Chapter 5
7.	d	Chapter 6
8.	a	Chapter 7
9.	b	Chapter 8
10.	c	Chapter 9
11.	d	Chapter 10
12.	b	Chapter 11
13.	c	Chapter 11
14.	a	Chapter 12
15.	d	Chapter 13
16.	a	Chapter 13
17.	b	Chapter 14
18.	c	Chapter 15
19.	d	Chapter 16
20.	b	Chapter 17

INTRODUCTION

COURSE OBJECTIVES

After completing this course, the learner will be able to:

1. Describe the epidemiology of substance use in the United States.
2. Discuss the concepts and principles of preventing substance abuse.
3. Describe components of a substance abuse assessment.
4. Distinguish among the various substances used.
5. Identify the effects of various substances on the body.
6. Describe the clinical considerations for clients with substance use disorders.
7. Summarize treatment approaches for a drug-dependent client.
8. Discuss the scope of substance use among health care professionals.

Substance abuse is a major public health concern that is directly linked to the top health problems in our country, including cancer, heart disease, and HIV/AIDS. The 2011 National Survey on Drug Use and Health reported that among the civilian, noninstitutionalized population of the United States aged 12 years old or older, 8.7% reported current use of illicit drugs; 26.5% currently used tobacco products; and 51.8% reported current alcohol use, with close to 6.2% reporting heavy drinking (Substance Abuse and Mental Health Services Administration, 2012).

Substance use is also directly related to America's top social problems, including drunk driving, violence, stress, and child abuse – at an estimated cost of more than $600 billion annually (National Institute on Drug Abuse [NIDA], 2012). It is a problem that affects individuals, families, and communities.

The overall purpose of this course is to provide healthcare professionals with a comprehensive overview of substance abuse and the addiction process, including the knowledge and skills necessary to comprehensively and holistically care for a substance-abusing patient; awareness of the prevalence of substance abuse problems; skills to identify substance-abusing patients; knowledge of strategies to prevent and treat substance abuse problems; and resources to further develop professional skills in providing care for patients with substance use disorder.

The recently published *Diagnostic and Statistical Manual of Mental Disorders*, 5th edition (*DSM-5*) organizes substance-related disorders in the diagnostic categories of substance use disorder, substance intoxication, substance withdrawal, and substance-induced disorder for each of the commonly used substances. Modifiers are also included to assess level of severity and stage of remission. These diagnoses replace the previously used terms substance abuse and substance dependence. The content of the course focuses on the epidemiology of addiction, sociocultural influences, commonly used substances, and current standards of care. Information is provided on prevention practices, assessment, and therapeutic treatment modalities, including pharmacological, psychological, group, and non-traditional therapies. Twelve types of substances are described, including their history, biochemistry, and effects on functioning.

References for Introduction

American Psychiatric Association. (2013). *Diagnostic and statistical manual of mental disorders* (5th ed.). Washington, DC: American Psychiatric Association.

Substance Abuse and Mental Health Services Administration. (2012). *Results from the 2011 National survey on drug use and health: Summary of national findings* (NSDUH Series H-44, HHS Publication No. (SMA) 12-4713.). Rockville, MD. Retrieved from http://www.samhsa.gov/data/NSDUH/2k11Results/NSDUHresults2011.htm#Fig3-1

National Institute on Drug Abuse. (2012). *Trends and statistics*. Retrieved from http://www.drugabuse.gov/related-topics/trends-statistics

CHAPTER 1

EPIDEMIOLOGY OF SUBSTANCE ABUSE

CHAPTER OBJECTIVE

After completing this chapter, the learner will be able to discuss the value and relevance of epidemiology for understanding substance use and abuse in the United States.

LEARNING OBJECTIVES

After studying this chapter, the learner will be able to:

1. Define epidemiology and related terms as they pertain to substance abuse.
2. Discuss the value of epidemiology in the field of substance abuse prevention.
3. Describe and compare methods for collecting epidemiological data on substance use and abuse patterns.
4. Define epidemiological trends of substance use and abuse in various populations.

OVERVIEW

Epidemiology is defined as a branch of medical science that deals with the incidence, distribution, and control of disease in a population. It is also the sum of the factors controlling the presence or absence of a disease or pathogen (Merriam Webster Online Dictionary, 2013). It is a field that is concerned with determining the nature of health problems, the characteristics of the population affected with these health problems, and the environmental conditions uniquely associated with such health issues or affected populations (Sloboda, 2002). The distinct difference between medical professionals (such as physicians) and epidemiologists is the focus of their efforts. Physicians are concerned with individuals, while epidemiologists gather data on the health of a population within an environmental context. Epidemiologists are often concerned with incidence rates (the rates at which people without a disease develop the disease during a specific time) and prevalence rates (the rate of people in a population who have a disease at a given time). The data gathered through the efforts of epidemiologists are used to plan prevention and treatment services.

Drug abuse epidemiology is a relatively new field that focuses on the type of drug used and the frequency of drug use in a certain period (Sloboda, 2002). Epidemiologists study risk factors associated with drug use and abuse, the identification of use and abuse phases, age at onset, and outcomes of use (such as overdoses and motor vehicle crashes). The purpose of this chapter is to describe the use of epidemiology in the study of substance use and abuse patterns in various populations. The chapter will compare various methods of collecting data and monitoring substance use and abuse; briefly discuss epidemiological trends of substance use; and discuss the value and uses of epidemiological data in the substance abuse field.

VALUE OF EPIDEMIOLOGY

Epidemiology is valuable because it helps us to identify risk factors and trends in use and abuse. This knowledge is critical in the decision-making process for resolving substance abuse problems. The U.S. Public Health Service and state health agencies use data to estimate the need for drug treatment facilities. Other federal, state, and local agencies use the information to support their drug use prevention programs and to monitor drug control strategies.

In many cases, combining data yields useful information. Combining information from such resources as the Monitoring the Future (MTF) survey regarding the use of a particular drug, and information from the Federal Bureau of Investigation's (FBI) Uniform Crime Reports regarding arrests for possession of that drug, may provide valuable data about the enforcement of laws. In other cases, information obtained from combining substance use levels with risk factor data can be used in prevention strategies. For example, the MTF survey asks about perceptions of harm from drug use. These data can be combined with information about actual use to determine if there are any relationships between the two. This may then help to guide prevention efforts.

Epidemiological studies inform us about the consequences of use. In many cases, developmental issues are of importance. For example, early onset of marijuana use is linked to more frequent use of marijuana, which is sustained by less time spent with parents and more time with drug-using peers (Best et al., 2005).

In other studies, the relevance of culture in understanding substance use is examined. In a study of 1,494 African American youth in grades 5 through 12 in Alabama, results suggest prevention efforts should include an emphasis on modeling attitudes, preventing gang and family violence, encouraging parental supervision, building positive teacher-student interactions and building positive school environments (Wright & Fitzpatrick, 2004). In a study of Mexican American, Puerto Rican, Cuban American, and other Latin American eighth-grade students, drug use was significantly higher in boys who did not live with both parents. Other risk factors included language first spoken, parental education, urbanicity, and region of the country (Delva et al., 2005).

MONITORING SUBSTANCE USE AND ABUSE

There are two approaches to monitoring drug abuse. These include collecting existing data to determine drug use patterns within drug using populations (surveillance) and using surveys to estimate the incidence and prevalence of abuse within a general population. Surveillance collects information from existing or archival data systems that reflect the consequences of drug abuse, such as drug abuse treatment, arrest reports for adults or adolescents, hospital emergency department visits, hospital discharge information, mortality information, and infectious disease reports (Slobada, 2002). Surveys are snapshots of drug abuse in a defined population.

Surveillance

The Community Epidemiology Work Group (CEWG) is one example of a surveillance system. Established in 1976, CEWG is a network composed of researchers from major metropolitan areas of the United States and selected foreign countries. Through this program, the CEWG provides current descriptive and analytical information regarding the nature and patterns of drug abuse, emerging trends, characteristics of vulnerable populations, and social and health consequences (National Institute on Drug Abuse [NIDA], 2009). The group meets biannually to review epidemiologic and ethnographic data from 20 U.S. metropolitan areas. They rely on multiple sources of data, including drug abuse treatment admissions and discharges; drug-related deaths; drug-exposed newborns; emergency department visits; public health data; acquired immunodeficiency syndrome (AIDS) cases associated with injection drug use; drug-related arrests; price and purity levels of drugs; survey findings; and ethnographic research data. Their most recent report, "Epidemiologic Trends in Drug Abuse: Highlights and Executive Summary," was published in 2009 and is available at http://www.drugabuse.gov/PDF/CEWG/CEWGJune09vol1_web508.pdf (NIDA, 2009).

Table 1-1 lists additional sources that can provide important information about trends in drug use.

National Surveys

There are three surveys that are used to monitor trends in the general population: Monitoring the Future (MTF), Youth Risk Behavior Surveillance System (YRBSS), and the National Survey on Drug Use and Health (NSDUH). Descriptions of these surveys are provided in Table 1-2. These surveys offer researchers, planners, and practitioners an understanding of the substance use and abuse trends in the United States. They also provide comparisons among various ethnic and racial groups.

MTF is an ongoing study of the behaviors, attitudes, and values of secondary school students, college students, and adults through age 50 in the United States. It began in 1975 and is conducted by the University of Michigan's Institute for Social Research. Each year, a total of 50,000 8th-, 10th-, and 12th-grade students are surveyed (twelfth graders since 1975, and eighth and tenth graders since 1991). The study focuses on the recent trends in the use of licit and illicit drugs, as well as the trends in the levels of perceived risk and personal disapproval associated with each drug (Johnston, O'Malley, Bachman, & Schulenberg, 2012a; 2012b; 2013). In addition, annual follow-up questionnaires are mailed to a sample of each graduating class for years after their initial participation.

TABLE 1-1: DRUG USE STUDIES

DATA	DESCRIPTION
National Epidemiologic Survey on Alcohol and Related Conditions (NESARC)	This is a longitudinal survey that consisted of a first wave (Wave I) from 2001 to 2002 and Wave 2 from 2004 to 2005 (Grant & Dawson, 2006). It is the largest comorbidity study conducted, with a sample size of 43,093. It also includes an oversampling of African Americans and Hispanics so it is a good mechanism to address race and ethnic disparities (NIAAA, n.d.).
Treatment Episode Data Set (TEDS)	This report provides information on the demographic and substance abuse characteristics based on annual admissions to alcohol and drug treatment facilities as reported to State administrative systems.
Drug Abuse Warning Network (DAWN)	This is a national probability survey of non-federal, short stay, general, surgical, and medical hospitals with 24-hour emergency departments (EDs) in all 50 states and the District of Columbia. The survey captures the episodes induced by or related to the use of an illegal drug or the nonmedical use of a legal drug. Of the more than 120 million ED visits in 2010, it is estimated that 2.3 million were drug-related (SAMHSA, 2012).
Uniform Crime Reports	Annual statistical publications, such as the comprehensive "Crime in the United States," are produced from data provided by nearly 17,000 law enforcement agencies across the United States (Federal Bureau of Investigation, n.d.).

TABLE 1-2: THREE NATIONAL SURVEYS FOR MONITORING TRENDS IN SUBSTANCE ABUSE

NAME OF SURVEY	DESCRIPTION
Monitoring the Future (MTF) – University of Michigan Institute for Social Research (Johnston, O'Malley, Bachman, & Schulenberg, 2012c, 2013; National Institute on Drug Abuse, 2012, 2013)	This is an ongoing study of the behaviors, attitudes, and values of secondary school students, college students, and adults up to 50 years of age in the United States. Each year, a total of 50,000 8th-, 10th-, and 12th-grade students are surveyed (twelfth graders since 1975, and eighth and tenth graders since 1991). The study focuses on the recent trends in the use of licit and illicit drugs, as well as the trends in the levels of perceived risk and personal disapproval associated with each drug.
National Survey on Drug Use and Health (NSDUH) – the Substance Abuse and Mental Health Services Administration (2012a)	This is the primary source of information on illicit drug use in the U.S. population aged 12 years and older. This report, conducted on an annual basis, provides national estimates of use, number of users, and other measures related to use of illicit drugs, alcohol, cigarettes, and other forms of tobacco, by population. It includes national estimates of trends in the initiation of substance use, as well as the extent of drug dependence and treatment in the United States.
Youth Risk Behavior Surveillance System (YRBSS) – Centers for Disease Control and Prevention (2012)	This survey monitors six categories of priority health-risk behaviors among children in grades 9 through 12. It tracks behaviors that contribute to unintentional and intentional injuries; tobacco use; alcohol and other drug use; sexual behaviors that contribute to unintended pregnancy and sexually transmitted diseases (including HIV infection); unhealthy dietary behaviors; and physical inactivity (including being overweight).

NSDUH is sponsored by the Substance Abuse and Mental Health Services Administration (SAMHSA). It is the primary source of information on illicit drug use by those in the U.S. population who are ages 12 and older; it was initiated in 1971 and is currently conducted on an annual basis. This report provides national estimates of use, number of users, and other measures related to the use of illicit drugs, alcohol, cigarettes, and other forms of tobacco by population. It includes national estimates of trends in substance use initiation, as well as the extent of both dependence and treatment in the country. The primary objectives of the NSDUH are to collect timely data on the magnitude and patterns of alcohol, tobacco, and illegal substance use and abuse; assess the consequences of substance use and abuse; and identify those groups at high risk for substance use and abuse. A scientific random sample of households throughout the United States is used and a professional field representative makes a personal visit to each household. Because the survey is based on a random sample, each selected individual represents approximately 3,000 other U.S. residents (SAMHSA, 2012b).

YRBSS is a means of monitoring health-risk behaviors among youth and young adults. It includes a national school-based Centers for Disease Control and Prevention (CDC) school survey for students in grades 9 through 12. The YRBSS monitors six categories of priority health-risk behaviors among youth and young adults – behaviors that contribute to unintentional and intentional injuries; tobacco use; alcohol and other drug use; sexual behaviors that contribute to unintended pregnancy and sexually transmitted diseases (STDs) (including HIV infection); unhealthy dietary behaviors; and physical inactivity (including being overweight) (CDC, 2012).

These surveys also monitor measures related to youth substance abuse prevention. The NSDUH, for example, includes items addressing attitudes about drug use, perceptions related to harm of use, perceived availability of drugs, and perceived parental disapproval of substance use. When perceptions of harm decrease, or a change of attitudes resulting in a more positive view about drug use occurs, concern about the efforts that need to take place to counteract these changes arises. Conversely, an increase in perceived risks of using a substance is positive and is shown to be associated with subsequent decreases in the use of certain substances. For example, the proportion of youths aged 12 to 17 who reported perceiving great risk from smoking one or more packs of cigarettes per day increased from 63.1% in 2002 to 66.2% in 2011. During that same period, the rate of past month cigarette smoking among this group decreased from 13.0% to 7.8% (SAMHSA, 2012b).

In looking at any of these data sets, it is clear that each one has its own set of biases. For example, in the national surveys, one has to look at whether the surveys are randomly chosen and the completion rates of those participating. The primary issue to consider overall is whether the data is representative of the country as a whole. Whether national data should be used in local planning is a common concern. In many cases, national data may not provide the information necessary to meet local needs; however, local surveys could be conducted to obtain more specific information. In these cases, national data should not be used to make decisions about states or communities that are not average in population distributions (in terms of, for example, race and ethnicity).

There are also differences in national survey results. These differences usually occur because of differences in sampling designs and weighting procedures used to make the sampling data nationally representative. Knowledge of the different sources of data and the potential biases is critical in making the best use of the data for planning purposes. In analyzing data, keep in mind that select groups of individuals may be missing. For example, by the time students get to the twelfth grade, many have dropped out of school. Therefore, the MTF will have an inherent bias in this respect.

EPIDEMIOLOGICAL TRENDS IN SUBSTANCE USE

Nationally representative surveys provide researchers, planners, and practitioners with an understanding of the substance use and abuse trends in the United States. For example, the 2012 MTF study found a substantive change in illicit drug use between 2001 and 2011 with 27%, 15%, and 2% declines in past month use among eighth, tenth, and twelfth graders, respectively. (In spite of this decline, however, there has been a slight increase in illicit drug use since 2007.) Other recent changes include a decline in lifetime use of cigarettes for all grades (cigarette smoking was at its lowest point in history in 2009, increased slightly in 2010 among 8th and 10th graders, and has since continued to decline among all three grades); a possible increase in Adderall misuse among 12th graders, with misuse holding steady below peak levels for 8th and 10th graders; and a significant decline in narcotics use (primarily Vicodin and OxyContin) among the three grades combined after several years of sharp increases (Johnston, O'Malley, Bachman, & Schulenberg, 2012a).

Consistent declines in marijuana use were seen from the mid-1990s until the mid-2000s; then, in 2006, prevalence rates once again began to increase. This trend continued until 2012, when rates of use for 10th and 12th graders halted (for 8th graders, prevalence has been declining since 2010). And because marijuana is much more prevalent than any other illicit drug, trends in its use tend to drive the index of "any illicit drug use" (Johnston et al., 2012a). The survey also found high rates of synthetic marijuana use. In

2011, the MTF survey began asking 12th graders about their synthetic marijuana (an herbal drug mixture that usually contains designer chemicals that fall into the cannibinoid family) use, with 11.4% of this population indicating past year use. In 2012, MTF included this question on the 8th and 10th grade surveys, to which 4.4% and 8.8%, respectively, confirmed past year use. The fact that as of early 2011 the Drug Enforcement Agency has synthetic marijuana as a Schedule I controlled substance (before then, it was readily available on the Internet, etc.) has not affected its use; prevalence rates among 12th graders remained steady through 2011 and 2012.

Another area of concern is use of smokeless tobacco. From the mid-2000s through 2010, smokeless tobacco use increased after a fairly long period of decline. As of 2010, the rates have been modestly decreasing among 8th, 10th, and 12th graders, but a recent and significant decline in perceived risk among both 8th and 10th graders threatens a future rise in use (Johnson et al., 2013). Additionally, for the first time in 2009, the non-medical use of Adderall (a stimulant commonly prescribed to treat ADHD) was measured. The survey found that over 5% of 10th and 12th graders had used the drug for non-medical purposes in the past year (NIDA 2009c). Survey results from 2012 indicated a decline since 2009 in use among 8th and 10th graders, but, as previously mentioned, use among 12th graders has increased (from 5.4% in 2009, to 7.6% in 2012).

Because alcohol is the drug of choice among teenagers, epidemiological trends of alcohol use are of particular concern. Drinking, for example, commonly begins at very young ages, and that early onset of alcohol use is a risk factor for the development of alcohol-related problems as adults. Another area of concern is the high prevalence of heavy episodic drinking, which is defined as five or more drinks in a row in the past 2 weeks. In 2012, binge-drinking rose significantly among 12th graders, from 22% to 24%. According to the MTF study, the perceived harmfulness in consuming one or two alcoholic beverages every day decreased among all three grades (Johnson et al., 2012a). The prevalence of being drunk at least once in the previous month was 4.4% for eighth graders, 13.7% for tenth graders, and 25.0% for twelfth graders (Johnston et al., 2012a).

The epidemiological studies allow some comparisons of various ethnic and racial groups. The results from the 2011 NSDUH study indicated that individuals reporting two or more races had the highest rates of illicit drug use at 13.5%, followed by American Indian and Alaskan American (13.4%), Native Hawaiians or other Pacific Islanders (11.0%), African Americans (10.0%), Whites (8.7%), Hispanics (8.4%), and finally, Asians at 3.8% (SAMHSA, 2012b).

Prevention science is built on the premise that identifiable precursors to health problems can be identified (Hawkins, Van Horn, & Arthur, 2004; Kellam, Koretz, & Moscicki, 1999; Coie et al., 1993). Approximately 20 years ago, Hawkins and colleagues produced a classic article identifying risk and protective factors for alcohol and drug problems in adolescence and early adulthood (Hawkins, Catalano, & Miller, 1992). These factors are important when studying epidemiological trends and "include but are not limited to family history and genetic vulnerability; comorbid conditions and their developmental antecedents; socio-demographic characteristics; social stressors, such as poverty and lack of social support; family characteristics; alcohol availability; temperament; and other individual factors" (Faden & Goldman, 2004/2005, p. 116). Risk and protective factors will be discussed in detail in Chapter 2.

SUMMARY

Epidemiology is a tool that helps public health officials and others to monitor the trends of substance use in the United States. Data is derived from researchers, practitioners, self-reports by substance users, or recorded events such as impaired driving arrests. The two most commonly used surveys that provide data about substance use among youth are MTF and YRBSS. Some data is also available from the NSDUH study, which monitors households with individuals ages 12 years and older. The value of epidemiological data to local areas will vary; however, it is generally agreed that the prevailing problems among young people can be identified with national data. Other sources provide overall surveillance data about the consequences of substance use for all ages.

EXAM QUESTIONS

CHAPTER 1

Questions 1-6

Note: Choose the one option that BEST answers each question.

1. The branch of medical science that deals with the incidence, distribution, and control of disease in a population is known as

   a. pathology.

   b. infection control.

   c. epidemiology.

   d. endocrinology.

2. A prevalence rate is defined as the

   a. rate at which people without a disease develop that disease.

   b. rate at which people in a population have a disease at a given point.

   c. control of a disease in a population.

   d. study of the determinants of disease.

3. The information generated by epidemiological studies is useful in the field of substance abuse prevention because it

   a. reduces the availability of illicit substances.

   b. describes the nature and monitors patterns of drug abuse trends.

   c. generates protocols for best practices.

   d. provides individual treatment plans for clients.

4. The survey that is the primary source of information on illicit drug use in the United States is the

   a. National Survey on Drug Use and Health (NSDUH).

   b. The Youth Risk Behavior Surveillance System (YRBSS).

   c. Monitoring the Future (MTF) survey.

   d. National Epidemiologic Survey on Alcohol and Related Conditions (NESARC).

5. The national survey that monitors six categories of priority health-risk behaviors among children in grades 9 through 12 is called

   a. Youth Risk Behavior Surveillance System (YRBSS).

   b. National Survey on Drug Use and Health (NSDUH).

   c. Monitoring the Future (MTF).

   d. National Epidemiologic Survey on Alcohol and Related Conditions (NESARC).

6. According to the most recent findings of the MTF survey, the most commonly abused substance among high school students is

   a. heroin.

   b. cocaine.

   c. methamphetamine.

   d. marijuana.

REFERENCES

Best, D., Gross, S., Manning, V., Gossop, M., Witton, J., & Strang, J. (2005). Cannabis use in adolescents: the impact of risk and protective factors and social functioning. *Drug and Alcohol Review, 24(*6), 483-488.

Centers for Disease Control and Prevention. (2012). Youth risk behavior surveillance – United States, 2011. Surveillance Summaries, June 8, 2012. *Morbidity and Mortality Weekly Report; 61* (No.4). Retrieved from http://www.cdc.gov/mmwr/pdf/ss/ss6104.pdf

Coie, J.D., Watt, N.F., West, S.G., Hawkins, J.D., Asarnow, J.R., Markman, H.J., et al. (1993). The science of prevention: A conceptual framework and some directions for a national research program. *American Psychologist, 48,* 1013-1022.

Delva, J., Wallace, J.M., O'Malley, P.M., Bachman, J.G., Johnston, L.D., & Schulenberg, J.E. (2005). The epidemiology of alcohol, marijuana, and cocaine use among Mexican American, Puerta Rican, Cuban American, and other Latin American eighth-grade students in the United States: 1991-2002. *American Journal of Public Health, 95*(4), 696-702.

Faden, V.B. & Goldman, M. (October 2005). The scope of the problem. *Alcohol Research and Health, 28*(3), 111-120. Available from http://pubs.niaaa.nih.gov/publications/arh283/111-120.htm

Federal Bureau of Investigation. (n.d.). *Uniform crime reports.* Accessed May 18, 2010, from http://www.fbi.gov/ucr/ucr.htm

Hawkins, J.D., Catalano, R.F., & Miller, J.Y. (1992). Risk and protective factors for alcohol and other drug problems in adolescence and early adulthood: Implications for substance abuse prevention. *Psychological Bulletin, 112*(112), 64-105.

Hawkins, J.D., Van Horn, M.L., & Arthur, M.W. (2004). Community variation in risk and protective factors and substance use outcomes. *Preventive Science, 5*(4), 213-220.

Johnston, L. D., O'Malley, P. M., Bachman, J. G., & Schulenberg, J. E. (2012a). *Monitoring the Future national survey results on drug use, 1975-2011.* Volume I: Secondary school students. Ann Arbor: Institute for Social Research, The University of Michigan.

Johnston, L. D., O'Malley, P. M., Bachman, J. G., & Schulenberg, J. E. (2012b). *Monitoring the Future national survey results on drug use, 1975-2011.* Volume II: College students and adults ages 19-50 Ann Arbor: Institute for Social Research, The University of Michigan.

Johnston, L. D., O'Malley, P. M., Bachman, J. G., & Schulenberg, J. E. (2012c). *The rise in teen marijuana use stalls, synthetic marijuana use levels, and use of 'bath salts' is very low.* University of Michigan News Service: Ann Arbor, MI. Retrieved 2/10/13 from http://www.monitoringthefuture.org

Johnston, L. D., O'Malley, P. M., Bachman, J. G., & Schulenberg, J. E. (2013). *Monitoring the Future national results on drug use: 2012 Overview, Key Findings on Adolescent Drug Use.* Ann Arbor: Institute for Social Research, The University of Michigan.

Kellam, S.G., Koretz, D., & Mosciki, E.K. (1999). Core elements of developmental epidemiologically based prevention research. *American Journal of Community Psychology, 27*(4), 463-482.

Merriam Webster Online Dictionary. (2013). *Epidemiology.* Retrieved from http://www.merriam-webster.com/dictionary/epidemiology

National Institute on Alcohol Abuse and Alcoholism. (n.d.). *NESARC: Findings on alcohol abuse and dependence.* Accessed May 18, 2010, from http://pubs.niaaa.nih.gov/-publications/arh29-2/152-156.htm

National Institute on Drug Abuse. (2009). *Epidemiologic trends in drug abuse: Highlights and executive summary.* Proceedings of the Community Epidemiology Work Group. NIH Publication No 10-7421. Accessed June 10, 2010, from http://www.drugabuse.gov/sites/default/files/cewgjune09vol1_web508.pdf

National Institute on Drug Abuse. (2012). *NIDA's 2012 Monitoring the Future survey shows rates stable or down for most drugs.* Accessed March 10, 2013, from http://www.drugabuse.gov/news-events/news-releases/2012/12/regular-marijuana-use-by-teens-continues-to-be-concern

National Institute on Drug Abuse. (2013). *2012 Monitoring the Future Results.* Accessed March 10, 2013 from http://www.drugabuse.gov/related-topics/trends-statistics/monitoring-future

Sloboda, Z. (2002). *Drug abuse epidemiology: An overview.* Offprint from Bulletin on Narcotics, LIV (1 and 2), 1-13.

Substance Abuse and Mental Health Services Administration. (2012a). *Highlights of the 2010 Drug Abuse Warning Network (DAWN) Findings on Drug-Related Emergency Department Visits.* Retrieved from http://www.samhsa.gov/data/2k12/DAWN096/SR096EDHighlights2010.htm

Substance Abuse and Mental Health Services Administration. (2012b). *Results from the 2011 National survey on drug use and health: Summary of national findings* (NSDUH Series H-44, HHS Publication No. (SMA) 12-4713). Rockville, MD. Accessed March 10, 2013 from http://www.samhsa.gov/data/NSDUH/2k11Results/NSDUHresults2011.htm

Wright, D.R. & Fitzpatrick, K.M. (2004). Psychosocial correlates of substance use behaviors among African American youth. *Adolescence, 39*(156), 653-667.

CHAPTER 2

PREVENTION OF SUBSTANCE ABUSE

CHAPTER OBJECTIVE

After completing this chapter, the learner will be able to discuss the concepts and principles of preventing substance abuse.

LEARNING OBJECTIVES

After studying this chapter, the learner will be able to:

1. Define the concept of prevention in the substance abuse field.
2. Describe risk and protective factors important in the substance abuse prevention field.
3. Identify risk and protective factors for substance use in adolescents.
4. Define principles of prevention and types of prevention programs.
5. Describe the effectiveness of prevention efforts in the substance abuse field.

OVERVIEW

"Prevention in the substance abuse field is understood as any activity designed to avoid substance abuse and reduce its health and social consequences" (Medina-Mora, 2005, p. 25). Prevention can include actions focused on reducing the supply of substances and actions that are aimed at decreasing the demand for substances. Reducing the supply of illegal substances include such interventions as destroying crops, substituting crops, prosecuting traffickers, and reducing illegal substances on the street. Demand reduction is focused on modifying factors that make individuals vulnerable to substance experimentation.

Goals for preventing substance abuse are clearly outlined not only in the National Drug Control Strategy (Office of National Drug Control, 2009) but also in the strategic plans of national agencies such as the Substance Abuse and Mental Health Services Administration (SAMHSA). The overall purpose of these types of action plans is to build the capacity of states, tribes, territories, and communities to decrease substance use and abuse, promote mental health, and reduce disability, co-morbidity, and relapse related to mental and substance use conditions (SAMHSA, 2012).

Epidemiological evidence suggests that there are continuous shifts between periods of increasing and decreasing abuse of substances and that prevention can modify the trend, generate or reinforce a downward shift, or help to diminish a rising trend (Medina-Mora, 2005).

CONCEPTUALIZATION OF PREVENTION

Levels of Prevention

Public health has long been concerned with prevention. In the field of epidemiology, there are three levels of prevention: primary prevention, which focuses on health promotion and protection before a problem arises; secondary prevention, which is generally concerned with early detection and prompt treatment; and tertiary prevention, which deals with limitation of disability and rehabilitation. In relation to substance use, primary prevention aims to reduce risks and prevent new cases, secondary prevention seeks to limit harm in the early stages of the disease, and tertiary prevention is focused on treating consequences of the disorder (Toumbourou et al., 2007).

There has been a tendency to consider primary prevention as the only true form of prevention (Medina-Mora, 2005). However, it is important to think of prevention in all three realms because effective prevention approaches are needed to address the nature of substance abuse disorders that are chronic and commonly recurring in nature. Therefore, the scope of prevention includes early intervention for individuals who have experimented with substances and treatment of their dependence, especially in relation to relapse prevention and social reintegration. It includes health promotion targeted at individuals, families, and communities, as well as efforts to reduce stigma and barriers to care (Medina-Mora, 2005).

Prevention Strategies

Another way of conceptualizing prevention work is based on the classification schema outlined by Gordon (1987) and discussed in an Institute of Medicine report (Mrazek & Haggerty, 1994; Kellam & Langevin, 2003). The classifications include universal, selective, and indicated prevention strategies.

Universal

Universal prevention strategies address the general population with messages and programs aimed at preventing or delaying the abuse of substances. Universal strategies deter the onset of substance abuse by providing all individuals – regardless of the degree to which they are at-risk – with the information and skills necessary to prevent the problem ((National Institute on Drug Abuse [NIDA], 2003). One of the advantages of universal programs is that they avoid labeling and stigmatizing. However, the major disadvantage of these programs is that they are most effective for those at lowest risk (Offord, 2000). An example of a universal program is "Life Skills Training," which was designed to teach general personal and social skills and resistance skills to middle or junior high school or elementary school children (Botvin, Baker, Dusenbury, Botvin, & Diaz, 1995; Griffin, Botvin, Nichols, & Doyle, 2003).

Selective

Selective prevention strategies are aimed at an at-risk subgroup within a larger population. Examples of these groups include adult children of alcoholics, dropouts, or students who are failing academically. The risk groups are identified on the basis of biological, psychological, social, or environmental risk factors. One advantage of these types of programs is the opportunity to address problems at an early stage; however, disadvantages include the difficulties of screening as well as the potential harm of labeling and stigmatizing participants (Offord, 2000). One example of a selective prevention program is "Focus on Families," a program for families with children ages 3 to 14 in which parents receiving methadone treatment were provided with supplemental family training sessions and support services (Catalano, Gainey, Fleming, Haggerty, & Johnson, 1999).

Indicated

Indicated prevention strategies are designed to prevent individuals with identified risk factors including substance use from progressing to the diagnosis of substance use disorder as defined in the *Diagnostic and Statistical Manual of Mental Disorders, 5th Edition* (DSM-5). The overall aim is to reduce first-time substance abuse, reduce the length of time problems continue, delay the onset of substance abuse, and reduce the severity of substance abuse. An example of an indicated prevention program is "Reconnecting Youth," which targets youth on a high school dropout trajectory with an increased vulnerability to drug involvement and suicide risk (Eggert, 2006).

A definition of prevention research, which was adopted by the Public Health Service, was developed by the National Institutes of Health (NIH) Bureaus, Institutes, and Divisions in 1984. It includes only research that is designed to yield results directly applicable to the identification of risk and to interventions that prevent the occurrence of disease or the progression of detectable but asymptomatic disease (Harlan, 1998). Prevention research strategies are multi-focused and are directed at strengthening individuals, families, classrooms, peers, or larger social environments.

RISK AND PROTECTIVE FACTORS

Factors associated with increased use of substances and factors that protect against the use or abuse of substances are not only important in studying epidemiological trends, but also in designing preventive efforts. The factors that affect the likelihood of substance use are called *risk and protective factors* (van den Bree & Pickworth, 2005). Risk factors are those that increase a vulnerability to the initiation, continuation, or escalation of use. Protective factors include individual resilience and other circumstances that reduce the likelihood to use substances. Previous research has identified risk and protective factors for adolescents across different contexts (Hawkins, Catalano, & Miller, 1992).

Many current studies use factors to identify individuals "at risk." One study examined at-risk students in 10 high schools in San Antonio, Texas, and San Francisco during the spring and fall of 2002. Attendance and grade point average data were used as screening protocols to identify high-risk students. "High risk" students were identified as being in the top quartile for absences and below the median grade point average, or teacher referred. Students identified as high risk were more likely to use cigarettes, alcohol, and marijuana; to exhibit suicide risk factors; and to engage in delinquent behaviors (Hallfors, Cho, Brodish, Flewelling, & Khatapoush, 2006).

Other studies have examined risk factors and their ability to predict changes in drug use. Using data from 13,718 middle school and high school students who participated in the Longitudinal Study of Adolescent Health, one study examined whether 21 risk factors could predict five stages of marijuana involvement (van den Bree & Pickworth, 2005).

These stages were:

1. initiation of experimental use
2. initiation of regular use
3. progression to regular use
4. failure to discontinue experimental use
5. failure to discontinue regular use.

In this study, three risk factors were predictive of all stages – own and peer involvement with substances, delinquency, and school problems. Other studies have tried to determine the role of genetics in relationship to the environment (Young, Rhee, Stallings, Corley, & Hewitt, 2006).

Risk factors can influence drug abuse in several ways. The more risks a person has, the greater the likelihood that he or she will abuse drugs. The protective factors can reduce risks; therefore, prevention programs should enhance protective factors and reverse risk factors (NIDA, 2003). An important goal of prevention is to change the balance between risk and protective factors so that the protective factors outweigh the risk factors. The impact of risk and protective factors changes with age; families have more of an influence with younger children, while peers have more of an impact on adolescents.

These risk factors and protective factors exist within six domains or settings: individual, family, peer, school, community, and society (Center for Substance Abuse Prevention, SAMHSA, 2010). Risk factors can exist within several domains and can overlap.

Individual Domain

Individual risk factors include personality factors, attitudes favorable toward drug use, decision-making skills, personal efficacy, lack of knowledge about consequences of use, antisocial behavior, sensation-seeking behavior, and a lack of adult supervision. Research has shown that social and personal skill-building can enhance individual capacities, influence attitudes, and promote positive behavior (Center for Substance Abuse Prevention, SAMHSA, 2010). These interventions usually include information about the negative effects of substance abuse, and consider race, ethnicity, age, and gender in their designs. It is clear that interventions must stress the immediate effects of use and social acceptance rather than the long-term effects of use. Such alternatives as sports programs, involvement in the arts, and community service can provide effective ways of reaching high-risk youth.

Family Domain

Family risk factors include low parental investment, low family cohesion, parental conflict, poor parent-adolescent communication, low parental monitoring of children, ineffective parental management, and parental drug use. Research evidence shows that interventions targeting the entire family can be effective in preventing adolescent substance abuse. Some selected strategies that are effective include focusing on developing parenting skills (and not just providing information about parenting); emphasizing family bonding; training parents to listen and interact in developmentally appropriate ways; and training parents to use positive and consistent discipline techniques and improve family communication through modeling, coaching, rehearsal, and role playing (Center for Substance Abuse Prevention, SAMHSA, 2010).

Peer Domain

The risk factors associated with the peer domain include peer use, peer norms that are positive to use, and peer activities that are conducive to use. Preventive strategies that relate to peers are structured alternative activities (such as a sober prom) in settings antithetical to drug use and that incorporate social and personal skills building. Other strategies include involving youth in developing alternative programs and peer-led interventions (Center for Substance Abuse Prevention, SAMHSA, 2010). However, a potential problem is including peers whose behavior is deviant into other groups.

School Domain

School risk factors include a lack of commitment to education, poor grades, school failure, a lack of attachment to school, negative school climate, and lenient school policies. School protective factors include academic achievement, school bonding, educational aspirations, and educational commitments. Research related to school-based approaches to prevention has found several important facts:

- Knowledge-oriented interventions alone do not produce measurable changes in behavior or attitudes and are considered the least effective educational strategy.
- Educational interventions that focus on correcting misconceptions about the prevalence of use can change attitudes that are favorable toward use. These are most effective when combined with other educational approaches such as fostering social skills.
- Interventions that are peer led or include some peer-led component are more effective than adult- or teacher-led approaches.
- Interactive approaches help to engage youth.
- Booster sessions help youth retain skills.
- Parental involvement and school policies that communicate a commitment to substance abuse prevention are important as effective strategies.

(Center for Substance Abuse Prevention, SAMHSA, 2010).

Prevention programs should be designed to intervene as early as preschool to address risk behaviors. The programs should target improving academic and social-emotional learning to address such risk factors as early aggression and academic failure. In middle school and high school, such skills as communication, self-efficacy, resistance skills, anti-drug attitudes, and peer relationships should be promoted to increase academic and social competence (NIDA, 2003). Prevention programs should be aimed at the general population.

Several reviews of school-based programs have been done over the past few decades. Hansen (1992) reviewed published prevention studies between 1980 and 1990 and found that comprehensive and social influence programs were the most successful. A more recent review of literature in June 2001 identified components critical to effective programs. These included timing and programming issues, content delivery issues, teacher training, and dissemination (McBride, 2003). A more recent meta-analysis of current practice in school-based prevention programs found that most providers taught effective content but few used effective delivery – illustrating the difficulty with the transfer of research knowledge into practice (Ennett et al., 2003).

Community Domain

Community risk factors include a lack of bonding to social and community institutions, lack of awareness of community substance abuse problems, community norms favorable to use, and insufficient community resources to support prevention efforts. Community institutions include churches, Boys and Girls Clubs, YMCA, and workplaces (Center for Substance Abuse Prevention, SAMHSA, 2010).

Researchers found that:

- controlling the environment around schools helps to reinforce strong community norms.
- mentoring programs can increase school attendance and create positive attitudes.
- community service can increase positive attitudes towards others.
- influencing increased worksite commitments to prevention efforts can be done by emphasizing decreased costs to employers.
- communicating a clear policy can help to change workplace norms.
- coalitions are important in formulating and implementing approaches to preventing substance abuse.

Lastly, it is recommended that the most effective approach to reaching populations in multiple settings is to present consistent, community-wide messages in each setting (NIDA, 2003). In planning for drug abuse prevention in the community, there are several steps involved. These steps are listed in Table 2-1 (NIDA, 2003).

TABLE 2-1: THE COMMUNITY PLAN

A well constructed community plan:

- identifies the specific drugs and other child and adolescent problems in a community
- builds on existing resources (such as current drug abuse prevention programs)
- develops short-term goals related to selecting and carrying out research-based prevention programs and strategies
- projects long-term goals so that plans and resources are available for the future
- includes ongoing assessments of the prevention program.

(NIDA, 2003)

Society and Environmental Domain

Risk factors in the society and environmental domains include norms tolerant of use, policies that enable use and abuse, a lack of enforcement of laws designed to prevent use and abuse, and inappropriate negative sanctions for use and abuse (Center for Substance Abuse Prevention, SAMHSA, 2010). The preventive approaches to addressing the society and environmental domain involve environmental interventions targeted to populations. Some selected findings from research indicate:

- Community awareness and media efforts can be effective in changing perceptions.
- Mass media can influence community norms about substance use.
- Audience perceptions and capacities to understand media messages are based on gender, culture, and stage of cognitive development.
- Effective mass media messages are broadcast through multiple channels.
- Counter advertising campaigns that disseminate information about the hazards of the product (tobacco) may help to reduce sales.
- Beverage server training to enforce laws against service to intoxicated patrons is effective in changing selling and service principles.
- Increasing the price of alcohol and tobacco through excise taxes can be an effective strategy.
- Increasing the minimum purchase age for alcohol to age 21 has been effective in decreasing alcohol use among youth.

Interventions at the societal or environmental level are a systems approach directed at public health concerns. Community-level problems include alcohol-related traffic crashes or non-traffic death and trauma with significant alcohol involvement. In the case of alcohol, policy change is an approach to addressing prevention and involves producing such structural changes in the environment as legal drinking ages, regulation of alcohol outlets, legal blood alcohol level for drinking and driving, advertising restrictions, and service to intoxicated persons and underage persons (Holder, 2000). There are three environmental prevention projects addressing alcohol that have shown significant efficacy: the Saving Lives project in Massachusetts, Communities Mobilizing for Change on Alcohol (CMCA) in Minnesota and Wisconsin, and the Community Trials Project in Northern California, Southern California, and South Carolina (Treno & Lee, 2002).

PRINCIPLES OF PREVENTION AND PROGRAMS

Research guides the development of prevention programs and principles of prevention. Sixteen principles have been outlined by the NIDA (2003). Many of these principles have already been discussed in relationship to risk and protective factors and family, school, and community programs. In addition, there are several principles related to program delivery: the core elements (structure, content, and delivery) of an original research-based intervention should be retained in the actual implementation; programs should be long term with repeated interventions; and the most effective interventions use interactive techniques, such as peer discussion or parent role playing (NIDA, 2003).

Table 2-2 lists the types, and examples of, programs focused on preventing drug abuse among children and adolescents and the characteristics of those programs. One of the best known programs is *Life Skills Training,* which is a universal program for middle school students focusing on risk and protective factors (Griffin, Botvin, & Nichols, 2006). Other versions of this program that focus on elementary and high school students have been developed.

Prevention in Special Populations

There are special populations that pose special concerns or challenges to clinicians in implementing effective preventive strategies. One of those groups is patients with co-morbid addiction and mental health problems (Selby & Vaccarino, 2005). Substance abuse, including smoking, is often associated with mental illness. A meta-analysis of worldwide studies for a 10-year literature search found that patients with schizophrenia have a higher prevalence of smoking than the general population and severely mentally ill patients (Leon & Diaz, 2005). Selby & Vaccarino (2005) stress that patients with co-morbid problems need additional screening for subclinical problems and

TABLE 2-2: TYPES OF PREVENTION PROGRAMS

TYPE OF PROGRAM	TARGET POPULATION	CHARACTERISTICS	EXAMPLES OF PROGRAMS
Universal	This includes general populations and sub populations (pregnant women, children, adolescents, and elderly persons).	Assesses the entire population as at-risk for substance abuse; administered to large groups without any prior screening.	Botvin's Life Skills (Griffin, Botvin, & Nichols, 2006) Classroom-centered and Family-school Partnership Intervention Project Star Project Alert
Selective	Risk groups are identified based on biological, psychological, social, or environmental risk factors known to be associated with substance abuse (children of alcoholics, dropouts, and students who are failing school).	Targets the entire subgroup, regardless of the degree of individual risk; the program is presented to the entire subgroup because the subgroup as a whole is at higher risk.	Adolescents Training and Learning to Avoid Steroids (ATLAS) Focus on Families (FOF) Strengthening Families Program (SFP)
Indicated	This includes individuals who do not meet *DSM-5* criteria but are showing early danger signs of substance abuse and other problem behaviors.	Addresses risk factors associated with individuals; aims are reduction in first-time use, reduction in length of time the symptoms continue, delay of onset of substance abuse, and/or reduction in the severity of substance abuse.	Project Towards No Drug Abuse Reconnecting Youth Progam

(Center for Substance Abuse Prevention, SAMHSA, 2010)

early interventions, such as immunizing patients at high risk for hepatitis A and B, counseling patients on safe injection practices, and recommending tobacco cessation, use of condoms, and avoiding high-risk sexual activity – all important in preventive care overall (Selby & Vaccarino, 2005). Iatrogenic drug dependence, which results when patients become addicted to medically prescribed drugs, is also of concern.

A recent study found that there were differences in the association of mental illness with substance abuse in different ethnic groups. Co-morbid substance abuse and mental health problems were more prevalent among non-Hispanic Whites and non-Hispanic Blacks, while Hispanics were more likely to have a substance abuse problem without co-morbid mental health problems (Karch, Barker, & Strine, 2007).

Another special group includes pregnant women. The adverse health effects of substance use on the developing fetus are significant – sometimes resulting in fetal alcohol syndrome and fetal alcohol spectrum disorders (Hankin, 2002). In an analysis of the Behavioral Risk Factor Surveillance System (BRFSS) for the years 2001 through 2003, the estimated binge drinking among childbearing-age women (age 18 to 44) increased from 11.9% to 13%. This estimated number rose from 6.2 million in 2001 to 7.1 million in 2003 (Tsai, Floyd, & Bertrand, 2006). In another study, based on self reports of 253 women, less than 20% of the pregnant women were abstinent in their first trimester and about one-half were abstinent for the duration of pregnancy (Chang, McNamara, Wilkins-Haug, & Orav, 2006).

Other groups in need of prevention efforts are adolescents and young adults. The prevalence of college students drinking alcoholic beverages is a serious concern because many students engage in heavy episodic or binge drinking (Larimer, Cronce, Lee, & Kilmer, 2004/2005). It is estimated that one in five college students engages in frequent episodic heavy consumption (binge drinking three or more times in the past 2 weeks) (National Institute on Alcohol Abuse and Alcoholism [NIAAA], 2002).

Cultural Considerations in the Design of Prevention Programs

Cultural considerations are important in addressing not only overall prevention but also primary prevention and recovery from substance abuse. Ethnic identity and its relationship to drug use has been a recent focus of study (Trimble, 1995; Marsiglia, Kulis, Hecht, & Sills, 2004; James, Kim, & Armijo, 2000). It is important to identify specific characteristics of various cultural groups overall to better design effective prevention programs.

A recent review of 18 prevention articles, which focused on Hispanic populations, resulted in recommendations for improving the effectiveness of interventions with this group. One such recommendation involved incorporating cultural factors into the research design. Many of these cultural variables, such as ethnic pride, machismo, or respect may be very important to outcomes (Castro et al., 2006). Previous studies found that strong family bonds and parental respect were additional protective factors among Latino youth (Pantin et al., 2003). For Mexican-American youth, a drug resistance strategies project called "Keepin it REAL," provides a culturally grounded drug prevention curriculum (Gosin, Marsiglia, & Hecht, 2003). A program called "Specific Event Drug and Alcohol Refusal Efficacy Scale" (SEDARE) is a culturally enhanced program for urban African-American girls (Belgrave, Reed, Plybon, & Corneille, 2004).

Impact of Prevention Strategies

How effective is substance abuse prevention? This question is increasingly viewed critically with an initiative to support only evidenced-based programs. Evaluating programs and efforts has become a part of evidenced-based policy. The Centers for the Application of Preventions Technologies (CAPT), which is supported through the Center for Substance Abuse Prevention, has a particular interest in evaluating effectiveness. A pyramid of effectiveness was developed by Drs. Peter Mulhall and Carol Hays for the Center for Prevention Research and Development, Institute of Government and Public Affairs at the University of Illinois that is now being used in the substance abuse field to guide thinking (Mulhall & Hays, n.d.). The levels of effectiveness are listed in Table 2-3. The least effective approaches are those evaluating effectiveness; the most effective are multiple site replications. However, despite all of the efforts to improve our knowledge about effective programs, criticisms about the method of evaluating these programs and an awareness that there continues to be a worldwide increase in substance use are ongoing issues (Gorman, 2003; Uchtenhagen, 2005).

Despite these limitations, there is evidence of the effectiveness of certain programs. Twenty-five long-term adolescent tobacco and other drug use prevention programs were reviewed (Skara & Sussman, 2003). This review provided empirical evidence, albeit with some reservations, of the effectiveness of programs in preventing or reducing substance use for up to 15 years after program completion. The strategies described in the study are primarily broad societal-level strategies focused on health promotion. In fact, laws that have deterred drinking and driving have resulted in an 18% reduction in drunk driving fatalities in Canada (Asbridge, Mann, Flam-Zalcman & Stoduto, 2004).

The most cost-effective strategies (taxation, conditioned availability, and reduced promotion) are usually political issues that are difficult to address. Tobacco use is one success story in this scenario (Uchtenhagen, 2005). The "war on drugs" is an approach that began more than 30 years ago. This approach, which is focused on addressing the supply of drugs, has run into problems. A recent study found that the primary focus of the war on drugs has shifted to low level marijuana offenses, resulting in law enforce-

TABLE 2-3: LEVELS OF EFFECTIVENESS OF SCIENCE-BASED PREVENTION

LEVEL OF EFFECTIVENESS	CHARACTERISTICS
Level 5 – Multiple site replication studies	• Evaluated using scientific methods • Program replications that require high fidelity • Published in more than one scientific peer-reviewed academic journal
Level 4 – Meta-analyses, expert review, and peer concensus	• Methods that synthesize prevention research and evaluation reports
Level 3 – Single trial effectiveness	• Must include pre- and posttests with either a comparison or control group to assess impact • Must have results published in at least one scientific peer-reviewed academic journal
Level 2 – Program evaluations and source documents	• Use evaluation methods such as pre- and posttest designs, qualitative analyses, and cohort evaluation • May be published in refereed or non-refereed publications
Level 1 – Testimonials, newspaper reports, and non-refereed publications	• Not considered research-based

(Mulhall & Hays, n.d.).

ment resources not being effectively allocated to offenses that are most costly to society. Instead, the funds are diverted away from other crime types (King & Mauer, 2006). The need for a rational approach to formulating a workable public policy for all drugs – not only alcohol – is needed (Trunkey & Bonnono, 2005).

Harm Reduction

Harm reduction is another approach to prevention (Medina-Mora, 2005). "Harm reduction is the term used to describe the goal and outcomes of interventions designed to protect and improve the medical, psychological, social, and occupational functioning of problem drinkers and drug takers, including those who continue to consume such substances" (Rosenberg, Melville, & McLean, 2004, p. 1125). Harm reduction is focused on a range of strategies to target consequences of alcohol and drug use. This type of strategy includes making sterile syringes available to I.V. drug users to reduce the risks of associated health issues and reducing such social consequences as crime. Other examples include education regarding safer drug ingestion methods, complementary and alternative therapies, and safe places where users can consume drugs and alcohol. There is evidence that harm-reduction strategies can be effective in saving lives and impacting measures at a population level (Toumbourou et al., 2007).

Future Directions of Prevention Strategies

The National Registry of Evidence-based Programs and Practices (NREPP) originated in 1997 in SAMHSA's Center for Substance Abuse Prevention (CSAP) as part of the Model Programs Initiative. More than 1,100 programs were reviewed and more than 150 were designated as model, effective, or promising programs. SAMHSA expanded the system and the new registry was launched in 2006. It provides ratings for each outcome targeted by the intervention. Several characteristics of evidence-based prevention have been formulated – a reliance on theory, addressing risk and protective factors, and representation in settings of influence (such as schools, community, and media).

Significant developments in prevention have been made over the past decade. It is critical that prevention programs address all forms of drug abuse, including legal drugs (cigarettes or alcohol), illegal drugs, and the inappropriate use of legally obtained substances (inhalants, prescription medications, and over-the-counter drugs). The programs should be targeted to the drug abuse problems in the local community and should be specific to the populations (age, gender, and ethnicity). Current and future challenges to school-based prevention research include:

- creating more rigorous designs with appropriate comparison groups
- developing meaningful school assessments
- studying the nature of the local adaptation of the programs ("the real world conditions")
- understanding the dissemination of evidence-based programs
- integrating school and community programs
- sustaining programs

(Greenberg, 2004).

At a community level, translating prevention science into community prevention systems is a priority in prevention research. A field-tested strategy is the Communities that Care system, which provides tools to help communities use local data on risk and protective factors to develop effective prevention systems (Hawkins, Catalano, & Arthur, 2002). This strategy was used to examine 28,091 students in 41 communities across the United States. Significant differences were found among the communities, providing an empirical foundation for tailoring community-wide efforts to prevent substance abuse (Hawkins, Van Horn, & Arthur, 2004).

Several issues are important when developing evidence-based preventions for the future. These include issues of diffusion, adaptability, and cost.

Diffusion

Pentz (2003) has characterized diffusion as adoption, implementation, sustainability, and dissemination. Rogers' *diffusion of innovation* theory hypothesizes that a program is most likely to be diffused if it is characterized by low complexity; observability of effects; trialability (or ability to try out a program on a small scale); compatibility of the program with existing programs; and a relative advantage over existing programs. Sustainability refers to the continued use of a prevention program after the initial research or grant support has ended (Pentz, 2003). There are three factors that are important in sustainability: individual community leaders and researcher characteristics, resources, and policy.

Program Adaptation

Cultural adaptation refers to modifications to programs that are culturally sensitive and tailored to a cultural group's traditional world views (Kumpfer, Alvarado, Smith, & Bellamy, 2002). *Program adaptation* is the modification of program content to accommodate consumer needs (Castro, Barrera, & Martinez, 2004). Both fidelity of implementation and program adaptation are essential, resulting in the need to develop hybrid prevention programs that build in adaptation and maximize fidelity of program implementation and effectiveness.

Cost

The effectiveness of programs and policies is important in considering cost. Holder (2000) stressed that effectiveness should be required before committing public or private funds to them. Consequently, the cost effectiveness of programs should be considered. This requires documentation of actual costs of design, implementation, and maintenance, as well as determining any reduction of alcohol and drug problems.

SUMMARY

An understanding of risk and protective factors is critical in designing effective prevention strategies. Risk factors can influence drug abuse in several ways. The more risk factors a person has, the greater the likelihood of that person abusing drugs. How these factors relate to one another is also critical in designing efforts for preventing substance use and abuse. For example, prevention efforts have broadened from individual factors only to the social world of the adolescent and macrolevel environmental factors (community and societal messages, norms, and availability) (Komro & Toomey, 2002).

Prevention of substance abuse is more than primary prevention efforts; it is a multitude of strategies directed toward the needs of populations for purposes of decreasing substance use and abuse. These strategies include affecting the supply and demand of drugs. Prevention efforts need to be comprehensive and principles need to be followed. Various programs, including universal, selective, and indicated programs have been designed. Other strategies include broad-based policy approaches, such as media campaigns or policy development. Evaluating all of these programs for their effectiveness will guide the field of substance abuse prevention in the future.

EXAM QUESTIONS

CHAPTER 2

Questions 7-11

Note: Choose the one option that BEST answers each question.

7. Primary prevention is focused on

   a. interventions before the onset of symptoms.
   b. harm reduction to reduce major health consequences.
   c. early identification of symptoms.
   d. treatment of dependence and relapse.

8. The type of prevention program that targets an individual who shows early signs of problem behavior is a(n)

   a. universal program.
   b. selective program.
   c. indicated program.
   d. primary prevention program.

9. Which statement regarding substance use in adolescents is true?

   a. The more risk factors a person has, the more likely he or she will abuse drugs.
   b. There is no direct correlation between risk factors and substance abuse.
   c. Protective factors cannot reduce the risk of substance abuse in adolescents.
   d. The goal of preventing substance abuse is to eliminate risk factors entirely.

10. A substance abuse counselor wants to decrease risk factors and increase protective factors. Which of the following is a risk factor?

    a. educational aspirations
    b. early anti-drug education
    c. parental conflict
    d. consistent discipline techniques

11. In evaluating the effectiveness of prevention programs, the highest level of scientific effectiveness is found in

    a. testimonials.
    b. meta-analyses.
    c. multiple site replications.
    d. a formal program evaluation.

REFERENCES

Asbridge, M., Mann, R.E., Flam-Zalcman, R., & Stoduto, G. (2004). The criminalization of impaired driving in Canada: Assessing the deterrent impact of Canada's first per se law. *Journal of Study of Alcohol, 65*(4), 450-459.

Belgrave, F.Z., Reed, M.C., Plybon, L.E., & Corneille, M. (2004). The impact of a culturally enhanced drug prevention program on drug and alcohol refusal efficacy among urban African American girls. *Journal of Drug Education, 34*(3), 267-79.

Botvin, G., Baker, E., Dusenbury, L., Botvin, E., & Diaz, T. (1995). Long-term follow up results of a randomized drug-abuse prevention trial in a white middle-class population. *Journal of the American Medical Association, 273*(14), 1106-1112.

Castro, F., Barrera, M., & Martinez, C.R. (2004). The cultural adaptation of prevention interventions: Resolving tensions between fidelity and fit. *Prevention Science, 5*(1), 41-45.

Castro, F., Barrera, M., Pantin, H., Martinez, C., Felix-Ortiz, M., Rios, R., et al. (2006). Substance abuse prevention intervention research with Hispanic populations. *Drug and Alcohol Dependence, 84*(Suppl 1), 529-542.

Catalano, R.F., Gainey, K.W., Fleming, C.B., Haggerty, K.P., & Johnson, N.O. (1999). An experimental intervention with families of substance abusers: One year follow-up of the Focus on Families Project. *Addiction, 94*(2), 241-254.

Center for Substance Abuse Prevention, Substance Abuse and Mental Health Services Administration, 2010. *Focus on Prevention.* HHS Publication No. (SMA) 10–4120. Rockville, MD: Center for Substance Abuse Prevention, Substance Abuse and Mental Health Services Administration. Accessed March 15, 2013 from http://store.samhsa.gov/shin/content/SMA10-4120/SMA10-4120.pdf

Chang, G., McNamara, T.K., Wilkins-Haug, L., & Orav, E.J. (2006). Estimates of prenatal abstinence from alcohol: A matter of perspective. *Addictive Behaviors, 31*(4), 419-424.

Eggert, L.L. (2006). *Reconnecting youth: An indicated prevention program.* Accessed June 11, 2010, from http://www.nida.nih.gov/MeetSum/CODA/Youth.html

Ennett, S.T., Ringwalt, C.L., Thorne, J., Rohrbach, L.A., Vincus, A., Simons-Rudolph, A., & Jones, S. (2003). A comparison of current practice in school-based substance use prevention programs with meta-analysis finding. *Prevention Science, 4*(1), 1-14.

Gordon, R. (1987). An operational classification of diseases prevention. In J.A. Steinberg & M.M. Silverman (Eds.), *Preventing mental disorders* (pp. 20-26). Rockville, MD: U.S. Department of Health and Human Services.

Gorman, D. (2003). Alcohol & drug abuse: The best practices, the worst of practices: The making of science-based primary prevention programs. *Psychiatric Services, 54*(8), 1087-1089.

Gosin, M., Marsiglia, F.F., & Hecht, ML. (2003). Keepin' it R.E.A.L.: A drug resistance curriculum tailored to the strength and needs of pre-adolescents of the southwest. *Journal of Drug Education, 33*(2), 119-142.

Greenberg, M.T. (2004). Current and future challenges in school-based prevention: The researcher perspective. *Prevention Science, 5*(1), 5-13.

Griffin, K.W., Botvin, G.J., Nichols, T.R. & Doyle, M.M. (2003). Effectiveness of a universal drug abuse prevention approach for youth at high risk for substance initiation. *Preventive Medicine, 36*(1), 1-7.

Griffin, K.W., Botvin, G.J. & Nichols, T.R. (2006). Effects of a school-based drug abuse prevention program for adolescents on HIV risk behavior in young adulthood. *Prevention Science, 7*(1), 103-112.

Hallfors, D., Cho, H., Brodish, P.H., Flewelling, R., & Khatapoush, S. (2006). Identifying high school students "at risk" for substance use and other behavioral problems: Implications for prevention. *Substance Use and Misuse, 41*(1), 1-15.

Hankin, J.R. (2002). Fetal alcohol syndrome prevention research. *Alcohol Research & Health, 26*(1), 58-65.

Hansen, W.B. (1992). School-based substance abuse prevention: A review of the state of the art in curriculum, 1980-1990. *Health education research, 7*(3), 403-430.

Harlan, W.R. (1998). Prevention research at the National Institutes of Health. *American Journal of Preventive Medicine, 14*(4), 302-307.

Hawkins, J.D., Catalano, R.F., & Arthur, M.W. (2002). Promoting science-based prevention in communities. *Addictive Behavior, 27*(6), 951-976.

Hawkins, J.D., Catalano, R.F., & Miller, J.Y. (1992). Risk and protective factors for alcohol and other drug problem in adolescence and early adulthood: Implications for substance abuse prevention. *Psychological Bulletin, 112*(1), 64-105.

Hawkins, J.D., Van Horn, and M.L., & Arthur, M.W. (2004). Community variation in risk and protective factors and substance use outcomes. *Prevention Science, 5*(4), 213-220.

Holder, H. (2000). Prevention of alcohol problems in the 21st century: Challenges and opportunities. *The American Journal on Addictions, 10*, 1-15.

James, W.H., Kim, G.K., & Armijo, E. (2000). The influence of ethnic identity on drug use among ethnic minority adolescents. *Journal of Drug Education, 30*(3), 265-280.

Karch, D.L., Barker, L., & Strine, T.W. (2007). Race/ethnicity, substance abuse, and mental illness among suicide victims in 13 U.S. states: 2004 data from the National Violent Death Reporting System. *Injury Prevention, 12* (Suppl II).

Kellam, S.G. & Langevin, D.S. (2003). A framework for understanding "evidence", in prevention research and programs. *Preventive Science, 4,* 137-153.

King, R.S.& Mauer, M. (2006). The war on marijuana: The transformation of the war on drugs in the 1990's. *Harm Reduction Journal, 3*(6).

Komro, K.A. & Toomey, T.L. (2002). Strategies to prevent underage drinking. *Alcohol Research & Health, 26*(1), 5-14.

Kumpfer, K.L., Alvarado, R., Smith, P. & Bellamy, N. (2002). Cultural sensitivity in universal family-based prevention interventions. *Prevention Science, 3*(3), 241-244

Larimer, M.E., Cronce, J.M., Lee, C.L., & Kilmer, J.R. (2004/2005). Brief interventions in college settings. *Alcohol Research and Health, 28*(2), 94-104.

Leon, J. & Diaz, F.J. (2005). A meta-analysis of worldwide studies demonstrates an association between schizophrenia and tobacco smoking behaviors. *Schizophrenia Research, 76*(2-3), 135-157.

Marsiglia, F.F., Kulis, S., Hecht, M.L., & Sills, S. (2004). Ethnicity and ethnic identity as predictors of drug norms and drug use among preadolescents in the US Southwest. *Substance Use and Misuse, 39*(7), 1061-94.

McBride, N. (2003). A systematic review of school drug education. *Health education research, 18*(6), 729-742.

Medina-Mora, M.E. (2005). Prevention of substance abuse: A brief overview. *World Psychiatry, 4*(1), 25-30.

Mrazek, P.J. & Haggerty, R.J. (Eds.). (1994). Reducing risks for mental disorders: Frontiers for preventive intervention research. Institute of Medicine, Committee on Prevention of Mental Disorders. Accessed March 10, 2013 from http://www.iom.edu/Reports/1994/Reducing-Risks-for-Mental-Disorders-Frontiers-for-Preventive-Intervention-Research.aspx

Mulhall, P. & Hays, C. (n.d.). *Research-based prevention: A pyramid for effectiveness.* Accessed April 3, 2013, from http://wweb.uta.edu/projects/sswtech/sapvc/resources/science_based_prevention.htm

National Institute on Drug Abuse. (2003). *Preventing drug abuse among children and adolescents: Prevention principles.* Accessed March 10, 2013, from http://www.drugabuse.gov/sites/default/files/redbook_0.pdf

Office of National Drug Control. (2013). *National Drug Control Strategy.* Accessed March 10, 2013, from http://www.whitehouse.gov/ondcp

Offord, D.R. (2000). Selection of levels of prevention. *Addictive Behaviors, 25*(6), 833-842.

Pantin, H., Coatsworth, J.D., Feaster, D.J., Newman, F.L., Briones, E., Prado, G., et al. (2003). Familias unidas: The efficacy of an intervention to increase parental investment in Hispanic immigrant families. *Prevention Science, 4*(3), 189-201.

Pentz, M.A. (2003). Evidence-based prevention: Characteristics, impact, and future direction. *Journal of Psychoactive Drugs, 35*(1), 143-152.

Rosenberg, H., Melville, J., & McLean, P.C. (2004). Nonpharmacological harm-reduction interventions in British substance-misuse services. *Addictive Behaviors, 29*(6), 1125-1229.

Selby, P. & Vaccarino, F.J. (2005). Substance abuse prevention: practical strategies for psychiatrists in the 21st century. *World Psychiatry, 4*(1), 32-33.

Skara, S. & Sussman, S. (2003). A review of 25 long-term adolescent tobacco and other drug use prevention program evaluations. *Preventive Medicine, 37*(5), 451-474.

Substance Abuse and Mental Health Services Administration. (2012). *Major programs: Strategic prevention framework and partnerships for success.* Accessed March 10, 2013, from http://www.samhsa.gov/About/

Toumbourou, J.W., Stockwell, T., Neighbors, C., Marlatt, G.A., Sturge, J., & Rehm, J. (2007). Interventions to reduce harm associated with adolescent substance use. *Lancet, 369*(9570), 1391-1401.

Treno, A.J. & Lee, J.P. (2002). Approaching alcohol problems through local environmental interventions. *Alcohol Research and Health, 26*(1), 35-40.

Trimble, J.E. (1995). Toward an understanding of ethnicity and ethnic identity, and their relationship with drug use research. In G. Botvin, S. Schinke, & M. Oralndi (Eds.), *Drug abuse prevention with multiethnic youth* (pp. 3-27). Thousand Oaks: Sage Publications.

Tsai, J., Floyd, R.L., & Bertrand, J. (2006). Tracking binge drinking among U.S. childbearing-age women. *Preventive Medicine, 44*(4), 298-302.

Trunkey, D.D. & Bonnono, C. (2005). A rational approach to formulating public policy on substance abuse. *Journal of Trauma, 59*(3 Suppl): S61-66.

Uchtenhagen, A. (2005). How effective is substance abuse prevention? *World Psychiatry, 4*(1), 33.

van den Bree, M.B. & Pickworth, W.B. (2005). Risk factors predicting changes in marijuana involvement in teenagers. *Archives of General Psychiatry, 62*(3), 311-319.

Young, S.E., Rhee, S.H., Stallings, M.C., Corley, R.P., & Hewitt, J.K. (2006). Genetic and environmental vulnerabilities underlying adolescent substance use and problem use: General or specific? *Behavioral Genetics, 36*(4), 603-15.

CHAPTER 3

ASSESSMENT OF SUBSTANCE USE DISORDERS

CHAPTER OBJECTIVE

After completing this chapter, the learner will be able to identify and describe the components of a comprehensive assessment for substance abuse.

LEARNING OBJECTIVES

After studying this chapter, the learner will be able to:

1. Identify goals of the comprehensive assessment.
2. Identify the detection limits of commonly used drugs.
3. Discuss the advantages and disadvantages of various methods of laboratory testing for the presence of drugs.
4. Identify the stages of an individual's readiness for change.
5. List assessment tools commonly used to screen for substance use disorders.
6. Describe problems that may arise when assessing special populations for substance abuse.

OVERVIEW

All individuals should be screened for substance abuse; however, it can be a challenging process due to the associated social stigma.

In addition to obtaining data from the general medical history, physical examination, and laboratory testing, the goals of a comprehensive substance abuse assessment are to:

- determine the presence and extent of substance use
- evaluate the individual's current level of functioning (such as cognitive capacity and social skills)
- identify problems that emerged consequent to substance use, such as adverse effects on the individual's medical and psychosocial status (including relationships with family and peers)
- identify areas of strength despite the problems
- establish a formal diagnosis
- determine the individual's readiness to change his or her behavior
- make initial decisions about the appropriate level of care.

Cultural considerations and the quality and amount of available social support should be incorporated into the assessment. It is important to rule out substance toxicity, withdrawal symptoms, or possible coexisting mental disorders, as well as indications that the individual is a potential danger to others or him- or herself. If danger is suspected, such persons should be promptly referred for crisis management. This interview should ideally be completed by a substance abuse specialist but may be conducted by other health care professionals after adequate training.

Substance abuse is the generic term that will be used in this chapter to refer to problem use of nicotine, alcohol, illicit, over-the-counter (OTC), or prescription drugs, and includes substance abuse, substance dependence, or drug addiction.

HISTORY OF SUBSTANCE USE

Specific inquiry must be made separately for each substance ever used and the drug primarily used. For OTC and prescribed drugs, direct questioning should include whether their use is other than what is recommended or prescribed. Additionally, individuals should be questioned about whether the medications were prescribed for them or someone else. Questions should include age at first use, duration, amount, route (such as inhalation or intravenous), and pattern of use.

Estimating the amount of drug used can be difficult. For example, practitioners can ask heroin users about the amount used and the associated cost. They can also ask about what source of funds supports their habit (including legal employment, money from significant others, stealing, or prostitution). If needles or other drug paraphernalia are employed, individuals should be asked if these items are shared and, if reused, if and how they are cleaned between uses.

GENERAL MEDICAL HISTORY

Screening

The goal of screening is to identify persons at risk for substance abuse. Periodic screening should be completed for all individuals presenting for care in all settings. "Red flag" signs, particularly associated with substance abuse, are listed in Table 3-1. Screening approaches should be brief and applicable to diverse populations in a wide range of clinical settings. Use of a standardized screening instrument is helpful to ensure consistency. The instrument selected should be easily administered by all categories of health professionals or easily self-administered within 10 to 15 minutes (Center for Substance Abuse Treatment, 1997).

TABLE 3-1: RED FLAGS FOR SUBSTANCE ABUSE PROBLEMS
• Frequently missed appointments
• Frequent absences from school or work
• History of frequent injuries
• Subjective concerns, such as pain, difficulty sleeping, anxiety, or depression
• Frequent requests for medication refills with the potential for abuse (such as opioids)
• Frequent changes in medical providers
• Periods of memory loss
• Tremors
• Alcohol odor on breath or clothing
• Red eyes
• Nicotine stains
• Unsteady gait
• Dilated or pin-point pupils
• Needle marks

If screening instruments are used as a self-report rather than an interview, results should be discussed with the individuals. If they appear to be under the influence of alcohol or drugs, the screen should be deferred until they are sober; otherwise, results are unlikely to be reliable. Unfortunately, no instruments have been found to be equally effective for all persons regardless of their gender, age, or culture. These factors should be kept in mind when selecting a screening instrument.

If individuals screen negative, the occasion should be used as an opportunity to focus on prevention of substance abuse problems, including maintaining safe levels of alcohol use.

If statements such as, "I never drink," are made, follow-up questions should be used to differentiate between abstinence as a life-long state or due to previous problems. If the latter is the response, such individuals would be at risk for relapse to substance abuse.

A positive screening is not a diagnosis. Instead, persons identified as being at-risk should then undergo a more comprehensive assessment. Individuals may be screened in primary care or other community settings, then referred for specialist care or screened, completely assessed, and treated.

Screening Instruments

The CAGE Questions Adapted to Include Drugs (CAGE-AID) presented in Table 3-2, is one example of a substance abuse screening instrument. If only a single question can be asked of adults, it might be, "Have you used street drugs more than five times in your life?" The question for adolescents might be, "Have you ever used street drugs, even once?"

TABLE 3-2: CAGE-AID

1. Have you felt you should cut down on your drinking or drug use?
2. Have people annoyed you by criticizing your drinking or drug use?
3. Have you felt bad or guilty about your drinking or drug use?
4. Have you ever had a drink or used drugs first thing in the morning (as an eye-opener) to steady your nerves or to get rid of a hangover?

One positive answer suggests the need for a comprehensive assessment; two positive answers strongly suggest a substance abuse problem.

Note. From *A Guide to Substance Abuse Services for Primary Care Clinicians.* Treatment Improvement Protocol (TIP) Series 24, by Center for Substance Abuse Treatment, 1997. DHHS Publication No. (SMA) 97-3139. Rockville, MD: Substance Abuse and Mental Health Services Administration.

The following selected instruments are also appropriate for screening (although longer than the CAGE-AID). Websites are included for additional information.

Alcohol

- Alcohol Use Disorders Identification Test (AUDIT) is a 10-item instrument designed as a brief health care clinician administered interview or self-report. The AUDIT has been validated cross-culturally.
  http://whqlibdoc.who.int/hq/2001/who_msd_msb_01.6a.pdf
- Michigan Alcoholism Screening Test (MAST) is a 22-question self-test focusing specifically on alcohol use.
  http://counsellingresource.com/lib/quizzes/drug-testing/alcohol-mast/

Other Drugs

- Drug Abuse Screening Tool (DAST) is a 28-item instrument focusing on lifetime drug behaviors.
  http://www.projectcork.org/clinical_tools/html/DAST.html
- Drug and Alcohol Problem Quick Screen (DAPQS) is a 30-item instrument that targets adolescent substance use disorders and behavior.
- Simple Screening Instrument for Alcohol and Other Drug Use (SSI-AOD) is a 16-item instrument recommended for adults and adolescents.
  http://www.dmhas.state.ct.us/cosig/pilot1.pdf

Withdrawal

When a substance has been used, clinicians should inquire if the individual has ever had withdrawal symptoms when they were not using the substance. For example, individuals may report hand tremors when not consuming alcohol. Common withdrawal symptoms are listed in Table 3-3. It is important to remember that reported withdrawal symptoms cannot

TABLE 3-3: COMMON WITHDRAWAL SYMPTOMS FOR SELECTED DRUGS

Alcohol	Opiods	Cocaine	Benzodiazepines
Hand tremors	Irritability	Irritability	Confusion
Grand mal seizures	Anxiety	Depression	Restlessness
Transient visual, or auditory hallucinations or illusions	Nausea	Suicidal thoughts	Insomnia
Sweating	Vomiting	Anxiety	Anxiety
Rapid heart rate	Abdominal cramps		Hallucinations
Agitation	Diarrhea		Tingling extremities
	Chills		Muscle cramps
	Yawning		Blurred vision
	Runny nose		
	Watery eyes		
	Problems sleeping		
	Bone or muscle pain		

be attributed to another medical condition. Withdrawal from alcohol can be assessed with the Addiction Research Foundation Clinical Institute Withdrawal Assessment for Alcohol (CIWA-AR). It evaluates orientation as well as the degree of nausea and vomiting, tremor, sweats, agitation, headache, and tactile, auditory, and visual disturbances or hallucinations. The tool takes about 5 minutes to administer. Persons who score lower than 10 may not need to be medicated for withdrawal symptoms. The CIWA-AR can be found online at http://www.chce.research.va.gov/apps/PAWS/content/quiz.htm.

Treatment History

Inquiries should include dates, lengths of stay, place and method of substance abuse treatment, including efforts directed at self-treatment. For each treatment episode, the clinician should ask about the degree of success – specifically, how long the individual was substance free, noting the longest substance-free period.

Consequences of Substance Use

Consequences of substance use may be grouped under medical, psychiatric, family, social, employment, and legal categories potentially affected by substance use. The Addiction Severity Index is a multidimensional 161-item structured interview on the areas potentially affected by substance abuse. It takes about 45 minutes to administer and can be found online at http://adai.washington.edu/instruments/pdf/Addiction_Severity_Index_Baseline_Followup_4.pdf

Medical illnesses related to substance use include hepatitis B and C, human immunodeficiency virus (HIV), sexually transmitted infections (STIs), esophagitis, gastrointestinal bleeding, pancreatitis, gastritis, thrombophlebitis, cellulitis, cardiomyopathy, and subacute endocarditis. Documentation of illnesses should include dates of hospital admissions (as applicable), name and dose of medications currently prescribed, and the frequency and amount actually used.

Psychiatric history includes psychiatric disorders and whether these disorders preceded or were subsequent to initiation of substance use; whether the person was ever under psychiatric care (and if so, the duration); whether such care occurred within inpatient or outpatient settings; and whether the person ever had thoughts of or attempted suicide. If the client gives permission to do so, alternate sources, such as close family members and friends, should be interviewed in an attempt to determine which came first – symptoms of the other psychiatric disorder or substance use.

Family history includes a history of substance abuse in other family members, including first- and second-degree relatives. It also includes information on the person's marital status, who they live with, the quality of their relationships with family members, and history of physical, emotional, and/or sexual abuse by a date, family member, or intimate partner.

Social history should include education, housing, and peer use of substances.

Employment and legal history should include whether substance use has ever affected job performance and whether the person was ever arrested or incarcerated as a result of substance use.

PHYSICAL EXAMINATION

Physical signs suggestive of substance abuse include the following:

- Alcohol: increased blood pressure, tremor, enlarged liver, diaphoresis, spider angiomas, flushed face, jaundice, nystagmus, odor of alcohol, excessive yawning, red palms, arrhythmias, gynecomastia, bloody stools, ataxia, and hyperactive reflexes.
- Opioids: needle marks, jaundice, goose bumps (piloerection), pinpoint or large pupils, excessive yawning, hoarse voice, and weight loss.
- Cocaine: irregular heart rhythm (arrhythmia), hoarse voice, wheezing, needle or track marks, weight loss, nasal irritation, and perforated nasal septum.
- Marijuana: conjunctivitis, increased appetite, rapid heart rate (tachycardia), and dry mouth.

Mental Status

A mental status evaluation is a critical part of the physical examination because the individual's cognitive level will guide treatment planning. Furthermore, diagnoses can be made for other conditions that present similarly to substance abuse, such as dementia. Another goal of the assessment process is to determine the potential presence of complications of drug use and refer for medical care as necessary. A neuropsychiatric assessment by a specialist should be an integral part of the assessment. Use of many substances, most notably alcohol, can cause brain injury. Results of this evaluation can then be matched to treatment, and rehabilitation is more likely to be successful. For example, individuals with significant cognitive impairment are less likely to benefit from counseling or insight-oriented therapy as their main treatment component.

LABORATORY TESTING

Laboratory testing can help distinguish between substance-related and non-substance-related psychiatric disorders. Due to the relatively short half-lives of most substances, a positive test result can usually confirm recent drug use only – depending on the method used – typically in the past 72 hours. Therefore, it is not possible to differentiate between a chronic user versus a first-time user when there is a positive result. Exceptions include fat-soluble drugs such as marijuana, which can be detected in the urine up to 30 days after the last use. However, with this extended detection time, recent use cannot be differentiated from use further back in time, particularly for chronic users.

Difficulties in interpreting drug results are further complicated by the lack of standardized measures. Unless the laboratory uses certified testing procedures, such as those from the National Institute on Drug Abuse or the

Department of Defense, what constitutes a positive test can vary from one laboratory to another. It is important to be aware of which drugs are tested at a given laboratory. For example, drugs typically tested in occupational settings as part of employment programs are typically limited to marijuana, cocaine, amphetamines, opiates, and phencyclidine (PCP). Test results support a substance abuse diagnosis but when used alone, they are inadequate to make a diagnosis. Limits of drug detection times for urine are listed in Table 3-4.

Steps for Drug Testing

Drug testing is often completed as a two-step process. The first step is the initial screen, followed by the second step, the confirmation test. Initial screening methodologies include immunoassay or thin layer chromatography (TLC). Both approaches yield a qualitative result that is reported as positive or negative based on a given range of detectable values. Therefore, only the *presence* or *absence* of the drug can be reported, not *the amount* of the drug in the sample. These screening tests, while more economical, are less sensitive. TLC is the least expensive screening method, however it does not reliably detect controlled substances, leading to more false-negative results compared to immunoassays. Additionally, it may yield false-positive results due to cross reaction with other similar chemical substances, such as cold and allergy medications and pain relievers. TLC is limited to detecting high levels of such drugs as methadone, cocaine, codeine, amphetamines, barbitu-

TABLE 3-4: DETECTION TIMES FOR COMMON DRUGS IN URINE TESTING

DRUG	DETECTION TIME
Amphetamines	1 to 3 days
Anabolic steroids – oral	Up to 3 weeks
Anabolic steroids – parenteral	Up to 1 year
Barbiturates – short acting	1 to 3 days
Barbiturates – long acting	1 to 3 weeks
Benzodiazepine	1 to 14 days
Cannabinoids	Occasional use: 1 to 3 days Chronic use: up to 30 days
Cocaine	1 to 3 days
Codeine	1 to 2 days
Cyclizine	1 to 2 days
Gamma hydroxybutyrate (GHB)	Up to 72 hours
Heroin/morphine	3 to 4 days
Ketamine	1 to 2 days
Lysergic acid diethylamide (LSD)	Up to 8 hours
Methadone	1 to 3 days
Methaqualone	1 to 7 days
Phencyclidine (PCP)	Occasional use: 1 to 5 days Chronic use: up to 30 days
Propoxyphene	1 to 3 days
Rohypnol	1 to 3 days

rates, morphine, and propoxyphene. TLC fails to detect common methamphetamines, such as 3, 4-methylenedioxyamphetamine (MDA) or 3, 4-methylenedioxymethamphetamine (MDMA), marijuana, PCP, fentanyl, or D-lysergic acid diethylamide (LSD) (Barron, Barron, & Barron, 2005).

Immunoassays include enzyme immunoassay (EIA) or radioimmunoassay analysis (RIA). These tests depend on antibodies that react with either the drug or its metabolites. They are more accurate and reliable than TLC and detect a greater variety of drugs. Unfortunately, it is easier to intentionally produce a false negative with this approach.

Gas chromatography mass spectroscopy (GC/MS) is a method used to confirm results of the initial screen. GC/MS is highly sensitive and considerably more expensive than other screening tests, but accurately distinguishes among similar chemicals, correctly identifying presence of the drug.

Validating Urine Samples

Drug users are often invested in submitting a "clean" sample and may add, substitute, or otherwise change the specimen to attain a negative test result. For example, drug users commonly dilute their urine by adding water or overhydrating themselves to reduce concentration of the drug to less than its detectable limit. Although GC/MS may be sensitive enough to detect the drug's presence, specimens that initially test negative are not routinely subjected to GC/MS testing. Therefore, it is important that urine samples be obtained under direct observation. To combat diluting, urine tested by laboratories is screened for additives and voided if specific parameters (such as specific gravity) are not met. Administratively, depending on the purpose for testing (such as criminal justice), it is critical that a chain of custody be verified. This is established when the sample is always within sight of a member of the drug testing team until its arrival at the testing laboratory.

Sources for Drug Testing

Sources for drug testing include blood, urine, breath, hair, saliva, and sweat. Urine testing is the most widely used and most cost-effective method. Urine is the source usually preferred due to higher drug concentrations obtained as compared to blood, saliva, and sweat. Generally, blood testing is most accurate but most expensive.

Saliva can also be used but, like urine, can only detect recent drug use. Saliva is commonly used because direct observation is easier than it is for urine, and it is more difficult to tamper with the sample. It is not without its disadvantages because recent smoking can contaminate the results.

Hair testing can detect drug use further back in time – 6 months or longer. The longer the hair, the farther back detection is possible; however, most laboratories only use hair within 3 to 5 cm from the scalp, limiting detection to 90 days. Variation can occur with the rate of hair growth, hair color (dark hair absorbs drugs more readily than lighter colored hair), and ethnicity (African American hair absorbs drugs more readily than other ethnic groups). Hair testing is used especially for cocaine dependence. Compared to urine, hair is less sensitive for marijuana.

Sweat tests can also be performed; patches are placed on the skin for a 10- to 14-day period to detect drug use while the patch is in place. Cocaine, morphine, amphetamine, and ethanol have all been detected in sweat; however, there is substantial variability among individuals in how the drug concentrates in sweat. Although it is a useful approach when urine testing is not practical, there is marked biologic variability in individuals' rate of sweat production leading to a greater variability of results and reliability of interpretation.

Testing for Alcohol Abuse

Blood alcohol concentration (BAC) reflects recent intake, measured in milligrams (mg) of alcohol per deciliter (dL) of blood and reported as a percentage. For example, 100 mg of alcohol in 1 dL of blood is reported as 0.10%. It then follows that two individuals with identical alcohol intake but different blood volumes (reflected in body weight) will have different BACs, with individuals having lower body weight testing at a higher BAC. This is part of the rationale for recommending lower safe drinking limits for women compared to men.

Breath analysis is the most common method to test for blood alcohol, even though it is less accurate and not as reliable as blood testing. Breathalyzers estimate BAC but cross reactions may occur with acetone; persons who have diabetes mellitus in ketoacidosis may be confused with individuals who have ingested alcohol. Furthermore, breathalyzer results can be affected by the subject's breathing pattern or hematocrit. Hyperventilation can produce falsely low readings and low hematocrits can produce falsely high readings.

Carbohydrate-deficient transferrin (CDT) is a marker for chronic alcohol use but is more accurate in men than women. It is capable of detecting consecutive daily intake of 60 grams of alcohol over a 7- to 10-day period. Gamma glutamyl transpeptidase (GGT) is a hepatic enzyme reflecting liver cell damage. The upper limit of normal for GGT is 30 to 50 international units (IU) and is considered abnormal when greater than 50 IU. It is also elevated with hyperthyroidism, anticonvulsant use, and nonalcoholic liver disease. Other laboratory tests supportive of alcohol abuse include increased mean corpuscular volume, increased mean corpuscular hemoglobin, hypercholesterolemia, and hyperglycemia. Although the latter tests are less sensitive than the GGT, such tests taken as a group should heighten the clinician's suspicions about alcohol abuse.

STAGES OF CHANGE

The Stages of Change, also known as the *Transtheoretical Model of Change* (DiClemente, Schlundt, & Gemmell, 2004), is one model commonly applied to substance abuse that can be used in the comprehensive assessment before treatment planning. Appropriate interventions can be planned based on the client's current stage of change. The model consists of six stages that individuals progress through toward making a behavioral change. However, rather than moving through the stages in a linear fashion, regressions to a previous stage can be common. Similarly, progression through one stage may be so rapid that it appears to have been skipped. The underlying rationale behind use of this model is to match the client's level of motivation to change with the appropriate treatment modality. The Stages of Change are as follows:

I. *Precontemplation.* In this initial stage, individuals do not want to change their behavior and offer several reasons why their substance use is not a problem. Behaviors reflective of this stage include arguing about the severity of their problem, not appropriately responding to the interviewer, or otherwise indicating a resistance or inability to change. Such behaviors have also been summarized as the four "R's": reluctant, rebellious, resigned, or rationalizing (Coombs & Howatt, 2005). Individuals in this stage may have a history of multiple substance abuse treatment episodes.

II. *Contemplation.* Individuals in this second stage are thinking about a change in their substance use behavior, suggesting the client's recognition of a serious problem. Such persons indicate they are listening and attending to what the interviewer is saying about their problem, even though they may still be ambivalent about acknowledging their problem.

III. *Preparation.* Individuals in the preparation stage express readiness to make a change in their behavior. They usually stop being argumentative and actively consider various options. These people admit they have a problem but are not yet entirely committed to the treatment plan.

IV. *Action.* Individuals in the action stage are ready to participate in a defined treatment program. They make observable steps toward change even though they may still be unstable. They are receptive to new ideas, but their motivation to implement change is inconsistent. Losses in areas affected by their substance use, such as employment forfeited during active substance use, begin to return.

V. *Maintenance and Relapse Prevention.* In this stage, individuals have accomplished their initial goals and have made changes in their lives. They have a starter set of coping strategies to draw upon when they are tempted to use substances. Individuals in the maintenance phase demonstrate that they possess the skills needed to avoid relapsing to substance use.

VI. *Termination.* In the final stage of termination, individuals have moved beyond their substance use, substituting other healthy life habits in its place.

An assessment instrument that clinicians can use to determine the client's location on this continuum is the Stages of Change Readiness and Treatment Eagerness Scale (SOCRATES) (Miller & Tonigan, 1996). Although it was originally designed to determine readiness for change in alcohol abusers, it has been adapted for use with drug abusers as well. This 19-item scale measures recognition, ambivalence, and taking steps. SOCRATES can be found online at http://casaa.unm.edu/inst/SOCRATESv8.pdf.

DIAGNOSTIC SUMMARY

Data from the comprehensive assessment is used for the diagnostic summary that evaluates individuals' substance use problems in the context of their unique life situations. By the end of the assessment, there should be sufficient data to make a formal substance use disorder diagnosis and formulate a treatment plan. There are two organizations with established diagnostic criteria for substance abuse. The American Psychiatric Association developed the *Diagnostic and Statistical Manual of Mental Disorders,* now in its 5th Edition (*DSM-5*), and is considered the national standard for the United States. The parallel system, the International Classification of Disease, now in its 10th revision (ICD-10), is used by the World Health Organization.

According to the *DSM-5,* the umbrella term *substance-related disorders* is subdivided between substance-induced disorders and substance use disorders. Substance-induced disorders are those that directly result from the pharmacologic effects of the drug, such as in withdrawal or intoxication. Other mental disorders can also be directly precipitated by drug effects.

Substance use disorders arise from the pattern of or consequences from substance use. Severity of the individual's problems is further described as mild, moderate, or severe, according to the number of symptoms met for the diagnosis. In general, mild is the presence of 2 or 3 symptoms listed in the criteria, moderate by 4 or 5 symptoms and severe by 6 or more symptoms. Severity can change over time to increase or decrease so it should be reassessed periodically. Because these criteria rely on the individual's behavior or functional impairment resulting from their substance use, these criteria apply to any drug. (See Table 3-5.)

There exist both similarities and differences between the DSM classifications of substance related disorders and those found in the ICD – 10 codes. Similarities include specific listing and codes for specific substances and the many similar criteria used for diagnosis. Differences relate to the categorization and labeling of symptom clusters.

ASSESSMENT OF SPECIAL POPULATIONS

Screening, recognition, and assessment of substance abuse can be challenging for such unique groups as adolescents, women, older adults, and persons with co-morbid conditions (in particular, mental disorders).

Adolescents

Adolescents are unique in that some substances that are legal for adults are illegal for them. It also may be difficult to differentiate between acting out and being affected by substance abuse. Further, they may be even less forthcoming than adults about their use. As with all people, screening should, at minimum, take place at all routine medical visits. However, many adolescents may not be seen regularly for such care; therefore, screening should occur whenever they present for care.

Because the number one cause of death among adolescents is accidents, with the largest subgroup being motor vehicle collisions (Medline Plus, 2012), it is crucial that screening for substance use, especially alcohol, occur. Caution must be used regarding screening instruments designed for adults being used with adolescents. Such tools are usually developmentally inappropriate. For example, the CAGE, while reliable for adults, should probably not be used to assess for adolescent substance use, and definitely not used as the sole screening tool. The CAGE eye-opener question, "Have you ever had a drink first thing in the morning to steady your nerves or to get rid of a hangover?" is not likely to be endorsed by a young adolescent. Knight, Goodman, Pulerwitz, and DuRant (2000) evaluated the reliability of

TABLE 3-5: SUMMARY OF *DSM-5* CRITERIA FOR SUBSTANCE USE DISORDER

Substance use disorder consists of a problematic pattern of substance use that may result in:

- The use of increased amounts of the substance
- The desire but lack of success in reducing or eliminating the use of the substance
- Excessive use of time related to the procurement, use, or recovery from effects of the substance
- A craving for the substance
- The use of the substance leads to decreased performance in various expected roles
- Use of the substance continues in spite of interpersonal, family or social problems related to its use
- Withdrawal from or decreased participation in other activities because of substance use
- Use of the substance in potentially hazardous circumstances
- Continued use of the substance regardless of negative physical or psychological consequences related to its use
- The need for increased amounts of the substance to achieve the desired effect or a decreased ability to achieve the desired effect with usual amounts of the substance
- Symptoms of withdrawal are experienced when the substance is decreased or eliminated.

brief substance use screening tests for a diverse group of adolescents including the SSI-AOD, recommended for use with both adolescents and adults. As part of this investigation, they adapted the CAGE for adolescents (CAGE-AA) and compared it to the SSI-AOD. The SSI-AOD was observed to be the most reliable, while the CAGE-AA could not be recommended for routine use. Additionally, adolescents should be routinely asked about anabolic steroids. The SSI-AOD can be found online at http://www.dmhas state.ct.us/cosig/pilot1.pdf.

The RAFFT is a brief, 5-question instrument developed specifically to screen for adolescent substance use (Bastiaens, Francis, & Lewis, 2000). Questions target whether friends or family members use substances, if they use substance alone, and whether substance use was ever problematic. A score of 3 is considered a positive screen. The RAFFT was also observed to be an effective screening tool for adult substance abuse. However, it is a less effective screen than the CAGE for alcohol abusers (Bastiaens, 2002).

The Problem Oriented Screening Instrument for Teenagers (POSIT) consists of 138 questions. It takes about 25 minutes to administer, and responses are "yes" or "no." It can be administered by an interviewer or self-administered using pencil and paper, audiotape, or computer. Adolescents may be more likely to respond truthfully to a computer-assisted or audiotaped version compared to a version administered by another person. The POSIT is also available in Spanish.

Older Adults

There are two groups of older adults at risk for substance use disorders associated with age of onset. The early-onset group had substance use problems as younger adults, which persisted as they aged. The late-onset group had their onset of problems begin after age 60. Typically, the substances involved are alcohol and prescription drugs. About 17% of adults older than 60 years of age have alcohol or prescription drug problems; however, they are frequently underdiagnosed (Volkow, 2006). Contributing to this under diagnosis is clinicians' belief that this group rarely has drug problems. In addition, symptoms from concurrent chronic illnesses may mask substance use disorders. Furthermore, it is important to consider *DMS-5* criteria as separate and distinct from biologic age-related changes in order not to miss an existing Substance Use Disorder in older adults. Such changes make substance problems more likely at smaller quantities compared to younger adults.

The CAGE has been noted to have overall good sensitivity and specificity and has also been validated for older adults. Sensitivity refers to a test's ability to detect "true positives;" that is, the percent of individuals with the disorder who screen positive with the test. Specificity refers to a test's ability to detect "true negatives," or the percent of individuals without the disorder who screen negative with the test. If the CAGE is used, a cut-off score of 1 should be used because this population is more likely to develop substance-related problems due to age-related changes. However, this tool is not as effective in discriminating between a current and previous drinking problem. The MAST has a geriatric version (MAST-G) for older adults wherein five or more "yes" answers suggests alcohol problems. Older adults should also be specifically screened for prescription drug abuse. The MAST-G can be found online at http://www.ncbi.nlm.nih.gov/books/NBK64829/#A46031.

Clients with HIV/AIDS

When assessing all persons, inquiries should include questions about HIV testing and results and assessment of high-risk behaviors. It is particularly important if the individual is known to be HIV-infected because substance abuse and its associated behaviors accelerate the progression of HIV (Volkow, 2006). Ask if they are on medications for HIV and, if so, the degree to which they adhere to their regimen.

Clients with Mental Illness

Drug use commonly coexists with other mental disorders. In the 1970s it was discovered that the combination of substance abuse and other mental disorders was associated with poorer treatment outcomes, including medical, social, and emotional problems. This comorbidity was so common that specific terminology named "dual diagnosis" emerged. It referred to any combination of mental disorders, such as a developmental disability and schizophrenia. The current term, "co-occurring disorders" (COD) refers to coexisting substance-related disorders with other mental disorders. Data from a number of epidemiologic studies suggests that up to 6 of every 10 persons who abuse substances also have at least one other mental illness (Volkow, 2006).

Drug use can precipitate, reduce, aggravate, mimic, or obscure psychiatric symptoms, complicating the diagnostic process for either the substance abuse or mental disorder. When drug use precipitates another mental disorder, it is then classified as a substance-induced disorder. Populations with increased COD prevalence compared to the general U.S. population include homeless people, criminal justice offenders, and those with a history of infectious disease (such as hepatitis C or HIV/AIDS). It is critical that persons with one disorder be screened for the other because treating only one can negatively impact both disorders. If the person has abstained from drug use for at least 30 days, clinicians should ask about the remaining mental health symptoms because symptoms from drug use should no longer be apparent.

Diagnosis of mental health disorders must be made by qualified professionals. There is no brief assessment for COD; however, the brief mental health assessment before the SSI-AOD may be used. Examples of instruments commonly used include the Structured Clinical Interview for *DSM-5* Disorders (SCID) and the Diagnostic Interview Schedule. The SCID is the interview most frequently used by psychiatrists.

Women

Substance abuse and domestic violence often co-occur. When women are asked about histories of domestic violence, it is important to do so privately, away from the abuser or other persons who may inform the abuser. If women endorse a history of or report current domestic violence, the assessment must address the safety concerns and their substance abuse.

Current practice encourages pregnant women to abstain from all alcohol, nicotine, or illicit drugs. Maternal alcohol use is evident in fetal alcohol syndrome and is the most common cause of mental retardation. About 9% of women in the United States drink alcohol at least once during pregnancy (Substance Abuse and Mental Health Administration, 2012). For alcohol screening, the T-ACE (Table 3-6) – a modification of the CAGE – is useful (Sokol, 1989). Alternatively, the TWEAK (Table 3-7), a 5-item instrument that uses questions from the CAGE, MAST, and T-ACE could be used (Center for Substance Abuse Treatment, 1997). Both instruments include a question on tolerance. Answers to this question appear to be positive more often for women – perhaps because it is less socially stigmatizing – encouraging more honest answers. For illicit drugs, the CAGE-AID could be used or this population could be asked directly, "Do you use street drugs?"

TABLE 3-6: T-ACE

T	**Tolerance:** How many drinks does it take to make you feel high?
A	Have people **Annoyed** you by criticizing your drinking?
C	Have you ever felt you ought to **Cut down** on your drinking?
E	**Eye opener:** Have you ever had a drink first thing in the morning to steady your nerves or get rid of a hangover?

The T-ACE is used to screen for pregnancy risk drinking, defined here as the consumption of 1 ounce or more of alcohol per day while pregnant. Scores are calculated as follows: a reply of more than two drinks to question T is considered a positive response and scores 2 points (0 points for two drinks or less), and an affirmative answer to question A, C, or E scores 1 point, respectively. A total score of 2 or more points on the T-ACE indicates a positive outcome for pregnancy risk drinking.

Note. From "The T-ACE questions: Practical prenatal detection of risk-drinking" by R.J. Sokol, S.S. Martier, & J.W. Ager, 1989, *American Journal of Obstetrics and Gynecology, 160,* p. 863-871.

TABLE 3-7: TWEAK

T	**Tolerance:** How many drinks can you hold?
W	Have close friends or relatives **Worried** or complained about your drinking in the past year?
E	**Eye-opener:** Do you sometimes take a drink in the morning when you first get up?
A	**Amnesia:** Has a friend or family member ever told you about things you said or did while you were drinking that you could not remember?
K (C)	Do you sometimes feel the need to **Cut down** on your drinking?

Scoring: A 7-point scale is used to score the test. The tolerance question scores 2 points if a woman reports she can consume more than five drinks without falling asleep or passing out. A positive response to the worry question scores 2 points. A positive response to the last three questions scores 1 point each. A total score of 2 or more indicates the woman is likely to be a risk drinker.

Note. From "New Assessment Tools for Risk Drinking During Pregnancy: T-ACE, TWEAK, and Others," by M. Russell, 1994. *American Journal of Obstetrics and Gynecology, 160*(4), 863-871.

CLIENT CONFIDENTIALITY

Eliciting honest answers from substance users can be challenging. All questions should be asked in a nonjudgmental manner. Clinicians should clearly explain why the questions are important and the potential consequences that may occur if information given is inaccurate. Before beginning the interview, all individuals should be informed about federal laws and regulations concerning confidentiality.

Federal law provides stringent requirements for disclosing client information related to substance use. The goal of the regulations in "Confidentiality of Alcohol and Drug Abuse Patient Records," 42 C.F.R. part 2 is to encourage people "to enter treatment without fear of stigmatization or discrimination as a result of information disclosure without the patient's express permission" (Center for Substance Abuse Treatment, 1997, p. 69). This law applies to facilities that provide substance abuse assessment and treatment as their primary mission. Ordinarily, federal regulations would not apply to general medical care facilities unless the clinician's primary function as part of providing care in that facility is substance abuse treatment and assessment, and if the facility receives federal assistance.

State laws may have additional requirements that vary among states. Some states may have stricter confidentiality laws; however, all states must adhere to federal requirements as a minimum standard. All clinicians should be explicitly aware of whether they must comply with federal regulations and what additional, if any, state requirements apply. Awareness of existing regulations to protect client information, along with communicating a genuine desire to help, should help convince individuals that truthful answers are in their best interest.

SUMMARY

Assessment for substance use disorders is far from simple; however, when an organized approach is taken, all individuals can be effectively assessed. After the initial screen, comprehensive assessment should include a detailed history, physical, and laboratory evaluation. Laboratory verification of substance use is commonly done with urine; however, its usefulness is limited because for most drugs, only very recent use can be confirmed.

Using the Stages of Change as a theoretical framework can assist clinicians in determining how ready the client is to change his or her behavior. At the end of this assessment, there should be adequate information to determine a substance use diagnosis.

Additional considerations should be made for such populations as adolescents, women, and older adults, and appropriate adjustments made. Doing so should make it possible to assess all individuals regardless of the health care setting.

EXAM QUESTIONS

CHAPTER 3

Questions 12-17

Note: Choose the one option that BEST answers each question.

12. Goals of the comprehensive assessment include

    a. determining the individual's readiness to change his or her behavior.
    b. determining the specific event that led to initiating substance use.
    c. limiting problem identification to events that preceded substance use.
    d. screening only individuals with highly suggestive signs and symptoms.

13. Which statement about laboratory testing for substance use is correct?

    a. Test results can be used as the sole source of information for diagnosing a substance abuse disorder.
    b. Marijuana can be detected in the urine for up to 72 hours after use.
    c. Results of drug tests are interpreted using universal, standardized measures.
    d. Blood test results cannot differentiate between a chronic user and a first-time user.

14. The most accurate laboratory method to determine the presence of drugs is

    a. enzyme immunoassay analysis (EIA).
    b. gas chromatography mass spectroscopy (GC/MS).
    c. radioimmunoassay analysis (RIA).
    d. thin layer chromatography (TLC).

15. Individuals in the precontemplation stage characteristically

    a. believe that they have a serious substance abuse problem.
    b. express tentative readiness to participate in a drug treatment program.
    c. express the belief that they do not have a drug problem.
    d. state, "It's time for me to do something about my problem."

16. A brief 5 question instrument developed specifically to screen for adolescent substance use is the

    a. CAGE
    b. CAGE-AA
    c. POSIT
    d. RAFFT

17. Diagnosing substance use disorders in older adults is difficult because

    a. older adults are less likely than younger adults to develop substance abuse problems.
    b. chronic illness and age-related biologic changes may mask symptoms.
    c. there are no assessment instruments currently available to evaluate substance abuse for this population.
    d. they rarely present to the clinic for screening.

REFERENCES

American Psychiatric Association. (2013). *Diagnostic and statistical manual of mental disorders* (5th ed.). Washington, DC: American Psychiatric Association.

Baron, D.A., Baron, D.A., & Baron, S.H. (2005). Laboratory testing for substances of abuse. In R.J. Frances, S.I. Miller, & A.H. Mack (Eds.), *Clinical textbook of addictive disorders* (3rd ed.). New York: Guilford Press.

Bastiaens, L., Francis, G., & Lewis, K. (2000). The RAFFT as a screening tool for adolescent substance use disorders. *American Journal on Addictions, 9*(1), 10-16.

Bastiaens, L., Riccardi, K., & Sakrhani, D. (2002). The RAFFT as a screening tool for adult substance use disorders. *American Journal of Drug and Alcohol Abuse, 28*(4), 681-691.

Center for Substance Abuse Treatment. (1997). *A guide to substance abuse services for primary care clinicians.* Treatment Improvement Protocol (TIP) Series 24. DHHS Publication No. (SMA) 97-3139. Rockville, MD: Substance Abuse and Mental Health Services Administration.

Center for Substance Abuse Treatment. (2005). *Substance abuse treatment for persons with co-occurring disorders.* Treatment Improvement Protocol (TIP) Series 42. DHHS Publication No. (SMA) 05-3922. Rockville, MD: Substance Abuse and Mental Health Services Administration.

Coombs, R.H. & Howatt, W.A. (2005). *The addiction counselor's desk reference.* Hoboken, NJ: John Wiley & Sons.

DiClemente, C.C., Schlundt, D., & Gemmell, L. (2004). Readiness and stages of change in addiction treatment. *American Journal of Addiction, 13*(2), 103-119.

Knight, J.R., Goodman, E., Pulerwitz, T., & DuRant, R.H. (2000). Reliabilities of short substance abuse screening tests among adolescent medical patients. *Pediatrics, 105*(4), 948-953.

Medline Plus. (2012). *Death among children and adolescents.* Accessed March 15, 2013, from http://www.nlm.nih.gov/medlineplus/ency/article/001915.htm

Miller, W.R. & Tonigan, J.S. (1996). Assessing drinkers' motivation for change: The Stages of Change Readiness and Treatment Eagerness Scale (SOCRATES). *Psychology of Addictive Behaviors, 10,* 81-89.

Russell, M.A. (1994). New assessment tools for risk drinking during pregnancy: T-ACE, TWEAK, and others. *Alcohol Health and Research World, 18*(1), 55-61.

Sokol, R.J., Martier, S.S., & Ager, J.W. (1989). The T-ACE questions: Practical prenatal detection of risk-drinking. *American Journal of Obstetrics and Gynecology, 160*(4), 863-871.

Substance Abuse and Mental Health Services Administration (2012). *Results from the 2011 National Survey on Drug Use and Health: Summary of national findings.* NSDUH Series H-44, HHS Publication No. (SMA) 12-4713. Rockville, MD: Substance Abuse and Mental Health Services Administration.

Tarter, R.E. (2005). Psychological evaluation of substance use disorder in adolescents and adults. In R.J. Frances, S.I. Miller, & A.H. Mack (Eds.), *Clinical textbook of addictive disorders* (3rd ed.). New York: Guilford Press.

Volkow, N.D. (2006). NIDA (National Institute on Drug Abuse) *Director's report to CPDD (College on Problems of Drug Dependence) meeting: Progress, priorities and plans for the future.* Problems of Drug Dependence 2005: Proceedings of the 67th Annual Scientific Meeting. NIH Publication No. 06-6014, 70-79.

Woody, G.E. & Cacciola, J. (2004). Evaluation and early treatment. In J.H. Lowinson, P. Ruiz, R.B. Millman, & J.G. Langrod (Eds.), *Substance abuse: A comprehensive textbook* (4th ed.). Philadelphia: Lippincott Williams & Wilkins.

CHAPTER 4

TREATMENT OF SUBSTANCE USE DISORDERS

CHAPTER OBJECTIVE

After completing this chapter, the learner will be able to discuss the different approaches and settings for treating substance use disorders.

LEARNING OBJECTIVES

After studying this chapter, the learner will be able to:

1. Describe the role of pharmacotherapy in treating substance use disorders.
2. Identify common medications used for substance disorder treatment.
3. Describe the current behavioral therapeutic approaches employed for substance use disorder.
4. Describe the advantages and disadvantages of various behavioral therapies.
5. Describe the results from the Project Match and the Drug Abuse Treatment Outcome Study (DATOS) clinical trials.

OVERVIEW

History has long documented the existence of substance use disorders and the attempts to treat them. Benjamin Rush, a physician from the Revolutionary War period, is credited with the origins of modern treatment approaches and is often called the "father of American psychiatry." He directed alcoholics to receive treatment in an asylum, family-type setting away from all responsibilities and access to alcohol. In the early 20th century, treatment attempts included substituting one opioid for another and detoxification trends that progressed to gradual reduction or non-use of the offending substance, isolation from other users, and use of non-addicting substances. Group support was fostered through religious conversion and various religious approaches to treatment in a supportive environment that exerted no demands on individuals (Westermeyer, 2005). Today's treatment methods can trace their beginnings to each of these approaches.

Beneficial treatment outcomes are closely related to treatment duration and setting – the longer the duration of treatment in the appropriate setting, the better the outcome. Overall, good outcomes are observed, particularly after 90 days of treatment. Other related critical factors include engagement and participation in treatment. There are three basic approaches to treatment of substance use disorders: pharmacotherapy, behavioral treatment, and a combination of the two. Settings vary and include inpatient, outpatient, residential, community, and office settings.

Perhaps the best source of national trends in treatment is the Treatment Episodic Data Set (TEDS) (Substance Abuse and Mental Health Services Administration [SAMHSA]), 2012b).

Data is collected annually from each state based on their substance abuse treatment system. It is a system based on admissions rather than individuals; therefore, one individual who was admitted for two treatment episodes would be represented twice in this data set. Additional limitations are that this data set excludes information from the Bureau of Prisons, Department of Defense, and Veteran's Administration. Further, the numbers do not represent demand for treatment or prevalence of substance use disorders.

HISTORICAL ASPECTS OF TREATMENT

In the 1800s, it was common to make medicines from opium (such as laudanum and paregoric) and, in 1832, morphine was extracted from crude opium. Morphine was followed by codeine and the introduction of commercial heroin in 1898. Consumption rapidly escalated until federal laws limited importation of opium, resulting in vast problems with opium smuggling. In 1912, the Hague Treaty, an international agreement to encourage nations to develop stringent laws restricting opioid consumption to medical purposes only, was instituted. In response, formal drug treatment emerged with clinics operated by police or health departments designed to maintain addicts on morphine. Two years later, the Harrison Act made non-medical opiate abuse illegal, representing the beginning of a federal role in addressing substance abuse. With opiate use solely under the control of medical care, it was observed that morphine-addicted individuals could be maintained on heroin in a manner permitting them to function in society. However, in 1919, it became illegal to prescribe opioid maintenance when addiction was the person's sole problem.

In the same year, an experiment by the New York City Health Department used heroin to recruit persons addicted to morphine into a 6-week inpatient detoxification and rehabilitation program. This experiment ended after about 1 year when it was observed that even after detoxification was complete, addicts usually relapsed to heroin use and all clinics were closed by 1925. With the subsequent incarceration of addicts, federal prisons quickly filled, necessitating the building of two opioid hospitals operated by the United States Public Health Service to treat addicts (Musto, 2005).

Treatment focusing on abstinence appeared first among organized religion, followed by the proliferation of self-help groups after World War II, permitting substance users to remain in their communities rather than relocating to asylums. Group support was given through structured meetings based on stepwise activities to encourage recovery. Membership in such groups required that individuals publicly identify themselves as an alcoholic or addict and declare their dependence on a "Higher Power." Alcoholics Anonymous (AA), established in 1935, is the prototype of this approach.

EPIDEMIOLOGY

According to the 2011 National Survey on Drug Use and Health (NSDUH), about 21.6 million people aged 12 years or older needed treatment for substance abuse or dependence (SAMHSA, 2012a). Unfortunately only 2.3 million received treatment – about 11% of those individuals needing it. In 2010, there were approximately 1.8 million admissions to state-certified treatment facilities (SAMHSA, 2012b). Five substances – alcohol (41%), opiates (23%), marijuana (18%), cocaine (8%), and stimulants (6%) – accounted for 96% of those admissions. Among alcohol admissions, 45% involved a secondary drug problem, demonstrating the frequency of polydrug abuse. Admissions for opiates refer primarily to heroin, and those for stimulants refer primarily to methamphetamines. Among all admissions for 2010, 63%

were for ambulatory treatment, 20% for detoxification, and 17% for residential facilities. Thirty three percent of admissions were by individual or self-referral and 37% by the criminal justice system (SAMHSA, 2012b).

TREATMENT

Two national organizations established guidelines for effective treatment programs and appropriate placement of individuals for those programs. The National Institute on Drug Abuse (NIDA) detailed key principles for effective treatment programs based on research conducted since the mid-1970s (NIDA, 2009). The American Society of Addiction Medicine (ASAM) recommends that six dimensions be constantly assessed to determine the appropriate level of drug treatment (ASAM, 2001). These dimensions evaluate the client's potential for having such acute problems as withdrawal, and such factors as his or her cognitive condition and readiness to change that could influence recovery from substance abuse. Treatment guidelines, dimensions, and intensity level of drug treatment are summarized in Tables 4-1 through 4-3.

Treatment can be divided into three phases: detoxification, treatment, and continuing care (also known as *after care*).

Detoxification with Pharmacotherapy

Pharmacotherapy can involve the use of medications to detoxify clients from the targeted drug or to provide a temporary or long-term substitute for the offending drug. Pharmacotherapy for substance abuse is based on the neurobiological changes in the brain affected by chronic substance use. For example, medications for opioid abuse (such as methadone, levo-alpha acetyl methadol [LAAM], buprenorphine, and naltrexone) all act on the same areas of the brain as the addictive substance.

TABLE 4-1: PRINCIPLES FOR EFFECTIVE TREATMENT PROGRAMS

- Addiction is a complex but treatable disease that affects brain function and behavior.
- No single treatment is appropriate for everyone.
- Treatment needs to be readily available.
- Effective treatment attends to multiple needs of the individual, not just his or her drug abuse.
- Remaining in treatment for an adequate period of time is critical.
- Counseling – individual and/or group – and other behavioral therapies are the most commonly used forms of drug abuse treatment.
- Medications are an important element of treatment for many patients, especially when combined with counseling and other behavioral therapies.
- An individual's treatment and services plan must be assessed continually and modified as necessary to ensure that it meets his or her changing needs.
- Many drug-addicted individuals also have other mental disorders.
- Medically assisted detoxification is only the first stage of addiction treatment and by itself does little to change long-term drug abuse.
- Treatment does not need to be voluntary to be effective.
- Drug use during treatment must be monitored continuously, as lapses during treatment do occur.
- Treatment programs should assess patients for the presence of HIV/AIDS, hepatitis B and C, tuberculosis, and other infectious diseases as well as provide targeted risk-reduction counseling to help patients modify or change behaviors that place them at risk of contracting or spreading infectious diseases.

Note. From *DrugFacts: Treatment Approaches for Drug Addiction* by National Institute on Drug Abuse, 2009. Accessed March 15, 2013, from http://www.drugabuse.gov/publications/drugfacts/treatment-approaches-drug-addiction

TABLE 4-2: DIMENSIONS OF CARE
1. Acute intoxication or withdrawal potential
2. Biomedical conditions and complications
3. Emotional, behavioral, or cognitive conditions and complications
4. Readiness to change
5. Relapse, continued use, or continued problem potential
6. Recovery environment
(ASAM, 2001)

TABLE 4-3: AMERICAN SOCIETY OF ADDICTION MEDICINE'S PATIENT PLACEMENT CRITERIA LEVELS OF SERVICE
Level 0.5: Early intervention
Level I: Outpatient treatment
Level II: Intensive outpatient/partial hospitalization treatment
Level III: Residential/Inpatient treatment
Level IV: Medically managed intensive inpatient treatment
(ASAM, 2001)

The goal of pharmacotherapy is normalizing brain function through direct reversal of changes incurred from chronic drug use. With drug therapy, most of the harmful effects in the brain are resolved in the first few weeks after addictive drug use has ceased. However, medications alone do not address other harmful effects of substances such as the environment in which drug use was initiated. It is within the social environment where drug cravings originated, that the risk for subsequent relapse to substance use increases. Nevertheless, for persons with substance dependence, medications are often the first approach to treatment, typically to address withdrawal symptoms.

Withdrawal occurs after the drug is abruptly stopped, usually among individuals who are substance-dependent. Generally, signs and symptoms of withdrawal are opposite those of intoxication. Substances potentially requiring detoxification include alcohol, opioids, anxiolytics, sedative-hypnotics, and stimulants. Depending on the severity of withdrawal, detoxification can occur in inpatient or outpatient settings. Behavioral therapies are often deferred due to notable client discomfort until the detoxification process is nearly complete.

Detoxification, often conceptualized as the first step in drug treatment, involves withdrawing clients from substances safely and effectively. First established in Eastern Europe, it became widely used in the mid-1900s. Generally, approaches to detoxification include medication use to prevent severe withdrawal symptoms, gradually reduce or taper the offending drug, or substitute for the offending drug.

Historically, drug substitution has been used, particularly for opioids. For example, laudanum (alcohol combined with opiates) was once prescribed for the treatment of alcoholism. Morphine, and later heroin, was prescribed for opium addiction in the mid-1800s. The latter approach has evolved to the current common use of methadone to substitute for heroin. Additional examples of the other approaches to detoxification include:

- alcohol – benzodiazepines are used to prevent severe alcohol withdrawal symptoms, including the likelihood of developing delirium or seizures
- anxiolytics or sedative-hypnotics – detoxification often focuses on medically supervised reductions.

Other medications used for detoxification include anticonvulsants, barbiturates, and neuroleptics.

Commonly used medications to treat alcohol and heroin abuse beyond detoxification are described in this section. Unfortunately, there is no medication approved by the Food and Drug Administration (FDA) specifically for cocaine abuse.

- *Disulfiram* interferes with the normal metabolism of alcohol and is perhaps the oldest drug used for alcohol treatment. When alcohol consumption follows disulfiram, individuals experience uncomfortable nausea, headaches, dizziness, flushing, and palpitations.
- *Naltrexone* is a long-acting opioid antagonist that blocks the effects of opioids to extinguish the conditioned cues that encourage drug use. It has also been observed to reduce alcohol craving. It is non-addicting with few adverse effects.
- *Acamprosate* was designed to reduce alcohol craving. Although its exact mechanism of action is not fully understood, it is believed to normalize brain function by affecting the activity of the neurotransmitters gamma aminobutyric acid (GABA) and glutamate.
- *Methadone* is a widely used drug for stabilization and maintenance of persons with opioid dependence. It is a long-acting opioid agonist that substitutes for the shorter-acting heroin. It is a broadly supported approach that permits clients who are opioid dependent to participate normally in their daily lives. *Methadone maintenance* programs may be located within comprehensive drug treatment centers, primary care clinics, or social service agencies. Regardless of location, treatment programs that include methadone dispensing are meticulously regulated by the federal and state government. Federal eligibility requires at least 1 year of opioid use and current evidence of opioid dependence. However, exceptions to eligibility criteria are made if the client is pregnant or recently discharged from a controlled facility such as prison. Methadone maintenance consists of these three phases:

  1. stabilization, wherein clients adjust to their methadone dose
  2. treatment planning, during which other problems affected by drug use are addressed, such as employment and physical health
  3. continued methadone at their maintenance dose with few other services, if any, associated with the previous phase.

  Attendance may be daily during the first phase and taper to once weekly in the maintenance phase.
- *Buprenorphine* is a partial mu agonist and kappa antagonist that is an alternative to methadone. It has a low risk of overdose and similar low potential for abuse. Buprenorphine is unique in that it can be prescribed by the primary care physician outside of formal, organized methadone maintenance programs.

Behavioral Therapy

Behavioral therapies constitute the bulk of treatment and include cognitive-behavioral, motivational interventions, and contingency management. Although not typically initiated during the detoxification period, if this period is extended, behavioral therapy can and should be initiated. Behavioral therapies are an important complement to pharmacotherapy because strategies learned are required to adhere to the medication regime and prevent substance abuse relapse.

Behavioral treatment can be delivered at an individual or a group level for a single session, such as a brief intervention, or for 1 year or more. This chapter will discuss brief interventions as a separate treatment approach based on *duration* of treatment rather than content. Additional treatment approaches that may supplement those previously mentioned or serve as the primary means of treatment include self-help or 12-step groups, family-based treatment, acupuncture, and faith-based groups.

No specific behavioral therapy appears to be more effective than another. For example, Project Match was a landmark multi-site research study of 1,726 alcohol-abusing or alcohol-dependent persons in which individuals were randomly assigned to individual level sessions of motivational enhancement therapy, 12-step facilitation, or cognitive behavioral therapy over a 12-week period (National Institute on Alcohol Abuse and Alcoholism [NIAAA], 1997). Before this study, it was commonly believed that clients should be matched to a specific treatment type based on their individual characteristics, such as the severity of other psychiatric problems or whether they had access to high social support. Hypotheses were made about a total of 16 individual characteristics. Only one – psychiatric severity – was significant, where study participants who were outpatients and had few or no psychological problems were more likely to have more abstinent days with 12-step facilitation versus cognitive behavioral therapy. While there was less than expected differential response to treatment, all participants demonstrated substantial and persistent reductions in alcohol intake regardless of the specific treatment they received.

Brief Intervention

Brief interventions have been constructed for clients whose substance use is not yet a major problem. A brief intervention may be all that is needed if individuals appear to have only mild substance abuse problems and if the goal is to prevent more severe problems. Brief interventions can be incorporated into non-specialist settings such as primary care. These settings may be the most suitable site for persons with mild to moderate substance problems because specialist settings normally are designed for persons with moderate to severe problems. Spontaneous remission of problematic substance use is not uncommon and a short intervention may be all that is required. Furthermore, treatment in a primary care or similar setting is less likely to be socially stigmatizing compared to drug treatment settings, and it may also be the ideal location to integrate drug treatment with other comorbid health problems. Components of brief interventions are listed in Table 4-4.

TABLE 4-4: COMPONENTS OF BRIEF INTERVENTIONS

COMPONENT	DEFINITION
Giving feedback	Giving feedback includes explaining screening results, impairment, and risks while clarifying the findings. Potential and actual health problems that likely developed or will develop from substance use should be stressed.
Informing about safe consumption	Advice on safe limits of consumption (such as no more than one alcoholic drink daily for women) should be tailored to and integrated with the client's unique health concerns.
Assessing the client's readiness for change	The client's preparedness to change his or her substance use behavior is assessed.
Negotiating goals and strategies	Negotiating for reductions in substance use as part of the continuum towards abstinence may be required.
Arranging for follow-up treatment	Progress should be monitored and, if not successful, the client should be referred to specialty addiction services.

Note. From *Brief Interventions and Brief Therapies for Substance Abuse.* Treatment Improvement Protocol (TIP) Series 34, by Center for Substance Abuse Treatment, 1999a. DHHS Publication Number 99-3353. Rockville, MD: Substance Abuse and Mental Health Services Administration.

Treatment duration can include one to several 10- to 15-minute sessions that aim to reduce or eliminate substance use. The focus might be limited to encouraging persons to recognize that they have a substance abuse problem. Content may not always be delivered directly and might consist of individuals reading self-help booklets. Alternatively, this may be the sole contact before referral for specialist care.

Research on this approach has been shown to be effective – more so for alcohol than illicit drug use for which fewer investigations have been conducted (Center for Substance Abuse Treatment [CSAT], 1999a). Specifically, brief interventions have been effective in reducing alcohol consumption up to 50% and are just as effective for women and persons from diverse cultures (CSAT, 1999a). However, these methods have not been well tested for adolescents or older adults. The ideal number of sessions or duration for each session is also unknown, although it is likely to vary with individuals and the severity of their substance problems. In addition to persons with mild to moderate substance abuse problems, persons who refuse to seek specialist care would also be appropriate candidates; part of the intervention could then include encouragement to obtain care in a more intensive setting.

For many individuals, a brief intervention serves as a good transition to specialist care where more comprehensive assessment and treatment can occur. Other individuals are better served through specialty services. Characteristics of clients less likely to benefit from brief interventions alone are listed in Table 4-5.

Contingency Management

Contingency management is an approach that emphasizes rewards for positive behavior versus punishment for negative behavior. This approach has four principles:

1. rapid and accurate detection of drug use
2. positive reinforcement of abstinence
3. loss of positive reinforcement upon detection of drug use
4. development of positive reinforcers to compete with drug use.

TABLE 4-5: CHARACTERISTICS OF CLIENTS LESS LIKELY TO BENEFIT FROM BRIEF INTERVENTIONS

- History of substance-related consequences (such as driving under the influence of alcohol)
- Evidence of physical tolerance (such as requiring higher amounts of the drug over time to obtain the same effects)
- Compulsive use of the substance
- History of withdrawal from the substance
- History of prior substance abuse treatment

Note. From *Brief Interventions and Brief Therapies for Substance Abuse.* Treatment Improvement Protocol (TIP) Series 34, by Center for Substance Abuse Treatment, 1999a. DHHS Publication Number 99-3353. Rockville, MD: Substance Abuse and Mental Health Services Administration.

Abstinence is reinforced with vouchers that can be redeemed for various desirable services or cash. Urine specimens are tested three times weekly with abstinence based on these urine results. Vouchers increase in value with each consecutive drug-free specimen. Drug-positive urine results in no receipt of vouchers and a reset of the next voucher to the initial baseline value. In numerous research trials, this approach has been highly accepted by clients with high rates of abstinence (Rounsaville, Carroll & Back, 2005). Abstinence occurred regardless of the cash value of the vouchers, implying that it is the reinforcement that is important, not the actual voucher. This approach has been effective for diverse populations, including homeless persons, pregnant women, and persons with mood disorders or schizophrenia. Contingency management has also been shown to improve attendance in occupationally-based and standard drug treatment settings (Carroll, 2004; Jones, Haug, Silverman, Stitzer, & Svikis, 2001).

Cognitive Behavioral Therapy

Cognitive behavioral therapy (CBT) is based on social learning theory and emphasizes modification of the client's thoughts and behaviors. The goal is to encourage abstinence by helping clients to learn and master effective coping skills that, in turn, help them to believe they can resist relapsing to substance abuse. The focus is on the exploration of positive and negative consequences of substance use. This approach is the foundation for relapse prevention, where clients are taught the skills needed to prevent a return to substance abuse after treatment.

Individual Psychotherapy

Individual psychotherapy is commonly combined with group and pharmacotherapy modalities. This approach emphasizes the psychosocial aspects of substance abuse, including motivation and dysfunctional thoughts. Individual psychotherapy is desirable when client privacy is important to facilitate effective treatment participation. It also provides more flexibility in that clients can proceed at their own pace while spending more time on their own unique issues, including repairing relationships with significant others. Clients who have a good capacity for introspection are more capable of making good alliances with their therapist and tend to benefit from this approach. Conversely, this approach is less successful when clients have little insight into their actions.

Group Therapy

Group therapy was developed when it was observed that the success of individual psychotherapy was limited and that positive peer support and reducing clients' feelings of isolation can best be accomplished with more than one person (CSAT, 2005b). These groups differ from self-help groups (such as AA) in that they are led by trained professionals. Typically, group size ranges from 5 to 12 persons and meetings occur from one to three times weekly. The basic models commonly applied to group therapy include emphases on:

- psychoeducation about substance use
- behavioral skills development needed for abstinence
- cognition and behavior therapy to change thoughts and actions leading to substance abuse
- social support to share information on managing day-to-day living characterized by abstinence
- interpersonal issues that interfere with abstinence

(CSAT, 2005b).

Persons with personality disorders (such as antisocial personality disorder) do not do as well in group therapy and tend to disrupt the group. Similarly, clients who are poorly motivated, unable to respect the need for confidentiality and privacy, have substantial cognitive deficits, are in the midst of a life crisis, or are psychotic, are also better served by other treatment approaches. Content focus varies with the group; as such, some groups may focus solely on relapse prevention while others include other topics. Group members should have similar needs in respect to the chosen content.

Self-help or 12-step Groups

Self-help or 12-step groups are widely available and most notably include AA and Narcotics Anonymous (NA). They are unique in that they do not rely on professional personnel to guide recovery. Twelve-step groups usually follow the same format and guidelines of "working through the steps." They are highly spiritual as a rule, but are not associated with a specific denomination or religion. The 12 steps espoused by AA and adapted for other groups are listed in Table 4-6.

These groups, also referred to as *mutual self-help groups,* involve a group of individuals with

TABLE 4-6: 12 STEPS OF ALCOHOLICS ANONYMOUS

1. Admitted we were powerless over alcohol and that our lives had become unmanageable.
2. Came to believe that a Power greater than ourselves could restore us to sanity.
3. Made a decision to turn our will and our lives over to the care of God as we understood Him.
4. Made a searching and fearless moral inventory of ourselves.
5. Admitted to God, to ourselves, and to other human beings the exact nature of our wrongs.
6. Were entirely ready to have God remove all these defects of character.
7. Humbly asked Him to remove our shortcomings.
8. Made a list of all persons we had harmed, and became willing to make amends to them all.
9. Made direct amends to such people wherever possible, except when to do so would injure them or others.
10. Continued to take personal inventory and when we were wrong promptly admitted it.
11. Sought through prayer and meditation to improve our conscious contact with God as we understood Him, praying only for knowledge of His will for us and the power to carry that out.
12. Having had a spiritual awakening as the result of these steps, we tried to carry this message to alcoholics, and to practice these principles in all our affairs.

Note. From A.A. World Services. (2002). *The twelve steps of Alcoholics Anonymous.* Retrieved April 2, 2013 from http://www.aa.org/en_pdfs/smf-121_en.pdf

similar problems who meet regularly (usually weekly) to share their experiences and offer support and encouragement with other group members. New group members are typically sponsored by another person who is further along in their recovery and who acts as a guide to the novice. This individual is commonly available to the novice 24 hours a day, 7 days a week. These support groups are free, characteristically anonymous, and confidential. They are open to anyone of any age desiring to stop using substances, regardless of the severity (or lack thereof) of their substance problem.

The goal is total abstinence – a drug-free existence whereby use of any medications including methadone is not supported for the long term. Proponents of the 12-step approach advocate staying drug-free "one day at a time" and expect clients to demonstrate a wish to cease substance use. Other groups based on the 12-step model, such as Al-Anon and Nar-Anon also exist and consist of the client's significant others affected by substance use. Twelve-step programs have been observed to be as effective as other perhaps more scientifically-based approaches (Coombs & Howatt, 2005).

Motivational Interventions

Motivational interventions (MI) are based on the Transtheoretical Model of Change previously discussed in Chapter 3 (Miller & Rollnick, 1991; CSAT, 1999b). MI strategies are adapted to each stage to meet clients in their current stage rather than presenting treatment options without considering the clients' current readiness to change. Strategies are premised on the concept that motivation is the key to changing clients' behavior. While it may seem obvious that motivation is critical to behavior change, what is different about the current interpretation is the nature of the concept. That is, motivation was formerly considered a behavioral trait that was static; for example, a client with "low motivation to change." In the present interpretation, motivation is dynamic and can be modified and enhanced by the clinician's style.

Treatment is viewed as a cyclical rather than a linear process. This approach can be incorporated into the clinician's interviewing style (then referred to as *motivational interviewing*) used for assessment and treatment. MI can be combined with other approaches, such as brief interventions and contingency management. It can also be used to directly address the client's stage of change. Examples of clinician approaches according to the client's stage of change are described in Table 4-7.

In addition to adapting the treatment approach to the stage of change, FRAMES is one of several similar approaches that are also used. FRAMES is a pneumonic that specifies the following components in one common way to implement MI:

- **F**eedback – after completing a comprehensive assessment, the clinician shares with the client his or her problems compared to the general population.
- **R**esponsibility – clients are explicitly given the choice to change or not change their behavior.
- **A**dvice – the clinician suggests rather than directs ways in which the client can change.
- **M**enu – the clinician offers various options for treatment.
- **E**mpathy – the clinician offers this essential component in counseling.
- **S**elf-efficacy – the clinician helps the client to feel he or she is capable of making the change.

Family-based Treatment

Family-based treatment acknowledges that the client's substance abuse has created problems with family members. It is widely recognized that the client's substance use adversely impacts his or her spouse or partner and children (CSAT, 2004). In the context of substance abuse treatment, the goals of family therapy are to minimize the impact of the client's substance use on the family and to use the family's strengths and resources to counsel the client on how to live a substance-free life (CSAT, 2004). About 60% to 95% of clients

TABLE 4-7: EXAMPLES OF CLINICIAN APPROACHES ACCORDING TO THE CLIENT'S STAGE OF CHANGE

STATE OF CHANGE	DEFINITION	EXAMPLE OF CLINICIAN APPROACH
Precontemplation	Client is not considering changing his or her behavior	• Explore the client's view of circumstances that led to his or her substance-related problems. • Praise the client for coming to treatment regardless of his or her reason.
Contemplation	Client is ambivalent but thinking about a change in substance use behavior	• Explain to the client that ambivalence is normal. • Stress the client's ability to make choices and inquire about his or her expectations of treatment.
Preparation	Client expresses readiness to consider a change in his or her substance abuse behavior	• Present various alternatives for treatment or behavior change. • Assist the client with obtaining help from supportive persons in his or her social network
Action	Client has started changing his or her substance use behavior treatment program	• Recognize the client's challenges in changing his or her behavior. • Highlight potential high-risk situations and possible coping behaviors.
Maintenance and relapse prevention	Client possesses skills needed to avoid replapse but may temporarily return to substance use	• Support coping behaviors and affirm the client's ability to experience pleasures without substances. • Inquire about the client's reasons for return to substance use, assess for stage of change, and respond as appropriate.

with substance abuse live with one or both parents or are in weekly contact with one or both parents. These rates are higher than those from the general population (Stanton & Heath, 2005).

Acupuncture

Acupuncture has been used primarily as an adjunct to more traditional substance abuse treatment. It is believed to work by moving energy in the body through channels referred to as *pathways*. Its use has been facilitated by the discovery that all meridians (a system of lines that connect points known as acupoints that are the specific sites for needle insertion) can be accessed through different points on the ear. Although not universally accepted as a legitimate treatment method, there have been a number of studies supporting reductions in withdrawal symptoms for alcohol, heroin, and cocaine when acupuncture is used (Brumbaugh, 1993).

Faith-Based Approaches

Unlike 12-step groups, faith-based approaches are religiously oriented. They emphasize the importance of faith in God and trust that God will deliver the individual from substance abuse. How drug treatment is translated into practice varies according to the specific religious orientation.

Harm Reduction

Harm reduction acknowledges that total abstinence is not effective for all clients. The goal of this approach is to reduce the negative effects of substance abuse. Examples may include needle exchange programs to reduce incidence of HIV, substituting methadone for heroin to facilitate healthier social functioning, and controlled alcohol drinking.

Treatment Settings

Treatment may take place in inpatient, outpatient, or residential settings. Within each setting, any of the previously discussed therapies can be used.

Inpatient

Inpatient hospitalization is the most intensive around-the-clock treatment with supervision by a multidisciplinary staff. It emphasizes medical management of detoxification or other medical and psychiatric crises, usually for a short period. *The Minnesota model of residential chemical dependency treatment* is an approach that is initially implemented in the inpatient setting. It focuses on abstinence as the primary treatment goal using the AA 12-step program as the major tool for recovery and relapse prevention. The Minnesota model requires a 28- to 30-day period of inpatient treatment followed by extensive community-based aftercare.

Residential

Residential treatment involves a live-in facility with 24-hour supervision. These settings use a structured living environment as an integral part of the clients' treatment plans. The primary advantage of these settings is that clients are away from their drug-related environment. Also known as *therapeutic communities* (TCs), these settings may be ideal for clients with a substance dependence diagnosis that is accompanied by severe psychosocial impairment and who do not meet clinical criteria for hospitalization. TCs employ two basic principles: the use of the residence as a microcosm of the larger community and the explicit expectation that clients will also assume partial responsibility for the recovery of their peers and that recovery is not solely achieved through treatment by staff. Traditionally, length of stay for TCs ranges between 18 to 24 months. However, with the advent of managed care, length of stay is now 12 months or fewer. This period may be as short as any number of consecutive full days, a variant also known as *intensive outpatient treatment*.

In this live-in environment, clients are referred to as "residents" who are expected to adhere to strict rules that promote commonly held behavioral norms. Adherence is reinforced with rewards for responsible social behavior and punishments for non-adherence. Varied individual and group therapy sessions using such approaches as CBT are also implemented within TCs. Treatment generally focuses on negative patterns of thinking and behavior that can be changed through reality-oriented individual and group therapy, intensive encounter sessions with peers, and participation in a therapeutic milieu. TCs can be established in independent settings such as a ranch, or within another physical environment such as a prison. Stages of TC treatment include:

- Stage I: Induction and early treatment – This period occurs over the first 30 days during which the resident learns TC procedures and to trust the other residents and treatment staff.
- Stage II: Primary treatment – Residents progress through increasing responsibilities, gaining additional privileges with consistent adherence to the rules.
- Stage III: Re-entry – Residents begin to separate from the TC environment and re-enter the outside larger community. Aftercare in the form of outpatient care and self-help groups should be part of the transition.

Outpatient

Outpatient treatment can be more or less intensive and may include medications for detoxification or maintenance. Less intensive outpatient treatment uses various individual, group or family counseling and therapeutic techniques, skills training, and educational support, including methadone maintenance treatment and drug-free approaches. This is the least standardized treatment approach. Most of these programs involve seeing clients only once or twice weekly and use some combination of counseling strategies, social work, and 12-step or self-help meetings.

Intensive outpatient treatment, also known as partial hospitalization, is typically a minimum of 9 hours of weekly attendance, usually in increments of 3 to 8 hours per day for 5 to 7 days per week, typically Monday through Friday. This setting is often recommended for patients in the early stages of treatment or those transitioning from residential or inpatient hospital settings.

Numerous and diverse therapeutic modalities and settings exist and, as Project Match (NIAAA, 1997) demonstrated, the type of modality is less important than the fact that clients are receiving treatment. Another pivotal clinical trial, the Drug Abuse Treatment Outcome Study (DATOS) suggests that for most clients, the amount of *time* in treatment is less important than the treatment *setting* (Simpson, Joe, Fletcher, Hubbard, & Anglin, 1999). This national longitudinal study involved 1,650 participants with cocaine dependence. Participants with problems of low severity had equivalent drug use outcomes regardless of time in treatment or setting. Participants with medium to high severity demonstrated better drug outcomes if they were in treatment for at least 3 months, regardless of treatment setting. However, a minimum of 3 months was required in an intensive setting, usually residential, for participants with the highest severity level.

Continuing Care

The final stage of treatment is continuing care, also referred to as *aftercare*. This stage is critical because, similar to high blood pressure and diabetes, substance abuse is a chronic illness that usually requires life-long management. From this perspective, it is not unusual for clients to be admitted to formal treatment multiple times for relapses, or *exacerbations* (the term frequently used for other chronic illnesses). The primary goal of continuing care is relapse prevention. Relapse prevention requires clients to master and solidify those strategies learned during the active treatment stage to maintain long-term change, reducing the risk of relapse.

A key component of continuing care is accomplished when clients recognize potentially high-risk situations that can precipitate substance abuse, including warning signs of relapse and management of the drug cravings elicited. Recognition of such warning signs is the central feature of relapse prevention because clients have been known to identify their warning signs sometimes weeks before they relapse (Daley & Marlatt, 2005). The simplest approach entails strict avoidance of people, places, and things associated with drug use. However, strict avoidance is rarely possible; therefore, clients must minimize exposure to such triggers, including removing all drug paraphernalia from their home.

Cue exposure therapy can be used, wherein clients are purposefully presented with cues specific to the client's drug cravings. This may be used for those situations associated with drug cravings that are difficult (if not impossible) to avoid. The goal of this therapy is to decrease the intensity of the client's cravings (Daley & Marlatt, 2005).

Other strategies clients might be taught to employ include:

- considering warning signs experienced by other persons in recovery
- daily journaling focused on connecting feelings or scenarios to relapse risk factors and warning signs
- devising an action plan on how to avoid substance use, who to ask for help, and when to ask for help

(Daley & Marlatt, 2005).

SPECIAL POPULATIONS

Adolescents

In 2010, adolescents between the ages of 12 and 19 years constituted 13.6% of all treatment admissions to publicly funded facilities (SAMHSA, 2012b). Adolescents between the ages of 15 and 19 were most commonly treated for the following substances (in order of decreasing frequency): marijuana, hallucinogens, inhalants, and stimulants other than cocaine or methamphetamines (such as methyl-phen-idate prescribed for attention deficit hyperactivity disorder). Indicators for inpatient treatment are listed in Table 4-8.

TABLE 4-8: INDICATORS FOR INPATIENT TREATMENT FOR ADOLESCENTS

1. History of failure in, or not qualifying for, outpatient treatment
2. Dual diagnosis with moderate or severe psychiatric disorders
3. Suicidal thoughts or behavior
4. History of intravenous drug use, drug dependence, or need for detoxification
5. Comorbid moderate or severe medical problems
6. Need for isolation from their community
7. Pregnancy

Note. From "Treating Adolescent Substance Abuse" (pp. 559-587) by Y. Kaminer & O. G. Bukstein, 2005. In R.J. Frances, S.I. Miller, & A.H. Mack (Eds), *Clinical textbook of addictive disorders,* 3rd ed. New York: Guilford Press.

Enrollment criteria for outpatient treatment includes:

- comorbid psychiatric disorders that do not require inpatient treatment
- previous successful outpatient treatment with follow-up
- agreement to a contingency contract that includes visit frequency, expected adherence to the curriculum including random urine drug screens, consequences of nonadherence to the contract, and participation in the community network together with self-help groups.

Behavioral treatments demonstrated to be successful with adolescents include family therapy, CBT, motivational interventions, contingency management, and 12-step programs (Kaminer & Bukstein, 2005). Research studies suggest that residential treatment programs yield better outcomes than outpatient programs (Pumariega, Kilgus, & Rodriguez, 2005). Selected medications for adolescents should ideally have a low abuse potential. Regrettably, no research has comprehensively evaluated the safety and effectiveness of any psychotropic medication to treat adolescent substance abuse. However, in the presence of comorbid psychiatric disorders, medications targeting the other psychiatric disorders may be used indirectly to treat substance use disorders. Fortunately, clinically significant withdrawal symptoms have rarely been observed in this age-group (Kaminer & Bukstein). Consequently, detoxification protocols for adolescents are not significantly different from those for adults.

Older Adults

In 2010, individuals age 50 or older constituted 38.6% of all treatment admissions to publicly funded treatment facilities, including 15.8% for individuals 65 years of age or older (SAMHSA, 2012b). Alcohol abuse was the most common reason for admission followed by prescription drugs – specifically tranquilizers and sedatives – and opiates (primarily heroin). For alcohol detoxification, reduced dosages of benzodiazepines have traditionally been used. If there are serious comorbid medical problems, detoxification should occur within the inpatient setting, preferably on a general medical floor, which is deemed to be a more acceptable setting by older clients (Zimberg, 2005). Disulfiram (in smaller doses) and naltrexone have both been found useful for older adults, although studies of safety for acamprosate have not been performed with this population. Both group and individual treatment modalities are effective within the older adult population (Zimberg, 2005).

Women

Women are more likely to seek treatment for substance abuse in mental health settings than traditional drug treatment settings because of the stigma attached to substance use.

Denial regarding the significance of their problem is compounded by the frequency with which substance abuse is missed in women. Many of the available treatment methods have been more effective for men. Consequently, women-only treatment was developed to address issues unique to women and to avoid the perception of harassment by men. However, little research specifically examines differential treatment outcomes (Ashley, Marsden, & Brady, 2003). What may be more important is that better treatment outcomes are observed with the delivery of specific services as part of treatment programming, regardless of a single or mixed gender environment. These services include child care, prenatal care, and women-focused topics (Ashley et al., 2003). Selection of women-only treatment versus mixed gender treatment should be individualized according to women's unique experiences. For example, women with a history of sexual victimization may fare better in women-only treatment. Additional special considerations that apply particularly to women, although they may apply to men as well, are summarized in Table 4-9.

TABLE 4-9: SPECIAL TREATMENT CONSIDERATIONS FOR WOMEN
• History of physical or sexual victimization
• Need for and access to obstetric or gynecologic care, including information on substance use during pregnancy
• Child care services
• Parenting education
• Stigma effects, including shame, guilt, and subsequent low self-esteem
• Sexual orientation
• History of commercial sex work

If domestic violence is present, a safety plan should be made with the client. The client should be advised to keep emergency phone numbers (such as police and domestic violence hotline and shelter) and critical items (such as money and birth certificates) on hand. She should also be guided to establish a code for trusted others so she can communicate if she is in impending danger.

Clients with HIV/AIDS

All clients, whether HIV-negative or positive should be given risk-reduction counseling to prevent HIV transmission or acquisition. Coordinated care and integrated treatment should be employed whenever possible. Individuals who are HIV-infected are best treated in settings that have a medical component on-site. Unfortunately, appropriate aftercare or outpatient settings can be difficult to find. If clients are on medications for HIV, particularly protease inhibitors, attention must be given to interaction with pharmacotherapies for substance use. Similar to older adult patients, consideration should be given to their cognitive status to rule out AIDS dementia that can influence selection of treatment modalities.

Occupational Settings

Ideally, coordination of treatment should occur within Employee Assistance Programs (EAP), if available. Rather than firing an individual (such as healthcare workers), treatment is coordinated from the work site. Models vary, but all provide communication between the employer and EAP regarding the employee's progress. Treatment is voluntary and success rates are favorable – close to 70% (Mack, Kahn, Frances, 2005).

Psychiatric Comorbidity

Due to recognition of poorer treatment outcomes when another psychiatric disorder is present, treatment approaches were devised to target both disorders. The Level of Care Quadrants Model, detailed in Figure 4-1, was developed to assist with effective service delivery depending on the severity of the combined disorders (CSAT, 2005a).

Historically, services were provided in sequential fashion; that is, treating either the substance abuse or mental health disorder first, depending on which one was deemed more severe

FIGURE 4-1: LEVEL OF CARE QUADRANTS

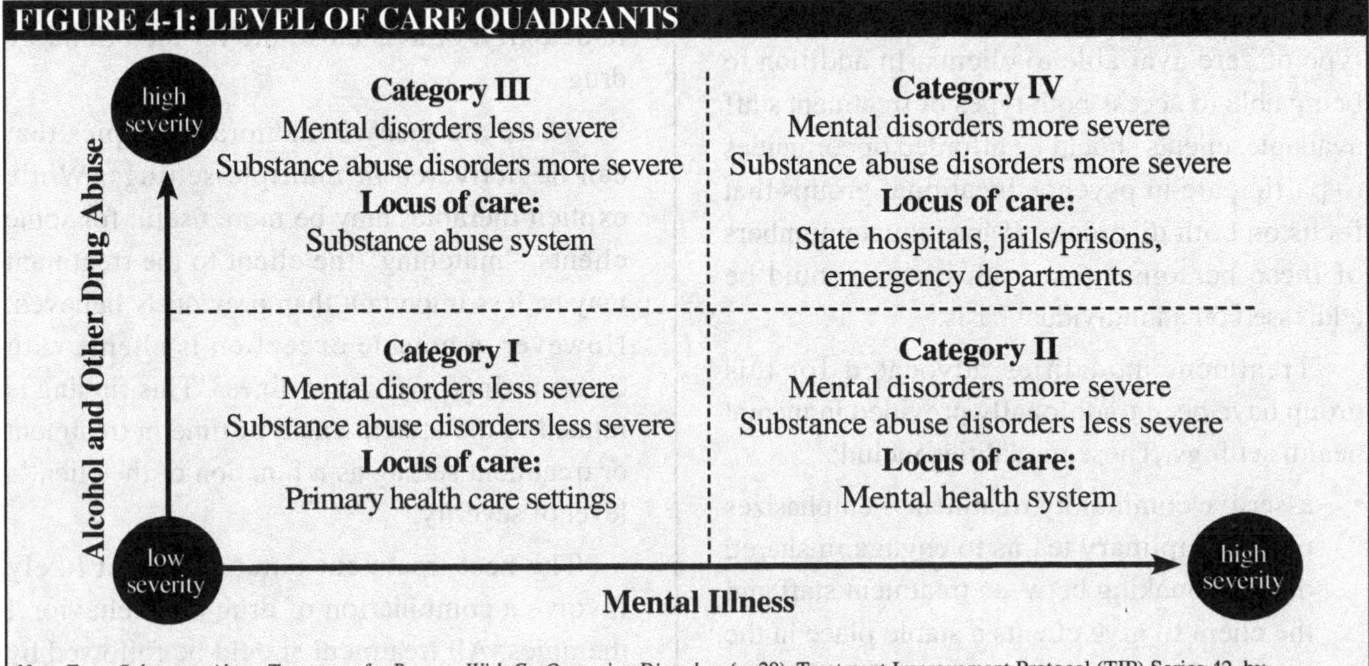

Note. From *Substance Abuse Treatment for Persons With Co-Occurring Disorders* (p. 29). Treatment Improvement Protocol (TIP) Series 42, by Center for Substance Abuse Treatment, 2005a. DHHS Publication No. (SMA) 05-3922. Rockville, MD: Substance Abuse and Mental Health Services Administration.

or which setting the person presented to first. For this approach, the other disorder was treated after the more severe one was stabilized. Typically, mental health disorders were treated in mental health settings and substance abuse problems in substance abuse treatment settings. Evaluated as ineffective for many clients, services were then provided in a parallel manner with both disorders treated simultaneously, but usually in separate treatment sites by separate treatment professionals (Mangrum, Spence, & Lopez, 2006). This approach was also recognized as frequently ineffective because of potential conflicting messages and the difficulty in adequately attending to both problems (CSAT, 2005a).

Integrated treatment of both disorders simultaneously and comprehensively by the same unified process and treatment staff or in the same treatment setting, is advocated as the ideal approach (CSAT, 2005a). However, choice of sequential, parallel, or integrated treatment should depend on the severity of each client's problems. For example, it would be more appropriate to sequentially address and treat the mental health disorder first for clients in Category II. Unfortunately, insurance and resource issues often dictate the type of care available to clients. In addition to being able to access both types of treatment staff available, clients should be afforded opportunities to participate in psychoeducational groups that focus on both disorders. If inadequate numbers of these persons exist, both issues should be addressed on an individual basis.

Treatment modalities advocated for this group have been traditionally provided in mental health settings. These modalities include:

- assertive community treatment – emphasizes multidisciplinary teams to engage in shared decision making between treatment staff and the client to give clients a stable place in the community
- intensive case management – involves standard case management but with fewer clients in the clinician's case load, permitting greater management intensity
- modified therapeutic community – adopts the principles of the standard therapeutic community (such as establishing the culture of mutual self-help and associating with the broader peer community to enact change) but making the following three important modifications: greater flexibility, reduced intensity, and additional individualization

(CSAT, 2005a).

SUMMARY

In 2010, only 11% of individuals needing substance abuse treatment received it. Over 1.8 million admissions were made to substance abuse treatment facilities – nearly half of them for alcohol abuse. Treatment comprises pharmacotherapy and behavioral therapy and should include continuing care after discharge from the formal treatment setting. Pharmacotherapy can be directly used to treat withdrawal symptoms, to detoxify, or as a substitute for the offending drug.

There are many behavioral therapies that can be delivered in multiple settings. While explicit therapies may be more useful for some clients, "matching" the client to the treatment may be less important than previously believed. However, a notable exception is clients with co-occurring psychiatric illness. This finding is related to the effectiveness of time in treatment or treatment setting as a function of the client's level of severity.

The best treatment outcomes most likely involve a combination of drug and behavioral therapies. All treatment should be followed by continuing care.

EXAM QUESTIONS

CHAPTER 4

Questions 18-23

Note: Choose the one option that BEST answers each question.

18. The use of medications in treating substance use disorders

    a. is restricted to long-term use.

    b. is restricted to temporary use.

    c. reverses the changes in the brain incurred from chronic drug use.

    d. should always be avoided.

19. Disulfiram

    a. interferes with the normal metabolism of alcohol.

    b. is a long-acting opioid antagonist.

    c. is a recently FDA-approved medication for alcohol dependence.

    d. is the drug of choice for cocaine dependence.

20. Behavioral therapy for substance abuse problems is appropriate

    a. if limited to a group of individuals.

    b. if more than one session is required.

    c. only for particular drugs of abuse.

    d. when used with pharmacologic treatment.

21. Research has shown an advantage of using contingency management is its effectiveness with

    a. homeless persons, pregnant women, and persons with mood disorders.

    b. people who use alcohol rather than illicit drugs.

    c. people who use illicit drugs rather than alcohol.

    d. adolescents and older adults.

22. A lesson learned from Project Match is that for most clients

    a. cognitive behavioral therapy is the most effective treatment.

    b. motivational enhancement therapy is the most effective treatment.

    c. participation in any treatment may be more important than the type of modality.

    d. personal characteristics are critical to their treatment outcome.

23. Findings from the Drug Abuse Treatment Outcome Study trial suggests that

    a. drug treatment should occur for at least 3 months for all clients.

    b. drug treatment should occur for longer than 3 months for clients with medium to severe problems.

    c. the amount of time in treatment is less important than the treatment setting.

    d. the amount of time in treatment is more important than the treatment setting.

REFERENCES

American Society of Addiction Medicine. (2001). *Patient placement criteria*, 2nd ed. revised. Accessed March 15, 2013, from http://www.asam.org/publications/patient-placement-criteria/ppc-2r

Ashley, O.S., Marsden, M.E., & Brady, T.M. (2003). Effectiveness of substance abuse treatment programming for women: A review. *The American Journal of Drug and Alcohol Abuse, 29*(1), 19-53.

Brumbaugh, A.G. (1993). Acupuncture: New perspectives in chemical dependency treatment. *Journal of Substance Abuse Treatment, 10*(1), 35-43.

Carroll, K.M. (2004). Behavioral therapies for co-occurring substance use and mood disorders. *Biological Psychiatry, 56*, 778-784.

Center for Substance Abuse Treatment. (1999a). Brief interventions and brief therapies for substance abuse. *Treatment Improvement Protocol* (TIP) Series 34. DHHS Publication No. (SMA) 99-3353. Rockville, MD: Substance Abuse and Mental Health Services Administration.

Center for Substance Abuse Treatment. (1999b). Enhancing motivation to change in substance abuse treatment. *Treatment Improvement Protocol* (TIP) Series 35. DHHS Publication No. (SMA) 99-3354. Rockville, MD: Substance Abuse and Mental Health Services Administration.

Center for Substance Abuse Treatment. (2004). Substance abuse treatment and family therapy. *Treatment Improvement Protocol, Series*, No. 39. DHHS Publication No. (SMA) 04-3957. Rockville, MD: Substance Abuse and Mental Health Services Administration.

Center for Substance Abuse Treatment. (2005a). Substance abuse treatment for persons with co-occurring disorders. *Treatment Improvement Protocol* (TIP) Series 42. DHHS Publication No. (SMA) 05-3922. Rockville, MD: Substance Abuse and Mental Health Services Administration.

Center for Substance Abuse Treatment. (2005b). Substance abuse treatment: Group therapy. *Treatment Improvement Protocol* (TIP) Series 41. DHHS Publication No. (SMA) 05-3991. Rockville, MD: Substance Abuse and Mental Health Services Administration.

Coombs, R.H. & Howatt, W.A. (2005). *The addiction counselor's desk reference.* Hoboken, New Jersey: John Wiley & Sons.

Daley, D.C. & Marlatt, G.A. (2005). Relapse prevention. In J.H. Lowinson, P. Ruiz, R.B. Millman, & J.G. Langrod (Eds.), *Substance abuse. A comprehensive textbook* (4th ed., pp. 772-786). Philadelphia: Lippincott Williams & Wilkins.

Jones, H.E., Haug, N., Silverman, K., Stitzer, M., & Svikis, D. (2001). The effectiveness of incentives in enhancing methadone-maintained pregnant women. *Drug and Alcohol Dependence, 61*(3), 297-306.

Kaminer, Y. & Bukstein, O.G. (2005). Treating adolescent substance abuse. In R.J. Frances, S.I. Miller, & A.H. Mack (Eds.), *Clinical textbook of addictive disorders* (3rd ed., pp. 559-587). New York: Guilford Press

Mack, A.H., Kahn, J.P., & Frances, R.J. (2005). Addictions in the workplace. In R.J. Frances, S.I. Miller, & A.H. Mack (Eds.), *Clinical textbook of addictive disorders* (3rd ed., pp. 340-353). New York: Guilford Press

Mangrum, L.F., Spence, R.T., & Lopez, M. (2006). Integrated versus parallel treatment of co-occurring psychiatric and substance use disorders. *Journal of Substance Abuse Treatment, 30*(1), 79-84.

Miller, W.R. & Rollnick, S. (1991). *Motivational interviewing: Preparing people to change addictive behavior*. New York: Guilford Press.

Musto, D. (2005). Historical perspectives. In J.H. Lowinson, P. Ruiz, R.B. Millman, & J.G. Langrod (Eds.), *Substance abuse: A comprehensive textbook* (4th ed., pp. 1-15). Philadelphia: Lippincott Williams & Wilkins

Nace, E.P. (2005). Alcoholics Anonymous. In R.J. Frances, S.I. Miller, & A.H. Mack (Eds), *Clinical textbook of addictive disorders* (3rd ed., pp. 587-599). New York: Guilford Press.

National Institute on Alcohol Abuse and Alcoholism. (1997). Patient-Treatment matching. *Alcohol Alert*, No. 36, United States Department of Health and Human Services, National Institutes of Health, National Institute on Alcohol Abuse and Alcoholism.

National Institute on Drug Abuse. (2009). *Drug Info Facts: Treatment approaches for drug addiction*. Accessed March 15, 2013, from http://www.drugabuse.gov/publications/drugfacts/treatment-approaches-drug-addiction

Pumariega, A.J., Kilgus, M.D., & Rodriguez, L. (2005). Adolescents. In J.H. Lowinson, P. Ruiz, R.B. Millman, & J.G. Langrod (Eds.), *Substance abuse: A comprehensive textbook* (4th ed., pp. 1021-1038). Philadelphia: Lippincott Williams & Wilkins.

Rounsaville, B.J., Carroll, K.M., & Back, S. (2005). Individual psychotherapy. In J.H. Lowinson, P. Ruiz, R.B. Millman, & J.G. Langrod (Eds.), *Substance abuse: A comprehensive textbook* (4th ed., pp. 653-671). Philadelphia: Lippincott Williams & Wilkins.

Simpson, D., Joe, G., Fletcher, B., Hubbard, R., & Anglin, D. (1999). A national evaluation of treatment outcomes for cocaine dependence. *Archives of General Psychiatry, 56*(6), 507-514.

Stanton, M.D. & Heath, A.W. (2005). Family/couples approaches to treatment engagement and therapy. In J.H. Lowinson, P. Ruiz, R.B. Millman, & J.G. Langrod (Eds.), *Substance abuse: A comprehensive textbook* (4th ed., pp. 680-690). Philadelphia: Lippincott Williams & Wilkins.

Substance Abuse and Mental Health Services Administration. (2012a). *Results from the 2011 National survey on drug use and health: Summary of national findings* (NSDUH Series H-44, HHS Publication No. (SMA) 12-4713). Rockville, MD. Accessed March 15, 2013 from http://www.samhsa.gov/data/NSDUH/2k11Results/NSDUHresults2011.htm

Substance Abuse and Mental Health Services Administration. (2012b). *Treatment Episode Data Set (TEDS) 2000-2010: National admissions to substance abuse treatment services*. Retrieved March 15, 2013 from http://www.samhsa.gov/data/2k12/TEDS2010N/TEDS2010NWeb.pdf

Westermeyer, J. (2005). Historical and social context of psychoactive substance use disorders. In R.J. Frances, S.I. Miller, & A.H. Mack (Eds.), *Clinical textbook of addictive disorders* (3rd ed., pp. 16-36). New York: Guilford Press.

Zimberg, S. (2005). Alcoholism and substance abuse in older adults. In R.J. Frances, S.I. Miller, & A.H. Mack (Eds.), *Clinical textbook of addictive disorders* (3rd ed., pp. 354-366). New York: Guilford Press.

CHAPTER 5

TOBACCO-RELATED DISORDERS

CHAPTER OBJECTIVE

After completing this chapter, the learner will be able to describe the clinical effects of tobacco use.

LEARNING OBJECTIVES

After studying this chapter, the learner will be able to:

1. Identify the prevalence of tobacco use in the U.S. adult and adolescent population.
2. Describe the health effects of tobacco use.
3. Discuss the role of nicotine as the causative agent of tobacco use disorder.
4. Discuss how to screen and treat a patient with a tobacco use disorder who wants to quit.
5. Discuss how to conduct a brief motivational interview with a patient who is not interested in quitting.

OVERVIEW

Cigarette smoking is the leading cause of preventable death and disability in the United States. Cigarette smoking results in 443,000 premature deaths each year and costs the nation more than $193 billion in direct medical costs and lost productivity (Centers for Disease Control and Prevention [CDC], 2011a; National Institute of Drug Abuse [NIDA], 2012a). Smoking and its associated illnesses decrease the life span of adults who smoke by 14 years (CDC, 2011a). Smoking cigarettes exposes the tobacco user to more than 50 cancer-causing chemicals. The tar in cigarettes increases the risk of lung cancer, emphysema, and bronchial disorders. The carbon monoxide gas from cigarettes markedly increases the risk of cardiovascular disease.

A national health objective described in Healthy People 2010 was to decrease the prevalence of cigarette smoking to less than 12% in the United States. This objective was not met, and was therefore retained in Health People 2020. Unfortunately, current data indicate that the target will once again fail to be met. In 2010, 19.3% of U.S. adults were current cigarette smokers, compared with 20.9% in 2005. While this does represent a decline, at this rate adult smoking percentages in the U.S. will only reach approximately 17% by 2020 – a rate considerably higher than the Healthy People 2020 target goal of ≤12%. Of the 19.0% (43.8 million adults) who were current cigarette smokers in 2011, 34.1 million (77.8%) smoked daily and 9.7 million (22.2%) smoke most days (CDC, 2012).

HISTORY

Tobacco (nicotine tobaccum) was first used by the pre-Columbian civilizations in the Americas for religious ceremonies. In the late

1400s, Christopher Columbus returned from his travels with a few tobacco leaves and seeds and described the use of tobacco in the Americas (Cable News Network, 2000; Hymowitz, 2005). By the mid-1500s, tobacco had been introduced to France, Spain, and England. In the United States, the first successful crop was cultivated in Virginia in 1612. By 1619, tobacco became the colonies' largest export and fueled the demand for slave labor (Cable News Network, 2000).

Initially, the most common method of use was smokeless tobacco, specifically snuff and chewing tobacco. However, the cigarette machine developed in the late 1800s allowed for mass production, and cigarettes became the most popular form of tobacco use. It was not until the late 1950s that the public became aware of the negative effects of smoking.

PREVALENCE

Initiation to tobacco use commonly occurs in adolescence, with tobacco abuse and dependence quickly following. In 2011, 2.4 million people 12 years of age and older smoked cigarettes for the first time (Substance Abuse and Mental Health Services Administration [SAMHSA], 2012). Nearly 56% of these new smokers were under 18 years of age. Cigarette smoking is by far the most common method of tobacco use, with less than 10% of adult and adolescents using cigars, pipes, and smokeless tobacco products (SAMHSA, 2012). Fifty percent of individuals who smoke for 1 month become chronically addicted. Recent research suggests that the majority of students in grades 6 through 10 who smoke meet the *Diagnostic and Statistical Manual for Mental Disorders (DSM-5)* criteria for tobacco use disorder. Surprisingly, 17% of students who smoked fewer than one cigarette per day and 13% who smoked only one per day also met the criteria for tobacco use disorder (Kandel et al., 2005; Polito, 2005) – specifically, tolerance, withdrawal, and impaired control (American Psychiatric Association [APA], 1996). Adolescents appear to be particularly vulnerable to the effects of nicotine, the substance in tobacco that is highly addictive.

Initiating cigarette smoking after ages 18 to 20 is unusual (Bigelow & Rand, 2003). Children and adolescents begin to smoke because their peers do, they have a desire to mimic adult or parent behavior, to rebel or feel independent, or they see it as a way to stay thin. In the past, tobacco advertisements have presented a strong risk factor for smoking by children and adolescents, but legislation enacted in 2009 (The Family Smoking Prevention and Tobacco Control Act) that places restrictions on tobacco products and their advertising has had an impact on public health (CDC, 2011b). Other predictors include use and abuse of alcohol and other drugs, attention deficit disorder, and depressive and anxiety disorders (APA, 1996). Currently 15.5% of eighth graders, 27.7% of tenth graders, and 39.5% of twelfth graders smoke (Johnston, O'Malley, Bachman, & Schulenberg, 2013). Most adolescents will smoke well into adulthood before they can finally quit.

The prevalence rate of cigarette smoking in the United States differs among gender and ethnic groups. Tobacco use is highest among men (32.3%), with the prevalence rate among women around 21.1% (SAMHSA, 2013). Indian and Alaskan natives have the highest rates of smoking at 43.0%, followed by 36.1% of persons reporting mixed races, 28.6% of Whites, and 26.2% of Blacks. The lowest rates of smoking are among Asians (13.0%) followed by Hispanics (20.4%) (SAMHSA, 2013).

Tobacco use also differs based on socioeconomic status and education. Adults who live below the poverty level have higher rates of smoking than those at or above the poverty level, 28.9% vs. 18.3% (CDC, 2011c). Adults with lower education levels smoke at greater rates than those with higher educational levels. The prevalence of smoking among adults who have only a General Educational Development (GED) diploma is 45.2%, compared to a prevalence rate of 18.8% among adults with college degrees (CDC, 2011c).

HEALTH EFFECTS

Tobacco users experience increased rates of cancer – particularly lung and oral cavity cancers, including cancer of the mouth, pharynx, larynx, esophagus, stomach, pancreas, cervix, prostate, kidney, ureter, and bladder. Cigarette smoking markedly increases cardiovascular disease, specifically cerebral vascular accidents (stroke), myocardial infarctions, angina, vascular disease, and aneurysms. In addition, cigarette smoking results in increased rates of emphysema, bronchial disorders, gastric ulcers, post-menopausal osteoporosis, diabetes mellitus, and macular degeneration. Cigarette smoking is linked to approximately 80% of all lung cancer deaths (American Cancer Society [ACS], 2013).

In pregnant women, carbon monoxide and nicotine interfere with the oxygen supply to the fetus. Nicotine crosses the placenta and is concentrated in the fetal blood, amniotic fluid, and breast milk. Nicotine levels in the fetus can be as much as 15% higher than maternal levels. As a result, pregnant women who smoke have higher rates of fetal death, decreased fetal growth, low birth weight infants and children with developmental delays. Smoking during pregnancy may also be associated with sudden infant death syndrome (SIDS), learning and behavioral problems and an increased risk of obesity in children (NIDA, 2012a).

Exposure to secondhand smoke can cause cardiovascular disease, lung cancer, respiratory disease, ear infections in children, asthma, and sudden infant death syndrome. The Environmental Protection Agency (EPA) defines secondhand smoke as "environmental tobacco smoke" (ETS). The EPA considers ETS a known human carcinogen in the Class A category, along with radon, benzene, and asbestos (Hymowitz, 2005). Studies suggest that nonsmokers exposed to ETS at work were 30% more likely to get lung cancer than non-exposed workers. The scientific evidence indicates that there is no risk-free level of exposure to secondhand smoke. According to *The Health Consequences of Involuntary Exposure to Tobacco Smoke: A Report of the Surgeon General* (USDHHS, 2006), evidence shows that:

- short exposures to secondhand smoke can cause blood platelets to become stickier, damage the lining of blood vessels, decrease coronary flow velocity reserves, and reduce heart rate variability, potentially increasing the risk of a heart attack
- secondhand smoke contains many chemicals that can quickly irritate and damage the lining of the airways; even brief exposure can result in upper airway changes in healthy persons and can lead to more frequent and more severe asthma attacks in children who already have asthma (USDHHS, 2006).

BIOCHEMISTRY

Nicotine is the drug in tobacco that causes addiction. It is a highly addictive substance that when inhaled quickly enters the brain with peak concentrations occurring in only a few seconds. The drug is readily absorbed by the brain, spleen, and liver and primarily metabolized in the liver. The nicotine molecule is shaped like the neurotransmitter acetylcholine and rapidly binds with the acetylcholine receptors, which are involved in muscle movement, respiration, heart rate, learning, and memory

(NIDA, 2013). Most importantly, acetylcholine and its receptors also cause the release of other neurotransmitters and hormones, specifically dopamine. Dopamine affects mood, pleasure, and reward. Researchers believe increased levels of dopamine play a critical role in the development of chemical addiction.

The rapid onset of the effects of nicotine clearly contributes to its high abuse potential (Schmitz & Delange, 2004). "Rapid delivery systems have a much higher abuse liability, or reinforcing efficacy, than slower delivering systems" (Schmitz & Delange, 2004, p. 390). The immediate "kick" from nicotine inhalation causes a release of epinephrine (adrenaline) which stimulates the body and causes blood pressure, respiration and heart rate to increase (NIDA, 2012b). At the same time, nicotine, mimicking the action of acetylcholine, increases the level of the neurotransmitter dopamine. Dopamine affects the brain pathways that control reward, pleasure, and motivation.

Within seconds of cigarette inhalation, the smoker experiences symptoms of pleasure and increased energy. These symptoms result in a positive reinforcement of the drug. A typical smoker will take 10 puffs on a cigarette during a period of 5 minutes in an attempt to continue the drug's pleasurable side effects and prevent withdrawal. The smoker will repeat this behavior throughout the day in the continued pursuit of reward and pleasure and to stave off the symptoms of withdrawal. NIDA (2012b) notes that, a person who smokes about 30 cigarettes a day (1½ packs) gets 300 hits of nicotine to the brain each day.

The initial feelings of pleasure and increased energy that occur after smoking are followed by feelings of depression and fatigue. The user will attempt to relieve these symptoms of depression and fatigue by increasing nicotine ingestion. Evidence suggests that chronic smokers who withhold nicotine for 24 hours experience increased anger, hostility, aggression, loss of cooperation, and impaired psychomotor and cognitive functions (NIDA, 2012b). This is termed *nicotine abstinence syndrome* or, more commonly, *nicotine withdrawal*.

Substance Use Disorder

The *DSM-5* describes tobacco use disorder as a problematic pattern of tobacco use leading to significant impairment or distress. Most smokers recognize the negative health effects of tobacco and have made multiple attempts to quit unsuccessfully. Similar to the diagnostic criteria for other substance use disorders, tobacco use disorder criteria include:

1. tolerance
2. withdrawal
3. substance is used in larger amounts or over a longer period than intended
4. persistent desire or unsuccessful efforts to cut down
5. a great deal of time spent in activities to obtain the substance
6. giving up or reducing important social, occupational, or recreational activities because of substance use
7. continued use despite knowledge of having persistent or recurrent health problems that are likely caused by the substance use

(APA, 2013).

To be diagnosed with tobacco withdrawal, the tobacco user must meet four of the following 7 criteria within 24 hours of decreased tobacco use or cessation:

1. depressed mood
2. insomnia
3. irritability, frustration, or anger
4. anxiety
5. difficulty concentrating

6. restlessness
7. increased appetite

(APA, 2013).

The most common withdrawal symptoms are impaired concentration and craving for nicotine.

SCREENING AND TREATMENT

Seventy percent of all smokers have expressed the desire to stop smoking. Since 1995, when smoking status was only identified during 65% of clinic visits, 90% of smokers are now reporting that they are being screened for smoking status during healthcare visits. According to the U.S. Department of Health and Human Services' Clinical Practice Guideline, *Treating Tobacco Use and Dependence* (Fiore et al., 2008), it is essential that clinicians and health care delivery systems institutionalize the consistent identification, documentation, and treatment of every tobacco user who is seen in a health care setting.

Treating Tobacco Use and Dependence suggests that all patients who use tobacco and are willing to quit should be treated using the "5 A's": *Ask, Advise, Assess, Assist,* and *Arrange*. Patients should be *asked* about tobacco use (Figure 5-1). If the patient is a current smoker or tobacco user, the clinician should strongly *advise* the patient to quit and *assess* the patient's willingness to quit. If the patient is willing to make a quit attempt, the clinician should *assist* the patient by offering appropriate treatment. This treatment includes helping the patient

FIGURE 5-1: ALGORITHM FOR TREATING TOBACCO USE

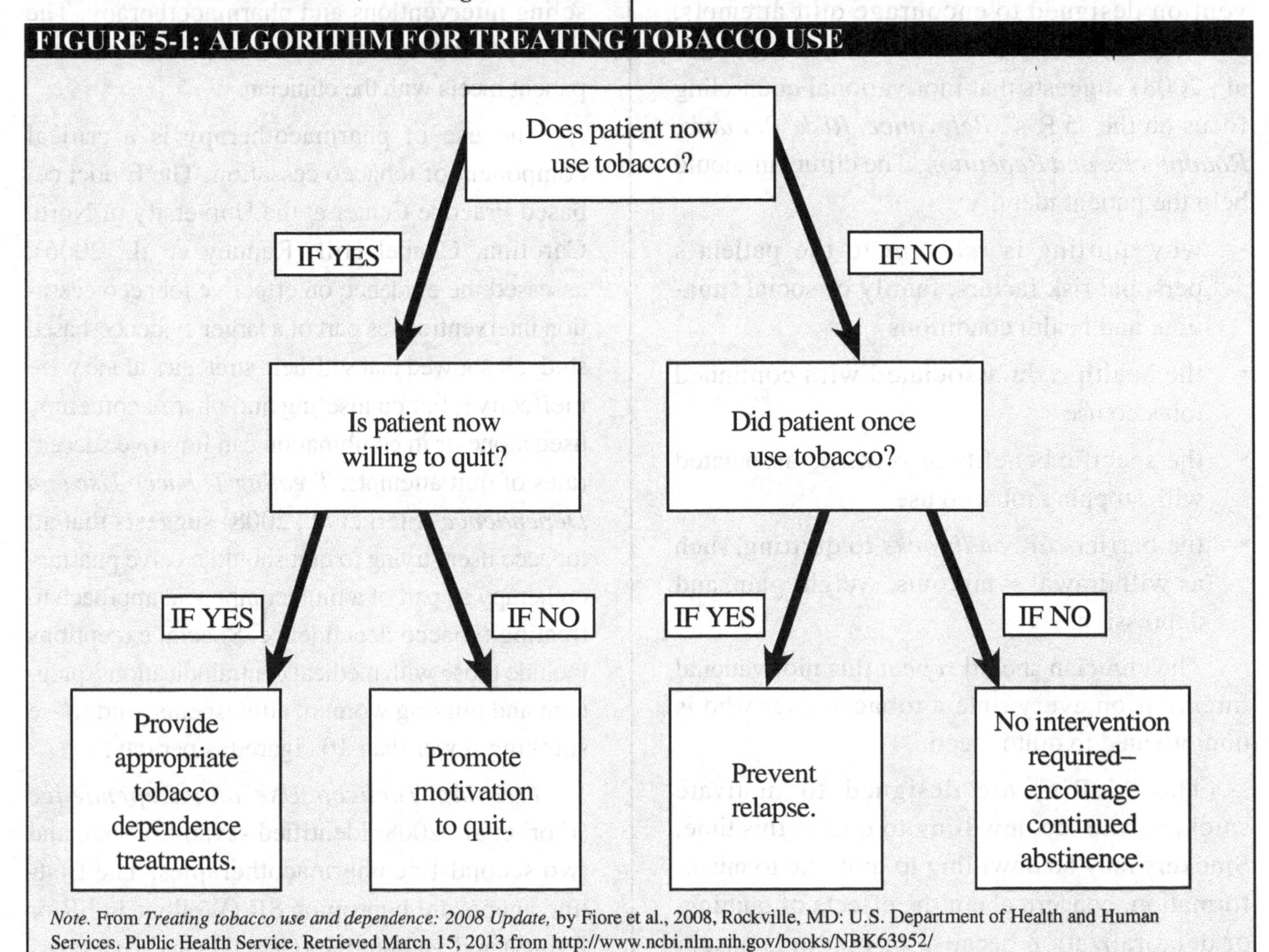

Note. From *Treating tobacco use and dependence: 2008 Update,* by Fiore et al., 2008, Rockville, MD: U.S. Department of Health and Human Services. Public Health Service. Retrieved March 15, 2013 from http://www.ncbi.nlm.nih.gov/books/NBK63952/

develop a quit plan; providing practical counseling and problem solving that addresses total abstinence, past quit experiences, and identification of triggers; helping the patient identify and develop a social support that will assist with the quit attempt; and, unless medically contraindicated, discussing, recommending, and referring the patient for the use of pharmacological options that increase success and decrease withdrawal symptoms. Lastly, the clinician should *arrange* for follow-up to monitor and facilitate the patient's quit attempt. Table 5-1 describes in detail the "5 A's" and the strategies that may be used for implementation.

If the patient has been assessed as a current tobacco user and is unwilling to stop, he or she should be offered a brief motivational intervention designed to encourage quit attempts. *Treating Tobacco Use and Dependence* (Fiore et al., 2008) suggests that motivational counseling focus on the "5 R's": *Relevance, Risk, Rewards, Roadblocks, and Repetition.* The clinician should help the patient identify:

- why quitting is *relevant* to the patient's personal risk factors, family or social situation, and health conditions
- the health *risks* associated with continued tobacco use
- the specific benefits or *rewards* associated with stopping tobacco use
- the barriers or *roadblocks* to quitting, such as withdrawal symptoms, weight gain, and depression.

The clinician should *repeat* this motivational intervention every time a tobacco user who is unmotivated to quit is seen.

The "5 R's" are designed to motivate smokers who are unwilling to quit at this time. Smokers may be unwilling to quit due to misinformation, concern about the effects of quitting, or demoralization because of previous unsuccessful quit attempts. Therefore, after asking about tobacco use, advising the smoker to quit, and assessing the willingness of the smoker to quit, it is important to provide the "5 R's" motivational intervention (Fiore et al., 2008). Table 5-2 describes in detail the "5 R's" and strategies for implementation.

Patients who have failed previous attempts to quit smoking should be reminded that it is common to experience repeated attempts to quit before being successful. If the patient has a history of tobacco use but is currently abstinent, the clinician should reinforce continued tobacco cessation and work with the patient to prevent relapse. Most relapses occur soon after the quit attempt; however, some people relapse months or even years after the quit date. Relapse prevention may include brief counseling interventions and pharmacotherapy. The key is to reinforce tobacco cessation each time the patient meets with the clinician.

The use of pharmacotherapy is a critical component of tobacco cessation. The Evidence-based Practice Center at the University of North Carolina, Chapel Hill (Ranney et al., 2006), assessed the evidence on effective tobacco cessation interventions as part of a larger evidence-based study. It showed that self-help strategies alone were ineffective, but counseling and pharmacotherapy used alone or in combination can improve success rates of quit attempts. *Treating Tobacco Use and Dependence* (Fiori et al., 2008) suggests that all tobacco users trying to quit should receive pharmacotherapy as part of a multicomponent approach to treating tobacco dependence. Special exceptions include those with medical contraindications, pregnant and nursing women, adolescents, and those smoking fewer than 10 cigarettes per day.

Treating Tobacco Use and Dependence (Fiori et al., 2008) identified seven first-line and two second-line pharmacotherapies. The first-line agents are bupropion SR (Wellbutrin SR or Zyban) and varenicline (Chantix) and five types

text continues on page 79

TABLE 5-1: THE "5 A'S" (1 OF 3)

ASK – ***Systematically identify all tobacco users at every visit.***

Action	Strategies for Implementation
Implement an office-wide system that ensures that, for every patient at every clinic visit, tobacco-use status is queried and documented. Repeated assessment is not necessary in the case of the adult who has never used tobacco or has not used tobacco for many years, and for whom this information is clearly documented in the medical record.	Expand the vital signs to include tobacco use or use an alternative universal identification system. Alternatives to expanding the vital signs are to place tobacco-use status stickers on all patient charts or to indicate tobacco use status using electronic medical records or computer reminder systems.

Vital Signs

Blood Pressure:______________________________

Pulse: _______________ Weight: _______________

Temperature: ______________________________

Respiratory Rate: ______________________________

Tobacco Use: (circle one) Current Former Never

ADVISE – ***Strongly urge all tobacco users to quit.***

Action	Strategies for Implementation
In a *clear, strong,* and *personalized* manner, urge every tobacco user to quit.	Advice should be: • *Clear* – "It is important for you to quit smoking (or using chewing tobacco) now and I can help you." "Cutting down while you are ill is not enough." "Occasional or light smoking is still dangerous." • *Strong* – "As your clinician, I need you to know that quitting smoking is the most important thing you can do to protect your health now and in the future. The clinic staff and I will help you." • *Personalized* – Link tobacco use to current health concerns, and/or its social and economic costs, and/or the impact of tobacco use on children and others in the household. "Continuing to smoke makes your asthma worse, and quitting may dramatically improve your health." "Quitting smoking may reduce the number of ear infections your child has."

ASSESS – ***Determine willingness to make a quit attempt.***

Action	Strategies for Implementation
Assess every tobacco user's willingness to make a quit attempt at the time.	Assess the patient's willingness to quit: "Are you willing to give quitting a try?" • If the patient is willing to make a quit attempt at this time, provide assistance. • If the patient will participate in an intensive treatment, deliver such a treatment or refer to an intensive intervention. • If the patient clearly states that he or she is unwilling to make a quit attempt at this time, provide an intervention shown to increase future quit attempts. • If the patient is a member of a special population (such as adolescent, pregnant smoker, or racial/ethnic minority), consider providing additional information.

continues on next page

TABLE 5-1: THE "5 A'S" (2 OF 3)	
ASSIST – ***Aid the patient in quitting (provide counseling and medication).***	
Action	**Strategies for Implementation**
Help the patient with a quit plan.	A patient's preparations for quitting should include the following: • *Set a quit date* – ideally, the quit date should be within 2 weeks. • *Tell* family, friends, and coworkers about quitting and request understanding and support. • *Anticipate* challenges to the planned quit attempt, particularly during the critical first few weeks. These include nicotine withdrawal symptoms. • *Remove* tobacco products from the environment before quitting and avoid smoking in places where a lot of time is spent such as work, home, or car. Make home smoke-free.
Provide practical counseling (problem solving/skills training).	• *Abstinence* – Total abstinence is essential. Not even a single puff after the quit date. • *Past quit experience* – Identify what helped and what hurt in previous quit attempts. Build on past success. • *Anticipate triggers or challenges in upcoming attempt* – Discuss challenges and triggers and how the patient will successfully overcome them (avoid triggers and alter routines). • *Alcohol* – Because alcohol can cause relapse, the patient should consider limiting and abstaining from alcohol while quitting. (Note that reducing alcohol intake could precipitate withdrawal in alcohol-dependent people.) • *Other smokers in the household* – Quitting is more difficult when there is another smoker in the household. Patients should encourage housemates to quit with them or to avoid smoking in their presence.
Provide intra-treatment social support.	• Provide a supportive clinical environment while encouraging the patient in his or her quit attempt. "My office staff and I are available to assist you." "I'm recommending treatment that can provide ongoing support."
Recommend the use of approved pharmacotherapy, except in special circumstances.	• Recommend the use of pharmacotherapies found to be effective. Explain how these medications increase smoking cessation success and reduce withdrawal symptoms. The first-line pharmacotherapy medications include bupropion SR, nicotine gum, nicotine inhaler, nicotine nasal spray, nicotine lozenge, nicotine patch and varenicline. Second line medications include clonidine and nortriptyline. There is insufficient evidence to recommend medications for pregnant women, smokeless tobacco users, light smokers and adolescents. (See Table 5-3.)
Provide supplementary materials, including information on quit lines.	• *Sources* – Federal agencies, nonprofit agencies, or local/state/tribal health departments/quitlines and the national quitline network (1-800-QUIT-NOW). • *Type* – Culturally/racially/educationally/age appropriate for the patient. • *Location* – Readily available at every clinician's workstation.

continues on next page

TABLE 5-1: THE "5 A'S" (3 OF 3)

ARRANGE – *Ensure followup contact.*	
Action	**Strategies for Implementation**
Arrange for follow-up contact, either in person or via telephone.	• *Timing* – Follow-up contact should occur soon after the quit date, preferably during the first week. A second follow-up contact is recommended within the first month. Schedule further follow-up contacts as indicated. • *Actions during follow-up contact* – Identify problems already encountered and anticipate challenges in the immediate future. Assess medication use and problems. Remind patients of quitline support (1-800-QUIT-NOW). Address tobacco use at next clinical visit (treat tobacco use as a chronic disease.) For patients who are abstinent, congratulate them on their success. If tobacco use has occurred, review circumstances and elicit recommitment to total abstinence. Consider use of or a referral to more intensive treatment.

Note. From *Treating tobacco use and dependence: 2008 Update,* by Fiore et al., 2008, Rockville, MD: U.S. Department of Health and Human Services. Public Health Service. Retrieved March 15, 2013, from http://www.ncbi.nlm.nih.gov/books/NBK63952/

of nicotine replacement therapy (NRT) – nicotine gum, nicotine inhaler, nicotine nasal spray, nicotine lozenge and the nicotine patch. All are approved by the Food and Drug Administration (FDA) for the first-line treatment of tobacco dependence. Currently there is insufficient data to order these medications in terms of efficacy; therefore, the choice of pharmacotherapy should be guided by the patient's characteristics, such as a history of depression or concerns about weight gain; the patient's previous experience with a specific pharmacotherapy (either positive or negative); the patient's and provider's preference; and the patient's insurance or pharmacy coverage. Specific indications for pharmacotherapy based on patient characteristics are found in Table 5-3.

The second-line pharmacologic agents for treatment of tobacco dependence are clonidine and nortriptyline. *Treating Tobacco Use and Dependence* (Fiori et al., 2008) suggests these second-line agents be considered for patients for whom first-line agents were not successful and for patients for whom first-line agents are contraindicated. Currently, these second-line agents are not FDA-approved for tobacco dependence.

Behavioral Counseling

There is a strong dose-response relationship between the intensity of tobacco dependence counseling and its effectiveness. Counseling that involves person-to-person contact either individually, in groups, or via telephone is consistently effective and its effectiveness increases with intensity. According to *Treating Tobacco Use and Dependence* (Fiori et al., 2008), two types of counseling and behavioral therapies have been found to be especially effective in nicotine-dependent patients who are attempting to quit. These therapies are providing practical counseling, such as problem-solving and skills training and providing clinician-focused social support (intra-treatment) as part of treatment, in which the health care provider encourages the patient in the quit attempt and communicates concern. Table 5-4 provides examples of these behavioral therapies.

Assisting the patient to quit tobacco use may be done as part of a brief intervention or an intensive treatment program. Evidence suggests that even a brief intervention counseling session of 3 minutes or fewer results in a significant increase in long-term abstinence.

text continues on page 82

TABLE 5-2: ENHANCING MOTIVATION TO QUIT TOBACCO – THE "5 R'S"

RELEVANCE – Encourage the patient to indicate why quitting is personally relevant, being as specific as possible. Motivational information has the greatest impact if it is relevant to a patient's disease status or risk, family or social situation (such as having children in the home), health concerns, age, gender, and other important patient characteristics (such as prior quitting experience or personal barriers to cessation).

RISKS – The clinician should ask the patient to identify potential negative consequences of tobacco use. The clinician may suggest and highlight those that seem most relevant to the patient. The clinician should emphasize that smoking low-tar/low-nicotine cigarettes or using other forms of tobacco (such as smokeless tobacco, cigars, and pipes) will not eliminate these risks.

Examples of risks are:

- Acute: Shortness of breath, exacerbation of asthma, harm to pregnancy, impotence, infertility, and increased serum carbon monoxide.
- Long-term: Heart attack and stroke, lung and other cancers (larynx, oral cavity, pharynx, esophagus, pancreas, bladder, cervix), chronic obstructive pulmonary diseases (chronic bronchitis and emphysema), long-term disability, and need for extended care.
- Environmental: Increased risk of lung cancer and heart disease in spouses, higher rates of smoking in children of tobacco users, and increased risk for low birth weight, sudden infant death syndrome, asthma, middle ear disease, and respiratory infections in children of smokers.

REWARDS – The clinician should ask the patient to identify potential benefits of stopping tobacco use. The clinician may suggest and highlight those that seem most relevant to the patient.

Examples of rewards include:

- improved health
- improved sense of taste
- improved sense of smell
- saving money
- improved self-esteem
- improved smell of home, car, clothing, and breath
- not worrying about quitting
- setting a good example for children
- having healthier babies and children
- not worrying about exposing others to smoke
- improved physical health
- performing better in physical activities
- reduced wrinkling and aging of skin and whiter teeth

ROADBLOCKS – The clinician should ask the patient to identify barriers or impediments to quitting and note elements of treatment (such as problem solving, or pharmacotherapy) that could address barriers.

Typical barriers include:

- withdrawal symptoms
- fear of failure
- weight gain
- lack of support
- depression
- enjoyment of tobacco
- being around other tobacco users
- lack knowledge of effective treatment options

REPETITION – The motivational intervention should be repeated every time an unmotivated patient visits the clinical setting. Tobacco users who have failed in previous quit attempts should be told that most people make repeated quit attempts before they are successful.

Note. From *Treating tobacco use and dependence: 2008 Update*, by Fiore et al., 2008, Rockville, MD: U.S. Department of Health and Human Services. Public Health Service. Retrieved March 15, 2013, from http://www.ncbi.nlm.nih.gov/books/NBK63952/

TABLE 5-3: CLINICAL GUIDELINES FOR PRESCRIBING MEDICATIONS FOR TOBACCO USE AND DEPENDENCE (1 OF 2)	
Who should receive medication for tobacco use? Are there groups of smokers for whom medication has not been shown to be effective?	All smokers trying to quit should be offered medication, except when contraindicated or for specific populations for which there is insufficient evidence of effectiveness (i.e., pregnant women, smokeless tobacco users, light smokers, and adolescents).
What are the first-line medications recommended in this Guideline update?	All seven of the FDA-approved medications for treating tobacco use are recommended: bupropion SR, nicotine gum, nicotine inhaler, nicotine lozenge, nicotine nasal spray, nicotine patch, and varenicline. The clinician should consider the first-line medications shown to be more effective than the nicotine patch alone: 2 mg/day varenicline or the combination of long-term nicotine patch use + *ad libitum* nicotine replacement therapy (NRT). Unfortunately, there are no well-accepted algorithms to guide optimal selection among the first-line medications.
Are there contraindications, warnings, precautions, other concerns, and side effects regarding the first-line medications recommended in this Guideline update?	All seven FDA-approved medications have specific contraindications, warnings, precautions, other concerns, and side effects. Refer to FDA package inserts for this complete information. (See information below regarding second-line medications.)
What other factors may influence medication selection?	Pragmatic factors also may influence selection, such as insurance coverage, out-of-pocket patient costs, likelihood of adherence, dentures when considering the gum, or dermatitis when considering using the patch.
Is a patient's prior experience with a medication relevant?	Prior successful experience (sustained abstinence with the medication) suggests that the medication may be helpful to the patient in a subsequent quit attempt, especially if the patient found the medication to be tolerable and/or easy to use. However, it is difficult to draw firm conclusions from prior failure with a medication. Some evidence suggests that re-treating relapsed smokers with the same medication produces small or no benefit, whereas other evidence suggests that it may be of substantial benefit.
What medications should a clinician use with a patient who is highly nicotine dependent?	The higher-dose preparations of nicotine gum, patch, and lozenge have been shown to be effective in highly dependent smokers. Also, there is evidence that combination NRT therapy may be particularly effective in suppressing tobacco withdrawal symptoms. Thus, it may be that NRT combinations are especially helpful for highly dependent smokers or those with a history of severe withdrawal.
Is gender a consideration in selecting a medication?	There is evidence that NRT can be effective with both sexes; however, evidence is mixed as to whether NRT is less effective in women than men. This may encourage the clinician to consider use of another type of medication with women, such as bupropion SR or varenicline.
Are cessation medications appropriate for light smokers (i.e., < 10 cigarettes/day)?	As noted above, cessation medications have not been shown to be beneficial to light smokers. However, if NRT is used with light smokers, clinicians may consider reducing the dose of the medication. No adjustments are necessary when using bupropion SR or varenicline.

continues on next page

TABLE 5-3: CLINICAL GUIDELINES FOR PRESCRIBING MEDICATIONS FOR TOBACCO USE AND DEPENDENCE (2 OF 2)	
When should second-line agents be used for treating tobacco dependence?	Consider prescribing second-line agents (clonidine and nortriptyline) for patients unable to use first-line medications because of contraindications or for patients for whom the group of first-line medications has not been helpful. Assess patients for the specific contraindications, precautions, other concerns, and side effects of the second-line agents. Refer to FDA package inserts for this information.
Which medications should be considered with patients particularly concerned about weight gain?	Data show that bupropion SR and nicotine replacement therapies, in particular 4 mg nicotine gum and 4 mg nicotine lozenge, delay – but do not prevent – weight gain.
Are there medications that should especially be considered for patients with a past history of depression?	Bupropion SR and nortriptyline appear to be effective with this population, but nicotine replacement medications also appear to help individuals with a past history of depression.
Should nicotine replacement therapies be avoided in patients with a history of cardiovascular disease?	No. The nicotine patch in particular has been demonstrated as safe for cardiovascular patients. See FDA package inserts for more complete information.
May tobacco dependence medications be used long-term (e.g., up to 6 months)?	Yes. This approach may be helpful with smokers who report persistent withdrawal symptoms during the course of medications, who have relapsed in the past after stopping medication, or who desire long-term therapy. A minority of individuals who successfully quit smoking use *ad libitum* NRT medications (gum, nasal spray, inhaler) long-term. The use of these medications for up to 6 months does not present a known health risk, and developing dependence on medications is uncommon. Additionally, the FDA has approved the use of bupropion SR, varenicline, and some NRT medications for 6-month use.
Is medication adherence important?	Yes. Patients frequently do not use cessation medications as recommended (e.g., they do not use them at recommended doses or for recommended durations); this may reduce their effectiveness.
May medications ever be combined?	Yes. Among first-line medications, evidence exists that combining the nicotine patch long-term (> 14 weeks) with either nicotine gum or nicotine nasal spray, the nicotine patch with the nicotine inhaler, or the nicotine patch with bupropion SR, increases long-term abstinence rates relative to placebo treatments. Combining varenicline with NRT agents has been associated with higher rates of side effects (e.g., nausea, headaches).

Note. From *Treating tobacco use and dependence: 2008 Update,* by Fiore et al., 2008, Rockville, MD: U.S. Department of Health and Human Services. Public Health Service. Retrieved March 15, 2013, from http://www.ncbi.nlm.nih.gov/books/NBK63952/

An intensive treatment intervention is appropriate for every tobacco user who has agreed to quit. Evidence has demonstrated that intensive interventions are more effective than brief interventions and should be used whenever possible. Table 5-5 lists the strategy components of an intensive intervention. Intensive interventions usually last longer than 10 minutes with four or more sessions. Individual, group, or proactive telephone counseling may be used. Multiple health care clinicians may provide counseling that focuses on health, financial, and psychosocial risks.

TABLE 5-4: ELEMENTS OF BEHAVIORAL COUNSELING AND THERAPIES

COMMON ELEMENTS OF PRACTICAL COUNSELING

Practical counseling (problem solving and skills training) treatment component	Examples
Recognize danger situations – Identify events, internal states, or activities that increase the risk of smoking or relapse.	• Negative affect and stress • Being around other smokers • Drinking alcohol • Experiencing urges • Smoking cues and cigarette availability
Develop coping skills – Identify and practice coping or problem-solving skills. Typically, these skills are intended to cope with danger situations.	• Learning to anticipate and avoid temptation • Learning cognitive strategies that will reduce negative moods • Accomplishing lifestyle changes that reduce stress, improve quality of life, and reduce exposure to smoking cues • Learning cognitive and behavioral activities to cope with smoking urges (such as distracting attention, changing routines)
Provide basic information – Provide basic information about smoking and successful quitting.	• Any smoking (even a single puff) increases the likelihood of full relapse. • Withdrawal typically peaks within 1 to 2 weeks after quitting, but may. persist for months. • Withdrawal symptoms include negative mood, urges to smoke, and difficulty concentrating. • Smoking is addictive in nature.

COMMON ELEMENTS OF SUPPORTIVE INTRA-TREATMENT

Supportive treatment component	Examples
Encourage the patient in the quit attempt.	• Note that effective tobacco dependence treatments are now available. • Note that one-half of all people who have ever smoked have now quit. • Communicate belief in the patient's ability to quit.
Communicate caring and concern.	• Ask how the patient feels about quitting. • Directly express concern and willingness to help as needed. • Be open to the patient's expression of fears of quitting, difficulties experienced, and ambivalent feelings.
Encourage the patient to talk about the quitting process.	Ask about: • reasons the patient wants to quit. • concerns or worries about quitting. • success the patient has achieved. • difficulties encountered while quitting.

Note. From *Treating tobacco use and dependence: 2008 Update,* by Fiore et al., 2008, Rockville, MD: U.S. Department of Health and Human Services. Public Health Service. Retrieved March 15, 2013, from http://www.ncbi.nlm.nih.gov/books/NBK63952/

The behavioral therapies, as well as previously discussed pharmacotherapies, should be used.

The literature includes alternative therapies to tobacco cessation, including acupuncture, exercise, hypnosis, bio-behavioral feedback, and herbal treatments. The current evidence is inconclusive regarding the effectiveness of these treatments with findings generally mixed or conflicting. Data regarding hypnosis and bio-behavioral feedback was insufficient to determine the efficacy of these treatments and that the findings related to acupuncture and exercise were mixed (Schmitz & Delange, 2004). Many nicotine-dependent patients express a desire to explore alternative treatments and this desire must be respected by the clinician. Alternative treatments may be considered as an adjunct to behavioral therapies and pharmacotherapies.

TABLE 5-5: STRATEGY COMPONENTS OF AN INTENSIVE INTERVENTION	
Assessment	Assessments should ensure that tobacco users are willing to make a quit attempt using an intensive treatment program. Other assessments can provide information useful in counseling (such as stress level or dependence).
Program clinicians	Multiple types of clinicians are effective and should be used. One counseling strategy would be to have a medical or health care clinician deliver messages about health risks and benefits and prescribe pharmacotherapy, and then nonmedical clinicians deliver additional psychosocial or behavioral interventions.
Program intensity	Because of evidence of a strong dose-response relationship, the intensity of the program should be: • session length – longer than 10 minutes. • number of sessions – four or more sessions. • total contact time – longer than 30 minutes.
Program format	Either individual or group counseling may be used. Proactive telephone counseling also is effective. Use of adjuvant self-help material is optional. Follow-up assessment intervention procedures should be used.
Type of counseling and behavioral therapies	Counseling and behavioral therapies should involve practical counseling (problem solving/skills training). See Table 5-4.
Pharmacotherapy	Every smoker should be encouraged to use pharmacotherapies endorsed in the guideline, except in the presence of special circumstances. Special consideration should be given before using pharmacotherapy with selected populations (such as pregnant women, or adolescents). The clinician should explain how these medications increase smoking cessation success and reduce withdrawal symptoms. The first-line pharmacotherapy agents include bupropion SR, nicotine gum, nicotine inhaler, nicotine nasal spray, and the nicotine patch. (See Table 5-3.)
Population	Intensive intervention programs may be used with all tobacco users willing to participate in such efforts.

Note. From *Treating tobacco use and dependence: 2008 Update,* by Fiore et al., 2008, Rockville, MD: U.S. Department of Health and Human Services. Public Health Service. Retrieved March 15, 2013, from http://www.ncbi.nlm.nih.gov/books/NBK63952/

SPECIAL CONSIDERATIONS AND ISSUES

Smokeless Tobacco

The two most common forms of smokeless tobacco in the United States are chewing tobacco and snuff. Chewing tobacco is generally a loose leaf product but also comes in the forms of plug and twist. Snuff is finely ground tobacco that can be dry or moist or come in sachets, similar to tea bags. Generally, smokeless tobacco users place the product between their gum and cheek and suck on the tobacco, frequently spitting out the juices (CDC, 2010). Smokeless tobacco is often a precursor to cigarette smoking and results in many of the same negative health consequences, such as nicotine dependence, an increased risk of oral cavity cancer, and gum disease. Smokeless tobacco contains 28 cancer-causing agents.

The population with the highest prevalence rate of smokeless tobacco use is White, male, high school students. It is estimated that 7.9% of all high school students are current smokeless tobacco users – males, 13.4%, and females, 2.3%. Estimates for race or ethnicity are 4.3% White, 1.3% Hispanic, and 0.7% African American. Nationally, 3.3% of all adults are smokeless tobacco users (CDC, 2010). Screening and treatment for smokeless tobacco users follows the same guidelines discussed in *Treating Tobacco Use and Dependence* (Fiori et al., 2008).

Mental Health Issues

The prevalence of tobacco use in adults 18 years of age and older with mental illness and substance use disorders is markedly higher than in the general population. As of January 2013, adults with a lifetime history of mental illness were noted to have a tobacco use prevalence rate of 36.1%, compared to 21.4% of adults in the general population with no history of mental illness (SAMHSA, 2013). Among adults with past year major depressive episode, the rate of daily cigarette use in January 2013 was 29.1%, while the rate was 15.2% among adults without past year major depressive episode (SAMHSA, 2013).

The prevalence of smoking in patients with other substance use disorders is even more impressive, with estimates ranging above 70%. Patients who are alcoholics are the heaviest smokers and have less success with smoking cessation than other patients with substance use disorders. Patients with co-morbid chemical dependence and tobacco dependence have much higher rates of morbidity and mortality. *Treating Tobacco Use and Dependence* (Fiori et al., 2008) recommends that tobacco users with chemical dependence be screened and treated using the "5 A's" protocol.

Older Smokers

All patients benefit from tobacco cessation, including patients older than age 65. Often, providers make the mistaken assumption that patients who continue to use tobacco into their 60's and 70's are not candidates for screening and treatment. Smoking cessation interventions that have been effective in the general population have been proven to be as effective with older adults. This includes counseling interventions, clinician advice, buddy support programs, age-tailored self-help materials, the nicotine patch and telephone counseling. The homebound older adult patient may especially benefit from proactive telephone counseling. Smoking cessation in older adults can reduce their risk of death from coronary heart disease, COPD, and lung cancer and decrease their risk of osteoporosis (Fiore et al., 2008).

SUMMARY

Tobacco use is the leading cause of preventable death and disability in the United States. Initiation of tobacco use most commonly occurs before age 18 and results in nicotine dependence that continues well into the patient's adult years. Nicotine is the drug in tobacco that causes addiction. It is a highly addictive substance that, when inhaled, quickly enters the brain. It is estimated that 26.5% of individuals 12 years of age and older in the U.S. smoke, and nearly 83% of them smoke daily (SAMHSA, 2012).

The Clinical Guideline *Treating Tobacco Use and Dependence* (Fiori et al., 2008) recommends that all adult and adolescent patients be screened for tobacco use (*ask*). If the patient is a current smoker or tobacco user, the clinician should strongly *advise* the patient to quit and *assess* the patient's willingness to quit. If the patient is willing to make a quit attempt, the clinician should *assist* the patient by offering appropriate treatment, and *arrange* for follow up. *"Ask, Assess, Advise, Assist and Arrange."*

If the patient is a current smoker but not interested in quitting, the clinician should provide motivational counseling that focuses on why quitting is *relevant,* the health *risks* associated with continued use, the *rewards* associated with stopping, the *roadblocks* to quitting, and *repeat* this motivational intervention every time a tobacco user is seen. *"Relevance, Risk, Rewards, Roadblocks and Repetition."*

Patients who are currently abstinent from nicotine should be offered counseling that reinforces their abstinence at every visit.

EXAM QUESTIONS

CHAPTER 5

Questions 24-28

Note: Choose the one option that BEST answers each question.

24. Increased health risk(s) caused from the tar when smoking cigarettes include

    a. lung cancer and respiratory disease.

    b. thyroid disease and kidney failure.

    c. diabetes mellitus in adulthood.

    d. dizziness and recurrent headaches.

25. Currently, the prevalence of tobacco use in the adult population in the United States is approximately

    a. 12%.

    b. 19%.

    c. 28%.

    d. 41%.

26. Nicotine has an onset of action in the brain that may be described as

    a. delayed; 6 hours before onset.

    b. moderately delayed; 4 hours before onset.

    c. moderately rapid; 2 hours before onset.

    d. rapid; seconds to minutes before onset.

27. According to *Treating Tobacco Use and Dependence* (2008), the best approach with a patient who wants to quit smoking is for the clinician to

    a. promote motivation for the patient to quit.

    b. encourage the patient to quit on his or her own.

    c. provide appropriate tobacco dependence treatment.

    d. discourage the use of adjunct alternative therapies.

28. Mr. Smith has smoked 1 pack per day for 20 years and is currently unwilling to stop. His medical history is significant for high blood pressure. The clinician begins a brief intervention stating, "Mr. Smith, I realize that you are not interested in stopping smoking today, but I am concerned that your smoking is increasing your blood pressure." This is an example of motivational counseling that focuses on personal

    a. repetition.

    b. rewards.

    c. roadblocks.

    d. health risks.

REFERENCES

American Cancer Society. (2013). *Lung cancer: Causes, risk factors, and prevention topics*. Retrieved March 15, 2013 from http://www.cancer.org/cancer/lungcancer-non-smallcell/detailedguide/non-small-cell-lung-cancer-risk-factors

American Lung Association. (2013). *Women and tobacco use*. Retrieved March 15, 2013 from http://www.lung.org/stop-smoking/about-smoking/facts-figures/women-and-tobacco-use.html

American Psychiatric Association. (1996). Practice guidelines for the treatment of nicotine dependence. *American Journal of Psychiatry, 153*(Suppl.), 1-31.

American Psychiatric Association. (2013). *Diagnostic and statistical manual of mental disorders* (5th ed.). Washington, DC: American Psychiatric Association.

Bigelow, G.E. & Rand, C.S. (2003). Tobacco use and dependence. In L.R. Barker, J.R. Burton, P.D. Zieve, N.H. Fiebach, D.E. Kern, P.A. Thomas, & R.C. Ziegelstein (Eds.), *Principles of ambulatory medicine* (6th ed.). Philadelphia: Lippincott Williams & Wilkins.

Cable News Network. (2000). *A brief history of tobacco*. Retrieved March 15, 2013, from http://www.cnn.com/US/9705/tobacco/history/

Centers for Disease Control and Prevention. (2010). *Smokeless tobacco*. Retrieved March 15, 2013 from http://www.cdc.gov/tobacco/data_statistics/by_topic/smokeless/index.htm

Centers for Disease Control and Prevention. (2011a). *Smoking & tobacco use: Tobacco-related mortality*. Retrieved March 15, 2013 from http://www.cdc.gov/tobacco/data_statistics/fact_sheets/health_effects/tobacco_related_mortality/

Centers for Disease Control and Prevention. (2011b). *Tobacco controls have public health impact*. Retrieved March 15, 2013 from http://www.cdc.gov/features/tobaccocontrols/index.html

Centers for Disease Control and Prevention. (2011c). *Vital signs: Current cigarette smoking among adults aged ≥18 years – United States, 2005-2010*. Retrieved from http://www.cdc.gov/mmwr/pdf/wk/mm6035.pdf#page=21

Centers for Disease Control and Prevention. (2012). Current cigarette smoking among adults – United States, 2011. *Morbidity and Mortality Weekly Report, 61*(44), 889-894. Retrieved March 15, 2013, from http://www.cdc.gov/mmwr/preview/mmwrhtml/mm6144a2.htm

Fiore, M.C., Bailey, W.C., Cohen, S.J., Dorfman, S.F., Goldstein, M.G., Gritz, E.R., et al. (2008). *Treating tobacco use and dependence: 2008 Update. Quick reference guide for clinicians*. Rockville, MD: U.S. Department of Health and Human Services. Public Health Service. Retrieved October 9, 2009, from http://www.ncbi.nlm.nih.gov/books/bv.fcgi?rid=hstat2.chapter.28163

Hymowitz, N. (2005). Tobacco. In R.J. Frances, S.I. Miller, & A.H. Mack (Eds.), *Clinical textbook of addictive disorders* (3rd ed., pp. 105-137). New York: Guilford Press.

Johnston, L. D., O'Malley, P. M., Bachman, J. G., & Schulenberg, J. E. (2013). *Monitoring the Future national results on drug use: 2012 Overview, Key Findings on Adolescent Drug Use*. Ann Arbor: Institute for Social Research, The University of Michigan.

Kandel, D., Schaffran, C., Griesler, P., Samuolis, J., Davies, M., & Galanti, R. (2005). On the measurement of nicotine dependence in adolescence: Comparisons of the mftq and a DMS-IV based scale. *Journal of Pediatric Psychology, 30*(4), 319-332.

Mayo Clinic. (2010). Nicotine dependence. Retrieved April 2, 2013 from http://www.mayoclinic.com/health/nicotine-dependence/DS00307/DSECTION=tests-and-diagnosis

National Institute on Drug Abuse. (2012a). *Smoking and pregnancy – what are the risks?* Retrieved March 15, 2013 from http://www.drugabuse.gov/publications/research-reports/tobacco-addiction/smoking-pregnancy%E2%80%94-what-are-risks

National Institute on Drug Abuse. (2012b). *Tobacco addiction*. Retrieved March 15, 2013, from http://www.drugabuse.gov/publications/research-reports/tobacco-addiction/how-does-tobacco-deliver-its-effects

National Institute on Drug Abuse. (2013). *Mind over matter: Nicotine*. Retrieved March 15, 2013 from http://teens.drugabuse.gov/mom/mom_nic1.php

Polito, J.R. (2005). Surveys suggest nicotine smoking extremely addictive. *Why quit news*. Retrieved May 13, 2006, from http://whyquit.com/pr/051305.html

Ranney, L., Melvin, C., Lux, L., McClain, E., Morgan, L., & Lohr, K. (2006). *Tobacco use: Prevention, cessation, and control.* Evidence Report/Technology Assessment No. 140. AHRQ Publication No. 06-E015. Rockville, MD: Agency for Healthcare Research and Quality. Retrieved August 8, 2006, from http://www.ahrq.gov/clinic/evrptpdfs.htm#tobacco

Schmitz & Delange. (2004) Nicotine. In J.H. Lowinson, P. Ruiz, R.B. Millman, & J.G. Langrod (Eds.), *Substance Abuse: A comprehensive textbook* (4th ed.). Philadelphia: Lippincott, Williams & Wilkins.

Substance Abuse and Mental Health Services Administration. (2012). *Results from the 2011 National survey on drug use and health: Summary of national findings* (NSDUH Series H-44, HHS Publication No. (SMA) 12-4713). Rockville, MD. Accessed March 10, 2013 from http://www.samhsa.gov/data/NSDUH/2k11Results/NSDUHresults2011.htm

Substance Abuse and Mental Health Services Administration. (2013). *Smoking and Mental Illness*. Retrieved March 15, 2013 from http://www.samhsa.gov/data/2k13/NSDUH093/sr093-smoking-mental-illness.htm

U.S. Department of Health and Human Services. (2006). *The health consequences of involuntary exposure to tobacco smoke: A report of the Surgeon General – Executive summary.* U.S. Department of Health and Human Services, Centers for Disease Control and Prevention, Coordinating Center for Health Promotion, National Center for Chronic Disease Prevention and Health Promotion, Office on Smoking and Health. Retrieved March 15, 2013 from http://www.surgeongeneral.gov/library/secondhandsmoke/report/executivesummary.pdf

CHAPTER 6

CAFFEINE

CHAPTER OBJECTIVE

After completing this chapter, the learner will be able to describe the history of caffeine use, its physiological effects, its clinical manifestations, and implications for treatment.

LEARNING OBJECTIVES

After studying this chapter, the learner will be able to:

1. Describe the epidemiology of caffeine use.
2. Identify common sources of dietary caffeine.
3. Describe the health effects associated with caffeine use.
4. Identify common adverse effects of caffeine use.
5. Describe clinical interventions used to assist the client in decreasing caffeine intake.

OVERVIEW

Caffeine, a mild central nervous system (CNS) stimulant, is the most commonly used mood-altering substance in the world. It occurs naturally as a plant alkaloid and is found in coffee, tea, the kola nut and, less commonly, in the guarana and mate plants.

The use of caffeine as a mild stimulant has been well documented. Coffee was first discovered in Ethiopia where Ethiopians would mix crushed dried coffee beans with fat that they rolled into balls for food. By the 14th century, the process of roasting and grinding coffee beans had been developed in Arabia. In addition, China has used tea for thousands of years.

Caffeine may also be produced synthetically, usually for soft drinks and medications. Caffeine may be found in multiple dietary sources and prescription and nonprescription drugs. Table 6-1 lists the content of caffeine in common food, beverages, and medications.

EPIDEMIOLOGY

Eighty percent of the world's population consumes caffeine in some form. In North America, it is estimated that 80% to 90% of adults and children use caffeine regularly (Juliano & Griffiths, 2005). While coffee is the most common source of caffeine for adults, caffeinated soft drinks is the most common source of caffeine in children. Not surprisingly, 70% of all soft drinks contain caffeine; the consumption of soft drinks in children and adolescents has skyrocketed in the past few decades, and 30-50% of children, adolescents and young adults are consuming caffeinated energy drinks (Substance Abuse and Mental Health Services Administration [SAMSHA], 2013).

It is very difficult to estimate the exact amount of caffeine intake because the amount

TABLE 6-1: CAFFEINE CONTENT IN COMMON FOODS AND MEDICATIONS

Substance	Serving Size (volume or weight)	Caffeine Content (range)	Caffeine Content (average)
Coffee			
Brewed/Drip	6 oz	77-150 mg	100 mg
Instant	6 oz	20-130 mg	70 mg
Espresso	1 oz	30-50 mg	40 mg
Decaffeinated	6 oz	2-9 mg	4 mg
Tea			
Brewed	6 oz	30-90 mg	40 mg
Instant	6 oz	10-35 mg	30 mg
Canned or Bottled	12 oz	8-32 mg	20 mg
Chocolate Drinks, Ice Cream and Yogurt			
Cocoa/Hot Chocolate	6 oz	2-10 mg	7 mg
Chocolate Milk	6 oz	2-7 mg	4 mg
Coffee Ice Cream or Yogurt	1 cup (8 oz)	8-85 mg	50 mg
Chocolate Bars, Chocolate and Gum			
Milk Chocolate	1.5 oz	2-10 mg	10 mg
Dark Chocolate	1.5 oz	5-35 mg	30 mg
Caffeinated Gum	1 stick	50 mg	50 mg
Soft Drinks			
7-up, Sprite	12 oz	0 mg	0 mg
Cola and Diet Cola drinks	12 oz	34-47 mg	37 mg
Mountain Dew, Mellow Yellow and Diet	12 oz	51-55 mg	51 mg
Sunkist Orange and Diet	12 oz	41 mg	41 mg
Sports/Energy Drinks			
Red Bull	8.5 oz	80 mg	80 mg
Full Throttle	16 oz	144 mg	144 mg
AMP Energy Drink	8.4 oz	75 mg	75mg
Caffeine-Containing Over-the-Counter Products			
Analgesics	2 tablets	64-130 mg	64 or 130 mg
Stimulants	1 tablet	75-350 mg	100 or 200 mg
Weight-loss Products	2-3 tablets	80-200 mg	80-200 mg
Sports Nutrition	2 tablets	200 mg	200 mg

often depends on the serving size and method of preparation. For example, "a serving of coffee can range from 17 mg for a small, 5 oz. cup of instant coffee to 500 mg for a large, 20 oz. cup of drip coffee" (Juliano & Griffiths, 2005, p. 406).

The Caffeine Awareness Alliance provides a Web site that is useful in estimating and calculating daily caffeine intake: http://www.caffeineawareness.org/calcu.php.

BIOCHEMISTRY

Caffeine is a lipid-soluble molecule (similar to alcohol and nicotine) that is rapidly and completely absorbed throughout the entire body, including such body fluids as saliva, amniotic fluid, breast milk, and semen (Juliano & Griffiths, 2005). The molecule quickly crosses the blood-brain barrier with peak blood levels occurring within 30 to 45 minutes and a half-life of 4 to 6 hours (Juliana & Griffiths, 2005). It is this rapid absorption that results in the stimulant effect of caffeine.

Caffeine is largely metabolized through the P450 liver enzyme system and results in three metabolites: paraxanthine, theophylline, and theobromine (Denaro & Benowitz, 1991). Paraxanthine acts to increase lipolysis elevating glycerol and free fatty acids; theobromine dilates blood vessels, increases urine volume, and contributes to the diuretic effect of caffeine; lastly, theophylline relaxes the smooth muscles of the bronchi. Tobacco increases the metabolism of caffeine, and several medications such as cimetidine and hormonal contraceptives decrease the rate of metabolism of caffeine.

HEALTH EFFECTS

Moderate amounts of caffeine, 20 to 200 mg, generally produce pleasant mood-altering effects, such as increased well-being and energy levels, alertness, happiness, and sociability (Johns Hopkins Bayview Medical Center, 2003). An 6-ounce cup of brewed coffee is generally equivalent to 100 mg of caffeine; a cup of brewed tea, 40 mg; and a 12-ounce cola, 40 mg (Johns Hopkins Bayview Medical Center, 2003). Among daily caffeine users, these pleasant mood-altering effects may have more to do with the suppression of such low-grade withdrawal symptoms as fatigue and sleepiness than with the direct effect of caffeine.

Significant amounts of caffeine, defined as higher than 200 mg may have negative mood-altering effects, such as nervousness, increased anxiety, jitteriness, and upset stomach. Energy drinks can contain about 80 to greater than 500 mg of caffeine (SAMSHA, 2013).These negative effects are mitigated by an individual's tolerance and are usually short in duration. Clients with anxiety disorders are particularly vulnerable to the effects of caffeine and many will self-limit their caffeine intake to decrease anxiety and panic symptoms. Other common health effects include insomnia, gastroesopheageal reflex disorder, mild increases in blood pressure, and urinary incontinence. Women who are pregnant or trying to become pregnant are counseled to decrease or abstain from caffeine intake.

Caffeine acts as a reinforcer. That is, individuals will continue to self-administer the drug if it is consumed in dosages that increase mood-altering effects. Tolerance, which describes the process of decreasing responsiveness of a drug after repeated exposures (Johns Hopkins Bayview Medical Center, 2003), occurs as well; however, it is often incomplete in nature with caffeine, most commonly interfering with sleep at night.

Withdrawal symptoms as a result of physical dependence have been well documented. These symptoms may begin 12 to 24 hours after the most recent dose of caffeine and peak at 48 hours (Juliano & Griffiths, 2005). The duration of withdrawal symptoms lasts between 2 to 7 days (Johns Hopkins Bayview Medical Center, 2003). The severity of withdrawal is usually reflective of the amount of daily consumption. Significant withdrawal symptoms occur with as little as 100 mg of caffeine per day – the equivalent of one cup of coffee. The most common withdrawal symptoms, in order of frequency, are:

- headache
- fatigue

- drowsiness
- difficulty concentrating
- work difficulty
- irritability
- depression
- flu-like symptoms

(Johns Hopkins Bayview Medical Center, 2003; Juliana L & Griffiths, 2005).

CLINICAL IMPLICATIONS

The *Diagnostic and Statistical Manual of Mental Disorders,* 5th Edition (*DSM-5*) (American Psychiatric Association [APA], 2013), lists three caffeine-induced psychiatric disorders – caffeine intoxication, caffeine-withdrawal, and unspecified caffeine –related disorder. The World Health Organization (ICD-10) recognizes caffeine dependence as a diagnosis; however, the *DSM-5* does not recognize the diagnosis of caffeine dependence.

Caffeine intoxication or caffeine poisoning is a result of a significant ingestion of caffeine – at least 250 mg but more likely more than 500 mg. Common signs of caffeine intoxication include: restlessness, nervousness (anxiety), excitement, insomnia, a flushed face, diuresis, gastrointestinal disturbance, twitching muscles, rambling thoughts and speech, tachycardia or cardiac arrhythmia, periods of inexhaustibility and psychomotor agitation. These symptoms cause impairment in functioning and are not due to another medical condition (APA, 2013).

Caffeine-induced anxiety disorder, sleep disorder, and NOS are caffeine-related symptoms that result in the diagnosis of anxiety, insomnia, or non-specific caffeine-related disorders. It is important to note that caffeine intoxication may mimic generalized anxiety disorder, panic disorder, bipolar disorder, and schizophrenia (Johns Hopkins Bayview Medical Center, 2003). As previously noted, caffeine ingestion, even at low doses, may exacerbate anxiety disorders.

When obtaining a client's history, it is important to elicit a thorough caffeine intake; this includes beverages, foods, and prescription and nonprescription drugs. Sensitivity to culture and ethnicity is also important in recognizing alternative methods of caffeine ingestion. Although it can be challenging to determine an accurate intake, if a client is consuming more than 200 mg of caffeine per day, he or she should be carefully questioned about the presence of physical symptoms and negative mood-altering symptoms and counseled to cut down on intake slowly.

In counseling a client on caffeine reduction, it is important to clearly identify the client's goal. Is the goal complete elimination of caffeine or a reduction in the amount consumed? If the goal is reduction, what is the reduction goal in terms of milligrams? First, educate the client on the dietary, pharmacological, and nonpharmalogical sources of caffeine. Estimate the current daily caffeine intake with the client. It is often helpful to have the client keep a food diary for 1 to 2 weeks to determine accurate caffeine intake. Provide handouts and client education materials with common sources of caffeine and milligrams associated with these sources. Encourage the client to slowly decrease caffeine by 10% to 25% every few days until the goal is reached. Suggest non-caffeinated alternatives to replace the usual sources of caffeine.

Similar to strategies used for substance use reduction and abstinence, employ motivational counseling techniques; encourage the client to set specific goals; share these goals with a close friend or significant other who can offer encouragement; identify potential barriers; reframe withdrawal as a temporary process; and follow up with the client to monitor progress.

SUMMARY

Caffeine is a mild CNS stimulant. Moderate amounts of caffeine (20 to 200 mg) generally produce a pleasant, mood-altering feeling. Significant amounts of caffeine (more than 200 mg) may have such negative, mood-altering effects as nervousness, increased anxiety, jitteriness, and upset stomach. Clients with anxiety disorders are particularly vulnerable to the effects of caffeine.

The most common symptoms of caffeine withdrawal are headache, fatigue, drowsiness, difficulty concentrating, difficulty working, irritability, depression, and flu-like symptoms (John Hopkins Bayview Medical Center, 2003; Juliano & Griffiths, 2005). There are four caffeine-induced psychiatric disorders (APA, 2004): caffeine intoxication, caffeine-induced anxiety disorder, caffeine-induced sleep disorder, and caffeine-related disorder NOS.

In obtaining a client's history, it is important to elicit a thorough caffeine intake. In counseling a client on caffeine reduction, it is important to clearly identify the client's goal. Encourage the client to slowly decrease caffeine by 10% to 25% every few days until the goal is reached.

EXAM QUESTIONS

CHAPTER 6

Questions 29-33

Note: Choose the one option that BEST answers each question.

29. Caffeine is a central nervous system

    a. depressant.
    b. stimulant.
    c. modifier.
    d. antagonist.

30. The average adult intake of caffeine in the United States is

    a. 180 mg per day.
    b. 220 mg per day.
    c. 280 mg per day.
    d. 320 mg per day.

31. The type of coffee with the highest caffeine content is

    a. 1 oz of espresso.
    b. 6 oz of brewed/drip.
    c. 6 oz of instant.
    d. 6 oz of decaffeinated.

32. The most common symptom of caffeine withdrawal is

    a. drowsiness.
    b. irritability.
    c. headache.
    d. flu-like symptoms.

33. When counseling a patient on decreasing his or her caffeine intake, the practitioner should recommend that caffeine be reduced by 10% to 25% every

    a. day until the goal is reached.
    b. other day until the goal is reached.
    c. few days until the goal is reached.
    d. 7 days until the goal is reached.

REFERENCES

American Psychiatric Association. (2013). *Diagnostic and statistical manual of mental disorders* (5th Ed.). Washington, DC: American Psychiatric Association.

Denaro, C.P. & Benowitz, N.L. (1991). Caffeine metabolism: Disposition in liver disease and hepatic-function testing. In R.R. Watson, (Ed.), *Drug and alcohol abuse reviews: Liver pathology and alcohol* (vol. 2, pp. 513-539). Totowa, NJ: Humana Press.

Johns Hopkins Bayview Medical Center. (2003). *Information about caffeine dependence.* Accessed Retrieved March 15, 2013, from http://www.caffeinedependence.org/caffeine_dependence.html

Juliano, L.M. & Griffiths, R.R. (2005). Caffeine. In J. H. Lowinson, P. Ruiz, R.B. Millman, & J.G. Langrod (Eds.), *Substance abuse: A comprehensive textbook* (4th ed.). Philadelphia: Lippincott Williams & Wilkins.

The Caffeine Awareness Alliance. (2010). *Caffeine calculator.* Accessed March 15, 2013, from http://www.caffeineawareness.org/calcu.php

Substance Abuse and Mental Health Services Administration. (2013). *Update on emergency department visits involving energy drinks: A continuing public health concern.* Retrieved April 2, 2013, from http://www.samhsa.gov/data/2k13/DAWN126/sr126-energy-drinks-use.pdf

CHAPTER 7

ALCOHOL

CHAPTER OBJECTIVE

After completing this chapter, the learner will be able to describe the screening process for and diagnosis and treatment of alcohol use disorders.

LEARNING OBJECTIVES

After studying this chapter, the learner will be able to:

1. Describe the prevalence of alcohol use disorders in the United States.
2. Differentiate between moderate and at-risk drinking behaviors.
3. Screen for alcohol use disorders.
4. Describe the health effects of alcohol use and abuse.
5. Discuss brief counseling interventions for moderate and at-risk drinkers and alcoholics.

OVERVIEW

Alcohol is the most widely used psychoactive substance in the world. Alcohol is consumed at meals, for medicinal or religious purposes, in celebrating special occasions, and as a social facilitator. Moderate use of alcohol appears to convey health benefits, while at-risk drinking behaviors and abuse result in significant morbidity and mortality. More than one-half of individuals in the U.S. ages 12 or older report being current drinkers (Substance Abuse and Mental Health Services Administration [SAMHSA], 2012). Identifying at-risk drinking with or without dependence is critical to help clients gain an understanding about the physical, social, and psychological risks associated with alcohol consumption.

HISTORY

The first known use of alcohol dates back to the Neolithic period (10,000 BC) when Stone Age people intentionally fermented beverages (Hanson, n.d.). The use of alcohol for medicinal and religious ceremonies is well documented. In the United States, alcohol was initially used for medicinal and religious purposes and was tolerated as a beverage in moderation. However, by the late 1800s, the Anti-Saloon League and the Temperance Movement became increasingly popular. By 1920, the U.S. Congress had passed the 18th Amendment, which prohibited the transportation, sale, and production of liquor (Hanson, n.d.; McGrew, 2006). The speakeasy replaced the local saloon and organized crime assumed control of the production and distribution of liquor with organized crime leaders such as Al Capone controlling the industry. By 1932, Franklin D. Roosevelt had accepted the

Democratic Party's nomination for president and urged the repeal of Prohibition. In 1933, the 21st Amendment was passed repealing prohibition (McGrew, 2006). Regulation of alcohol occurs at the local, state, and federal level. Nationally, the minimum age of drinking is age 21.

EPIDEMIOLOGY AND PREVALENCE

The most common type of alcohol consumed in the United States is beer, followed by spirits and wine. Figure 7-1 shows a historical trend by beverage type. Among people in the U.S. aged 12 years and over, 51.8% report being current drinkers. (A current drinker is defined as a person who has consumed at least one drink or more in the past 30 days.) This translates to an estimated 133.4 million people in the U.S. population. These numbers are unchanged from 2010 (SAMHSA, 2012). Figure 7-2 details current alcohol use by age group.

The National Survey on Drug Use and Health (NSDUH) is a survey that benchmarks alcohol consumption in the United States. Administered annually, the survey includes specific and detailed questions about the consumption of alcoholic beverages. A standard drink is defined as a can or bottle of beer, a glass of wine or a wine cooler, a shot of liquor, or a mixed drink with liquor in it (SAMHSA, 2012). Figure 7-3 shows the National Institute on Alcohol Abuse and Alcoholism's (NIAAA) definition of a standard drink. In 2011, heavy drinking (defined as five or more drinks on the same occasion on each of 5 or more days in the past 30 days) was reported by 6.2% of the population age 12 or older (15.9 million people). Binge drinking, which includes heavy drinking and is defined as five or more drinks on the same occasion on at least 1 day in the past 30 days, was reported by 22.6% of the population age 12 or older. In addition to current alcohol use, Figure 7-2 describes binge and heavy alcohol use among persons age 12 or older in 2011. The highest rates of current alcohol use, as well as binge drinking, occur

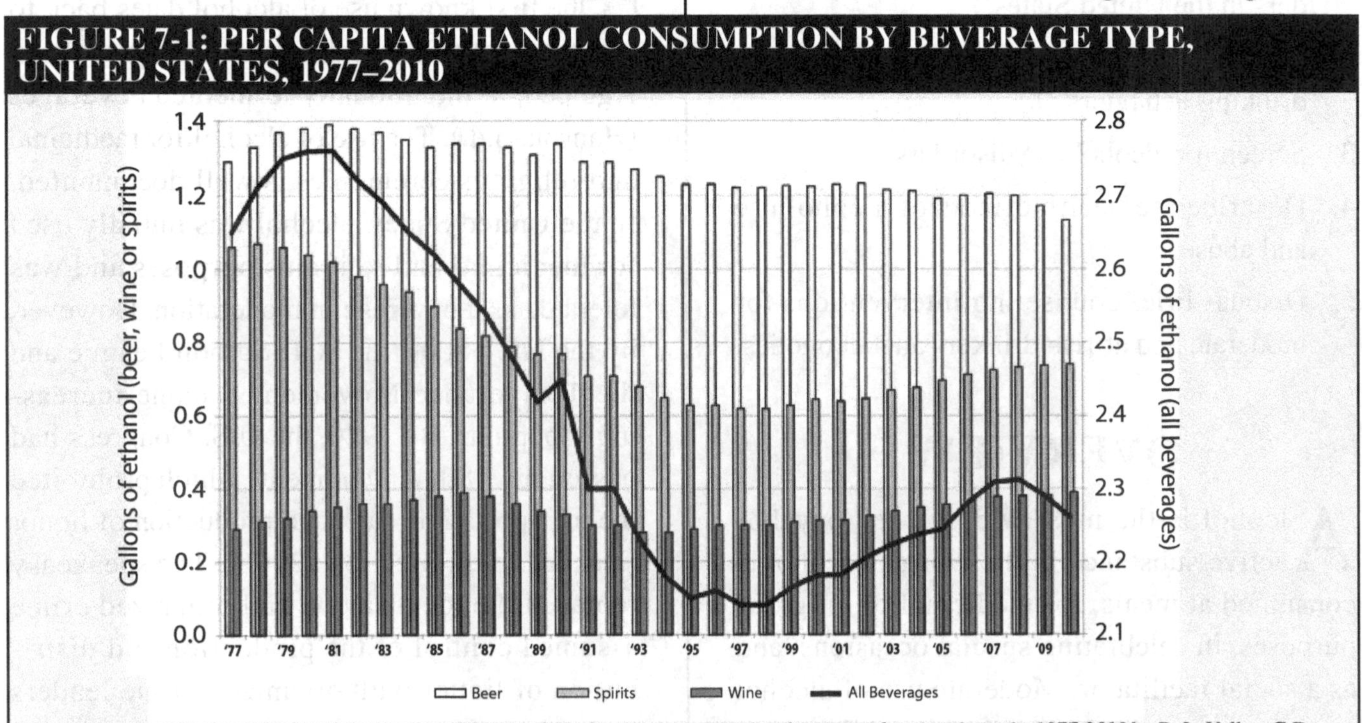

FIGURE 7-1: PER CAPITA ETHANOL CONSUMPTION BY BEVERAGE TYPE, UNITED STATES, 1977–2010

Note. From *Surveillance Report #95: Apparent per capita alcohol consumption: national, state, and regional trends, 1977-2010* by R. LaVallee, G.D. Williams, & H. Yi, 2012, Bethesda, MD: National Institute on Alcohol Abuse and Alcoholism, Division of Epidemiology and Prevention Research. Retrieved April 4, 2013, from http://pubs.niaaa.nih.gov/publications/Surveillance95/CONS10.htm

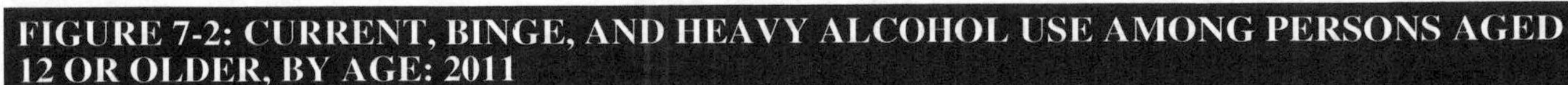

FIGURE 7-2: CURRENT, BINGE, AND HEAVY ALCOHOL USE AMONG PERSONS AGED 12 OR OLDER, BY AGE: 2011

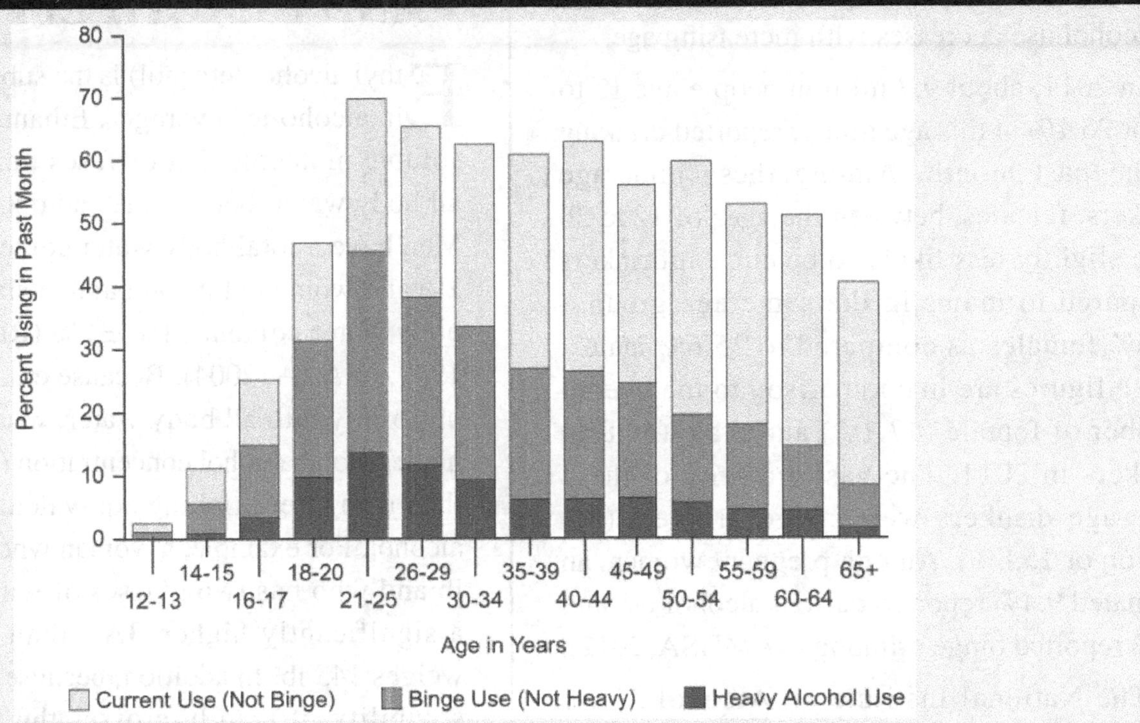

Note. From *Results from the 2011 National Survey on Drug Use and Health: Summary of National Findings* (Office of Applied Studies, NSDUH Series H-44, HHS Publication No. (SMA) 12-4713) by Substance Abuse and Mental Health Services Administration, 2012. Rockville, MD. Retrieved April 3, 2013, from http://www.samhsa.gov/data/NSDUH/2k11Results/NSDUHresults2011.htm#3.1

FIGURE 7-3: WHAT IS A STANDARD DRINK?

A standard drink is any drink that contains about 14 grams of pure alcohol (about 0.6 fluid ounces or 1.2 tablespoons). Below are standard drink equivalents. These are approximate because different brands and types of beverages vary in their actual alcohol content.

12 oz. of beer or cooler	8–9 oz. of malt liquor 8.5 oz. shown in a 12-oz. glass that, if full, would hold about 1.5 standard drinks of malt liquor	5 oz. of table wine	3–4 oz. of fortified wine (such as sherry or port) 3.5 oz. shown	2–3 oz. of cordial, liqueur, or aperitif 2.5 oz. shown	1.5 oz. of brandy (a single jigger)	1.5 oz. of spirits (a single jigger of 80-proof gin, vodka, whiskey, etc.) Shown straight and in a highball glass with ice to show the level before adding a mixer*
~5% alcohol	~7% alcohol	~12% alcohol	~17% alcohol	~24% alcohol	~40% alcohol	~40% alcohol
12 oz.	8.5 oz.	5 oz.	3.5 oz.	2.5 oz.	1.5 oz.	1.5 oz.

Note. From *Helping Patients Who Drink Too Much: A Clinician's Guide, 2005 Edition* by National Institute on Alcohol Abuse and Alcoholism, NIH Publication No. 07-3769, 2005a. Accessed March 15, 2013, from http://pubs.niaaa.nih.gov/publications/Practitioner/CliniciansGuide2005/guide.pdf

in the 21 to 25 year-old age-group (SAMHSA, 2012). Among older age-groups, the prevalence of alcohol use decreases with increasing age.

In 2011, about 9.7 million people age 12 to 20, or 25.1% of this age group, reported drinking in the past month. Among these underage drinkers, females, between the ages of 12 to 20 were slightly less likely to be current drinkers compared to males in the same age group – 24.6% females as compared to 25.6% males. These figures are in comparison to the overall number of female (47.1%) and male (56.8%) drinkers in 2011. The vast majority of these underage drinkers were binge drinkers (6.1 million or 15.8%). Among pregnant women, an estimated 9.4% reported current alcohol use and 2.6% reported binge drinking (SAMHSA, 2012).

The National Institute on Alcohol Abuse and Alcoholism (NIAAA, 2007) estimates that about 3 in 10 adults in the United States drink at levels that increase their risk for physical, mental health, and social problems. Of these heavy drinkers, about 1 in 4 meets the American Psychiatric Association's (APA) *DSM-5* criteria for alcohol use disorder (2013). According to NIAAA (2007), men may be at risk for alcohol-related problems if their alcohol consumption exceeds 14 standard drinks per week or 4 drinks per day, and women may be at risk if they have more than 7 standard drinks per week or 3 drinks per day.

Recommendations for moderate drinking are as follows:

- Healthy men – no more than 2 drinks in a day and no more than 14 drinks in a week.
- Healthy women – no more than 1 drink in a day and no more than 7 drinks in a week.
- Healthy people over the age of 65 – no more than 1 drink in a day and no more than 7 drinks in a week.

(NIAAA, 2007)

BIOCHEMISTRY AND HEALTH EFFECTS

Ethyl alcohol (ethanol) is the substance found in alcoholic beverages. Ethanol is a water-soluble molecule that diffuses uniformly into all body water, both inside and outside of cells. Men have a total body water content of 65% ± 2% and women of a comparable size have total body water content 51% ± 2% (Randall et al., 1999; NIAAA, 2004). Because ethanol diffuses uniformly into all body water, women achieve higher blood alcohol concentration (BAC) levels than men after drinking equivalent amounts of alcohol. For example, a woman who weighs 145 lb and who has two glasses of wine will have a significantly higher BAC than a man who weighs 145 lb. In addition, because of ethanol's solubility, it readily crosses the blood-brain barrier, profoundly affecting the central nervous system (CNS); it crosses the placenta to affect fetal development and affects every organ in the body.

Ethanol is primarily absorbed from the stomach (about 20%) and the small intestine (about 80%) (Muthusamy, 2008). The age-old recommendation of "eat before you drink" is based on the fact that food in the stomach delays gastric emptying and the absorption of ethanol into the system. An empty stomach increases gastric emptying and, therefore, absorption is increased. Thus, drinking on an empty stomach increases BAC levels. Other factors that appear to affect ethanol absorption include medications, illicit drugs, nicotine, and estrogen levels.

Ethanol is considered to be a CNS depressant with both protective and harmful qualities. According to the World Health Organization (WHO: 2004), the link between alcohol consumption and consequences depends on the amount consumed and patterns of drinking and toxic and beneficial biochemical effects. An example of beneficial biochemical effects in a moderate drinker would be the protection against blood clot formation and prevention of coronary artery disease. Moderate drinking also appears to confer benefits against diabetes, gallbladder disease, and ischemic stroke (due to blood clots) and improve lipid levels.

The harmful effects of alcohol in clients who drink heavily, abuse alcohol, or are alcohol dependent are profound and significant. Several recent meta-analysis studies have linked more than 60 disease conditions to the toxic effects of alcohol (WHO, 2004). Alcoholic gastritis, alcohol abuse and dependence, alcoholic cardiomyopathy and polyneuropathy, alcoholic liver cirrhosis and hepatitis, and alcoholic psychosis are all directly associated with alcohol. In addition, alcohol is associated with cancers of the mouth, esophagus, liver, and breast (in women). Alcohol increases the risk for cancers of the stomach, pancreas, colon, rectum, prostate, salivary glands, ovaries, endometrium, prostate, and bladder (WHO, 2004). Prenatal exposure to alcohol increases the risk for infant low birth weight, prematurity, intrauterine growth retardation, and spontaneous abortion. Fetal alcohol spectrum disorders, which include fetal alcohol syndrome, are the most common preventable causes of mental retardation in the United States.

The evidence also indicates that "a clear and consistent association exists between alcohol dependence and depressive disorders" (WHO, 2004, p. 43). It is often unclear whether the alcohol problems precede the depression or the depression precedes the alcohol problems. However, the presence of co-morbid depression must be considered in every client who presents with an alcohol use disorder.

Alcohol use is a major contributing factor to accidents, injuries, and trauma (including motor vehicle accidents, head injuries, spinal cord injuries, burns, and drowning) (WHO, 2009). Alcohol use is also associated with assault, homicide, and family violence. According to the U.S. Department of Justice, alcohol use is reported to have been a factor in the crimes of more than 4 out of 10 convicted murderers. Nearly one-half of those convicted of assault and sentenced to probation had been drinking when the offense occurred (Greenfeld & Henneberg, n.d.).

The disease of alcoholism is characterized by a cycle of denial, minimization, and multiple failed quit attempts that result in negative consequences that affect every aspect of a person's life. Alcoholics *involuntarily* and *unintentionally* acquire an *inconsistent inability to control* alcohol intake and have a *persistent urge to drink.* This intermittently controlled drinking produces personality changes. Drinking no longer is a conscious activity; the alcoholic demonstrates a persistent inability to control drinking coupled with significant negative consequences. These consequences affect the individual's personal, professional, emotional, physical, and economic life (see Table 7-1).

About 50% to 60% of the risk for alcoholism is genetically determined. Identical twins, who share the same genes, are twice as likely as fraternal twins, who share only 50% of their genes, to resemble each other in terms of alcoholism (Tonigan, 2003).

The neurotransmitters gamma-aminobutyric acid and serotonin are likely involved in this process. In addition, personal stressors, family risk factors, and environmental factors are important contributors to the development of an alcohol use disorder.

Research suggests that women exhibit a "telescoped" or more rapid development to alcoholism, with fewer drinking years than men (NIAAA, 2004; Randall et al., 1999). The morbidity and mortality data on alcoholism reflects these phenomena. Female alcoholics have death rates 50% to 100% higher than those

TABLE 7-1: EFFECTS OF ALCOHOL ABUSE AND ALCOHOL DEPENDENCE

Family	• Withdrawal from family activities • Marital conflict • Acting out of children • Sexual problems
Community	• Withdrawal from community activities • Embarrassing behaviors at community functions
Financial and Legal Difficulties	• Legal problems • Driving under the influence • Financial difficulties
Spiritual and Emotional Difficulties	• Changes in emotional health • Mood swings • Anger • Denial and rationalization • Depression, anxiety, and panic disorders • Forgetfullness
Physical Problems	• Poor personal hygiene • Weight loss • Sniffing, sneezing, watery eyes • Cough • Unexplained bruises • Frequent visits for health care • Multiple prescriptions • Chronic pain
Job Performance	• Deteriorating performance • Excessive use of sick time • Calling in sick on Fridays and/or Mondays • Poor judgment • Disorganization • Withdrawal from co-workers

of male alcoholics. They develop alcoholic liver disease at lower levels of intake and over shorter periods when compared to men (NIAAA, 2004). Their liver disease progresses from alcoholic hepatitis to cirrhosis at a faster rate than in men. Further, a greater percentage of female alcoholics die from suicides, alcohol-related accidents, circulatory disorders, and cirrhosis of the liver than men.

SCREENING

General Considerations

Screening for alcohol use and alcohol-related problems enables the clinician to identify people who are likely to have an alcohol problem. Screening can be done: as part of a routine examination, before prescribing a medication that interacts with alcohol, in the emergency department or urgent care center or when seeing women who are pregnant or trying to conceive; people who are likely to drink heavily, such as smokers, adolescents, and young adults; people who have health problems that may be alcohol induced; and people who have a chronic illness that is not responding to treatment as expected. Screening can occur as part of the pre-examination interview, as part of a routine examination, and/or before prescribing medications (NIAAA, 2007).

The NIAAA (2007) recommends that screening follow these steps: ask about alcohol use, assess for alcohol use disorders, advise and assist, and follow up with continued support (see Table 7-2).

TABLE 7-2: SCREENING FOR ALCOHOL USE

Step 1:	Ask about alcohol use.
Step 2:	Assess for alcohol use disorders.
Step 3:	Advise and Assist – for at-risk drinking – for alcohol use disorders.
Step 4:	At follow-up, continue support – for at-risk drinking – for alcohol use disorders.

(NIAAA, 2007)

One study has shown that a positive response to the question, *"On any single occasion during the past 3 months, have you had more than five drinks containing alcohol?"* identifies the client who either meets the NIAAA criteria for at-risk drinking or the *DSM-5* criteria for alcohol abuse or dependence (Taj, Devera-Sales, & Vinson, 1998; NIAAA, 2007; APA, 2013). NIAAA (2007) has recommended that the clinician begin by asking the client, *"Do you sometimes drink beer, wine or other alcohol beverages?"*

If the client answers "no," then the screening is complete. If the client answers "yes," the clinician should ask, *"How many times in the past year have you had five or more drinks in a day?"* (for men) or *"...four or more drinks in a day?"* (for women). If the client responds that he or she drinks at these levels, the screening is considered positive and the client should be asked, *"On average, how many days per week do you have an alcoholic drink, and on a typical drinking day, how many drinks do you have?"* From this information, the clinician should determine the weekly average of drinking by multiplying the number of days per week the client drinks by how many drinks the client consumes (see Figure 7-4).

The Alcohol Use Disorders Identification Test (AUDIT) provides a reliable and valid baseline in which to assess alcohol use and may be completed by the client before seeing a clinician. Table 7-3 provides information on the AUDIT.

Adolescents

In 2011, current alcohol use was reported by 2.5% of 12-13 year olds; 11.3% of 14-15 year olds; and 25.3% of 16-17 year olds in the United States (SAMHSA, 2012). "Many young people are experiencing the consequences of drinking too much, at too early an age. As a result, underage drinking is a leading public health problem in this country" (NIAAA, 2006, p. 1). The average age of first alcohol use in 2003 was 14 years. This statistic is important because adolescents who begin to drink alcohol before age 15 experience a four-fold increased risk for alcohol dependence in their lifetime (NIAAA, 2006).

Adolescents drink for a multitude of reasons including risk-taking and impulsivity; environmental factors such as the influence of parents and peers; hereditary and genetic risk factors; and because of psychiatric disorders or at-risk personality characteristics (NIAAA, 2006). There also appears to be significant differences between the adolescent brain and the adult brain. These differences result in an increase tolerance to alcohol and a corresponding decrease in the experience of negative consequences for the adolescent.

Health effects of alcohol on the adolescent include brain effects, liver effects and growth, and endocrine effects. Studies in animals suggest that alcohol use during stages of critical brain development results in long-lasting effects (NIAAA, 2006). "It is simply not known how alcohol will affect the long-term memory and learning skills of people who begin drinking heavily as adolescents" (NIAAA, 2006, p. 4). Other health effects include the risk at which the adolescent places himself during periods of drinking. According to the NIAAA (2006), each year, approximately 5,000 adolescents younger than age 21 die as a result of drinking. Fatal motor vehicle accidents, homicides, suicides, falls, burns, and drownings comprise the majority of these deaths. Other consequences of adolescent alcohol use include trauma related to drinking and driving, risky sexual behaviors, and victimization.

Screening for adolescent alcohol and drug use should be done at every opportunity. A brief screening tool that has demonstrated sensitivity in identifying alcohol and drug problems in adolescents is the CRAFFT tool. These questions take only a few minutes and a positive response to two or more is highly predictive of an alcohol-related disorder.

- **C** Have you ever ridden in a **CAR** driven by someone (including yourself) who was "high" or had been using alcohol or drugs?
- **R** Do you ever use alcohol or drugs to **RELAX,** feel better about yourself, or fit in?
- **A** Do you ever use alcohol or drugs while you are by yourself, **ALONE**?
- **F** Do you ever **FORGET** things you did while using alcohol or drugs?
- **F** Do your family or **FRIENDS** ever tell you that you should cut down on your drinking or drug use?
- **T** Have you gotten into **TROUBLE** while you were using alcohol or drugs?

(Knight, Sherrit, Shrier, Harris & Chang, 2002).

text continues on page 110

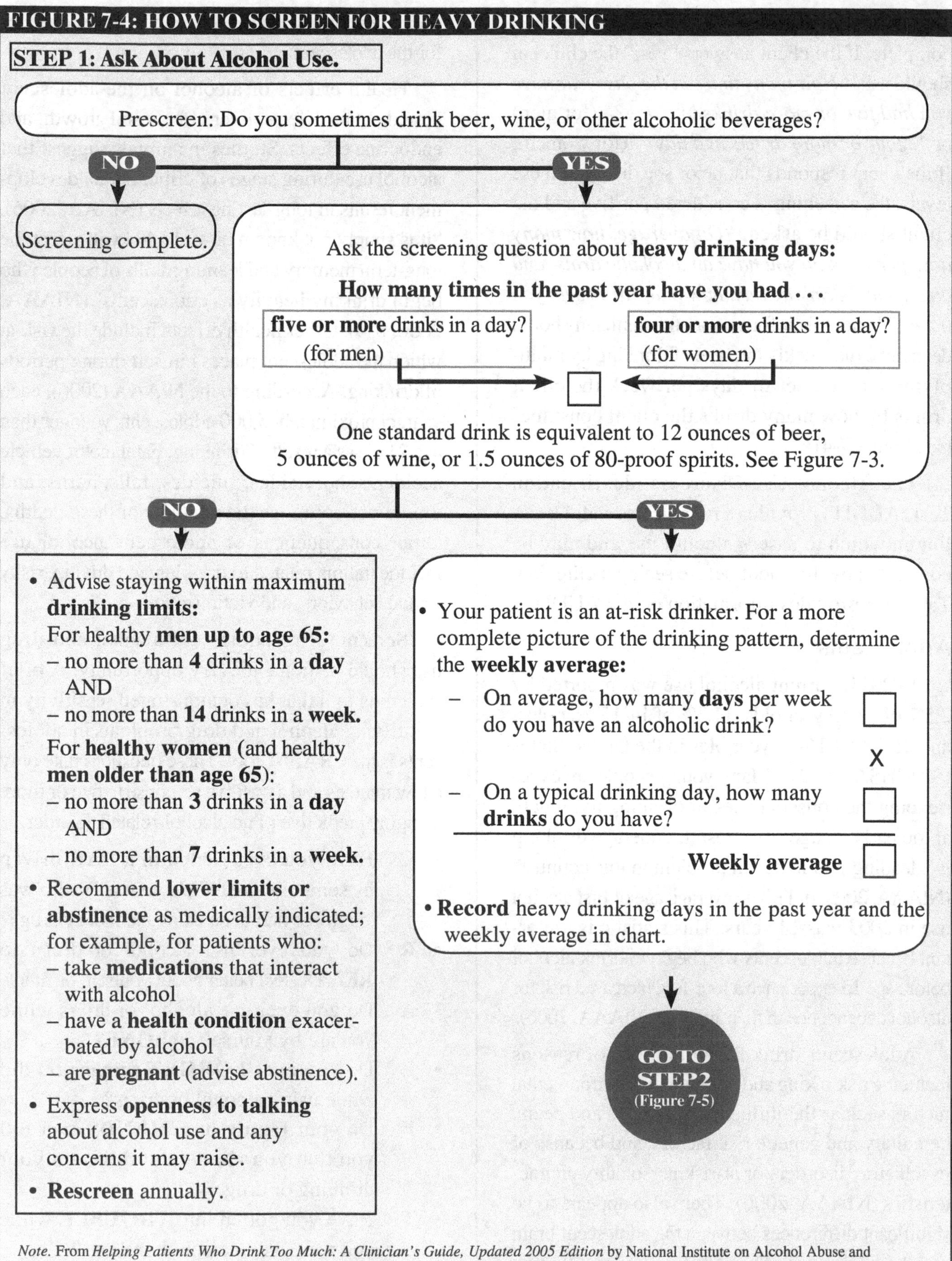

FIGURE 7-4: HOW TO SCREEN FOR HEAVY DRINKING
STEP 1: Ask About Alcohol Use.
Prescreen: Do you sometimes drink beer, wine, or other alcoholic beverages?
NO
YES
Screening complete.
Ask the screening question about heavy drinking days:
How many times in the past year have you had . . .
five or more drinks in a day? (for men)
four or more drinks in a day? (for women)
One standard drink is equivalent to 12 ounces of beer, 5 ounces of wine, or 1.5 ounces of 80-proof spirits. See Figure 7-3.
NO
YES
• Advise staying within maximum drinking limits:
For healthy men up to age 65:
– no more than 4 drinks in a day AND
– no more than 14 drinks in a week.
For healthy women (and healthy men older than age 65):
– no more than 3 drinks in a day AND
– no more than 7 drinks in a week.
• Recommend lower limits or abstinence as medically indicated; for example, for patients who:
– take medications that interact with alcohol
– have a health condition exacerbated by alcohol
– are pregnant (advise abstinence).
• Express openness to talking about alcohol use and any concerns it may raise.
• Rescreen annually.
• Your patient is an at-risk drinker. For a more complete picture of the drinking pattern, determine the weekly average:
– On average, how many days per week do you have an alcoholic drink?
X
– On a typical drinking day, how many drinks do you have?
Weekly average
• Record heavy drinking days in the past year and the weekly average in chart.
GO TO STEP 2
(Figure 7-5)

Note. From *Helping Patients Who Drink Too Much: A Clinician's Guide, Updated 2005 Edition* by National Institute on Alcohol Abuse and Alcoholism, NIH Publication No. 07-3769, 2007. Accessed March 15, 2013, from http://pubs.niaaa.nih.gov/publications/Practitioner/CliniciansGuide2005/guide.pdf

TABLE 7-3: ALCOHOL USE DISORDERS IDENTIFICATION TEST (AUDIT)

PATIENT: Because alcohol use can affect your health and can interfere with certain medications and treatments, it is important that we ask some questions about your use of alcohol. Your answers will remain confidential so please be honest.

Place an X in one box that best describes your answer to each question.

Questions	0	1	2	3	4	
1. How often do you have a drink containing alcohol?	Never	Monthly or less	2 to 4 times per month	2 to 3 times per week	4 or more times per week	
2. How many drinks containing alcohol do you have on a typical day when you are drinking?	1 or 2	3 or 4	5 or 6	7 to 9	10 or more	
3. How often do you have five (four if assessing a woman) or more drinks on one occasion?	Never	Less than monthly	Monthly	Weekly	Daily or almost daily	
4. How often during the past year have you found that you were not able to stop drinking once you had started?	Never	Less than monthly	Monthly	Weekly	Daily or almost daily	
5. How often during the past year have you failed to do what was normally expected of you because of drinking?	Never	Less than monthly	Monthly	Weekly	Daily or almost daily	
6. How often during the past year have you needed a first drink in the morning to get yourself going after a heavy drinking session?	Never	Less than monthly	Monthly	Weekly	Daily or almost daily	
7. How often during the past year have you had a feeling of guilt or remorse after drinking?	Never	Less than monthly	Monthly	Weekly	Daily or almost daily	
8. How often during the past year have you been unable to remember what happened the night before because of your drinking?	Never	Less than monthly	Monthly	Weekly	Daily or almost daily	
9. Have you or someone else been injured because of your drinking?	No		Yes, but not in the past year		Yes, during the past year	
10. Has a relative, friend, doctor, or other health care worker been concerned about your drinking or suggested you cut down?	No		Yes, but not in the past year		Yes, during the past year	
Total						

Note: To reflect standard drink sizes in the United States, the number of drinks in question 3 was changed from six to five.

Note. From *The Alcohol Use Disorders Identification Test: Guidelines for use in primary care* by T.F. Babor, J.C. Higgins-Biddle, J.B. Saunders, & M.G. Monteiro, 2001, World Health Organization. Accessed March 15, 2013, from http://whqlibdoc.who.int/hq/2001/who_msd_msb_01.6a.pdf

Every opportunity should be taken to counsel adolescents on risks associated with alcohol use and methods to reduce harm. Adolescents who have been identified as having an alcohol use disorder should be referred to treatment. However, according to the NIAAA (2006), "a major unmet need exists in the treatment of alcohol use disorders. In 2002, 1.4 million youth met the criteria for alcohol abuse or dependence, but only 227,000 actually received any treatment for these problems" (p. 2). Compounding this lack of available treatment, treatment programs generally do not address the specific needs of adolescents. Youth perceive traditional services, such as Alcoholics Anonymous and alcohol treatment programs, as less helpful. Adolescents prefer easy access to treatments that allow them to remain in their home and school and that specifically address their needs (NIAAA, 2006). The health care provider should also be mindful of the fact that adolescents may have comorbid drug disorders along with alcohol use disorders.

BRIEF INTERVENTIONS

Brief interventions, as described in the following scenario, that are tailored to specific concerns are preferred.

Ms. Jones, a 35-year-old mother of two children, presents to the emergency department complaining of a headache, heartburn, and a stomachache. The clinician completes her history and then **asks** specific questions.

Example 1

Clinician: Ms. Jones, do you sometimes drink alcohol, such as beer, wine, or spirits."

Ms. Jones: "Yes, I do, but I'm not sure how that relates to why I'm here today."

Clinician: "Ms. Jones, the reason it is important is that it helps me get a better understanding of your health history, so...in the past year, has there been an occasion when you have had four or more drinks in one day?"

Ms. Jones: "Yes...generally just for special occasions like weddings and New Year's Eve, and then just sometimes during the week."

Clinician: "Ok, so on how many days per week do you have a drink?"

Ms. Jones: "Oh...maybe 1 to 2 days per week."

Clinician: "And on those days, how many drinks do you have?"

Ms. Jones: "Probably one or two glasses of wine."

In this example, Ms. Jones is drinking at the maximum, 2 days a week with two glasses of wine, which is a weekly total of four alcoholic beverages per week. The NIAAA considers this a moderate and safe drinking level for women. The clinician has **asked** and **assessed** Ms. Jones's alcohol use. However, if Ms. Jones had responded differently, it may have led to further discussion.

Example 2

Ms. Jones: "Oh, I usually have a drink with my husband when the kids go to bed."

Clinician: "Ok, so how many days per week do you have a drink?"

Ms. Jones: "I probably drink 5 or 6 nights a week and no more than two or three glasses of wine."

Ms. Jones is drinking at the maximum 6 nights per week with three glasses of wine, which is a weekly total of 18 alcohol beverages. At this point, she is meeting the criteria for at-risk and heavy drinking and the clinician should assess Ms. Jones for an alcohol use disorder. To determine this, the clinician should carefully assess whether Ms. Jones has experienced any significant negative consequences related to her drinking in the past 12 months. This includes consequences related to role failure, risk of bodily harm, run-in with the law, and relationship trouble (see Figure 7-5).

FIGURE 7-5: HOW TO ASSESS FOR ALCOHOL USE DISORDERS

STEP 2: Assess for Alcohol Use Disorders.

Next, determine whether there is a *maladaptive pattern of alcohol use,* causing *clinically significant impairment* or *distress.* It is important to assess the severity and extent of all alcohol-related symptoms to inform your decisions about management.

Determine whether, in the past 12 months, your patient's drinking has **repeatedly** caused or contributed to

- ☐ **risk** of bodily harm (drinking and driving, operating machinery, and swimming).
- ☐ **relationship** trouble (family or friends).
- ☐ **role failure** (interference with home, work, or school obligations).
- ☐ **run-ins** with the law (arrests or other legal problems).

If yes to **one or more** → your patient has **alcohol abuse.**

In either case, proceed to assess for dependence symptoms.

Determine whether, in the past 12 months, your patient has

- ☐ **not been able to stick to drinking limits** (repeatedly broke them).
- ☐ **not been able to cut down or stop** (repeated failed attempts).
- ☐ **shown tolerance** (needed to drink a higher quantity to get the same effect).
- ☐ **shown signs of withdrawal** (tremors, sweating, nausea, or insomnia when trying to quit or cut down).
- ☐ **kept drinking despite problems** (recurrent physical or psychological problems).
- ☐ **spent a lot of time drinking** (or anticipating or recovering from drinking).
- ☐ **spent less time on other matters** (activities that had been important or pleasurable).

If yes to **three or more** → your patient has **alcohol dependence.**

Does the patient meet the criteria for abuse or dependence?

NO → **Your patient is still at risk for developing alcohol-related problems.** → **GO TO STEPS 3 & 4 for AT-RISK DRINKING See Fig. 7-6**

YES → **Your patient has an alcohol use disorder.** → **GO TO STEPS 3 & 4 for ALCOHOL USE DISORDERS See Fig. 7-7**

Note. From *Helping Patients Who Drink Too Much: A Clinician's Guide, Updated 2005 Edition* by National Institute on Alcohol Abuse and Alcoholism, NIH Publication No. 07-3769, 2007. Accessed March 15, 2013, from http://pubs.niaaa.nih.gov/publications/Practitioner/CliniciansGuide2005/guide.pdf

Ms. Jones: "Well, yes, it seems that sometimes my husband and I get into fights – not physical or anything – after we've been drinking. It's hard on the kids because I think they can hear us. Sometimes after the fights, I have a hard time getting to sleep and I don't get the kids to school on time the next day."

In this case, Ms. Jones's positive response suggests that she has a maladaptive pattern of alcohol use, is drinking heavily and at-risk levels, and may meet the *DSM-5* criteria for alcohol use disorder. The clinician must then assess the extent and severity of her alcohol-related symptoms and determine if Ms. Jones has any of the cardinal signs of alcohol use disorder.

Questions that assess alcohol dependence focus on the presence of three or more of these symptoms: tolerance, withdrawal, inability to stick to drinking limits, inability to stop or cut down, spending a lot of time drinking and less time on other matters, and drinking despite problems.

Clinician: "Have you had a period when your drinking interfered with your relationship with your kids or husband or some of your responsibilities?"

Ms. Jones: "You know, I'm a good mother but I seem to have trouble in the morning with the kids, getting them up, dressed, fed, and getting them to school after one of those nights. I just seem to move slowly sometimes." (Time spent related to drinking or recovering)

Clinician: "I see. So when you and your husband have been drinking and fight, have you ever been frightened or concerned for your safety?"

Ms. Jones: "No, my husband is a good man; he would never hurt me or the kids." (Physical problems)

Clinician: "Oh, that's good to know. So, have you ever wanted to stop or cut down on your drinking, but tried and found that you couldn't?" (Impaired control)

Ms. Jones: "No, not really."

Clinician: "Have you ever found that you have to drink much more than you once did to get the effect you want?"

Ms. Jones: "No, I'm sort of a cheap date – two drinks is usually all I can handle." (Tolerance)

Ms. Jones does not clearly fit the *DSM-5* criteria for alcohol dependence but it does appear that she is drinking at at-risk and heavy drinking levels. She also does not clearly meet the criteria for alcohol use disroder yet. She should be counseled to cut down on her drinking.

In Example 1, Ms. Jones was assessed to be drinking at moderate levels – four drinks per week. Again, the guidelines for safe drinking for healthy women is no more than three drinks in a day and no more than seven drinks in a week. Following the NIAAA (2007) guidelines, the clinician should now advise Ms. Jones that she should stay within the maximum drinking limits.

Clinician: "Ms. Jones, safe drinking levels for healthy women is considered to be no more than three drinks per day or no more than seven drinks in a week. You are currently drinking about four alcoholic beverages per week and are drinking at safe levels. I advise you to stay within these limits. Are there any questions or concerns you have about this?"

In Example 2, Ms. Jones was drinking a maximum of 18 alcoholic beverages and assessed to be drinking heavily at at-risk levels. Ms. Jones does not have an alcohol use disorder but is certainly at very high risk for developing one. The clinician should use professional judgment in determining whether to advise cutting down or abstaining.

Such factors as a family history of alcohol problems, advanced age, and injuries related to drinking, or such symptoms as sleep disorders or sexual dysfunction, should be considered in determining the recommendation to abstain or cut down (NIAAA, 2007). If Ms. Jones is willing to consider changing her drinking habits and engage in a discussion, the clinician could consider several options. Option 1 may be to advise that she cut down to recommended limits. Option 2 may be to abstain completely for perhaps 2 months, then reconsider future drinking. If Ms. Jones attempts to cut down and drink at moderate levels but is not successful, then abstinence should be recommended. In advising a client who is drinking heavily or at at-risk levels, it is important to state your conclusion and recommendations clearly. Be matter-of-fact and nonconfrontational and relate to the client's concerns to medical findings and your advice (see Figure 7-6).

FIGURE 7-6: ASSESSING FOR AT-RISK DRINKING (NO ABUSE OR DEPENDENCE) (1 OF 2)

STEP 3: Advise and Assist.

- **State your conclusion and recommendation clearly:**
  - "You are drinking more than is medically safe."
    Relate to patient's concerns and medical findings, if present.
  - "I strongly recommend that you cut down (or quit) and I'm willing to help."
- **Gauge readiness** to change drinking habits:
  - "Are you willing to consider making changes in your drinking?"

Is the patient ready to commit to change at this time?

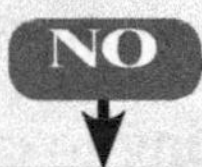

Do not be discouraged – ambivalence is common. Your advice has likely prompted a change in your patient's thinking, a positive change in itself. With continued reinforcement, your patient may decide to take action. For now,

- **Restate your concern** about his or her health.
- **Encourage reflection**: Ask patients to weigh what they like about drinking vs. their reasons for cutting down. What are the major barriers to change?
- **Reaffirm *your* willingness to help** when he or she is ready.

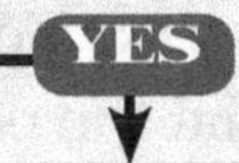

- **Help set a goal:** Cut down to within maximum limits or abstain for a period of time.
- **Agree on a plan,** including:
  - what specific steps the patient will take (such as not go to a bar after work, measure all drinks at home, drink alternate alcoholic and non-alcoholic beverages)
  - how drinking will be tracked (diary, kitchen calendar)
  - how the patient will manage high-risk situations
  - who might be willing to help, such as significant others or nondrinking friends.
- **Provide educational materials.**

continued

FIGURE 7-6: ASSESSING FOR AT-RISK DRINKING (NO ABUSE OR DEPENDENCE) (2 OF 2)

continued

STEP 4: At Follow-up: Continue Support.

REMINDER: Document alcohol use and review goals at each visit.

Was the patient able to meet and sustain the drinking goal?

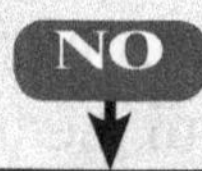

- **Acknowledge that change is difficult.**
- **Support any positive change** and address barriers to reaching the goal.
- **Renegotiate the goal and plan;** consider a trial of abstinence.
- **Consider engaging significant others.**
- **Reassess the diagnosis** if the patient is unable to either cut down or abstain. (Go to Step 2.)

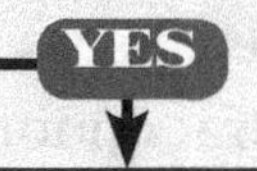

- **Reinforce and support continued adherence** to recommendations.
- **Renegotiate drinking goals** as indicated (such as if the medical condition changes or if an abstaining patient wishes to resume drinking).
- **Encourage to return** if unable to maintain adherence.
- **Rescreen** at least annually.

Note. From *Helping Patients Who Drink Too Much: A Clinician's Guide, Updated 2005 Edition* by National Institute on Alcohol Abuse and Alcoholism, NIH Publication No. 07-3769, 2007. Accessed March 15, 2013, from http://pubs.niaaa.nih.gov/publications/Practitioner/CliniciansGuide2005/guide.pdf

Clinician: "Ms. Jones, you are drinking more than is medically safe. Moderate drinking for women is one drink per day or no more than seven drinks per week. You are drinking 18 drinks per week and I'm concerned that you are experiencing some symptoms related to your heavy drinking. Physically, your insomnia at night and even your symptoms today of a headache, stomachache, and heartburn may be related to the amount of alcohol you are consuming. I'm also concerned about the arguments you are having at night and the difficulty you're having the morning after with your children. Alcohol lowers your inhibitions and is actually a depressant – it affects your behavior, and perhaps those night time arguments."

"I strongly recommend that you consider cutting down to one drink per night with no more than seven drinks per week or you can consider stopping drinking for a couple months. See if you can do it and how that affects the night time arguments and these symptoms you're having."

"Are you willing to consider changing your drinking habits?"

Ms. Jones: "I didn't realize I was drinking so much. Sure, I can cut down to one per day."

If a client is willing to commit to changing his or her drinking habit, the clinician should provide a brief intervention. This intervention focuses on the following:

- State your concern and recommendations clearly. Be straightforward and nonconfrontational and relate to the client's concerns to medical findings and your advice.
- If the client agrees to change his or her drinking habits, mutually set a goal. Recommend that the client cut down to

within maximum limits or abstain from alcohol for a period of time.

- Agree on a plan. Define what specific steps the client will take, how drinking will be tracked, how the client will manage high-risk situations, and who may be willing to help.
- Provide educational materials to support the client.
- Lastly, provide follow up

(NIAAA, 2007).

Brief interventions are relatively simple counseling strategies that may occur one or more times. Clinical trials have demonstrated that brief interventions can decrease alcohol use significantly among those who drink more than the recommended limits but who are not alcohol dependent (NIAAA, 2007). Research studies, which followed clients who were drinking at at-risk levels and who received brief interventions, have demonstrated up to a 33% reduction in alcohol consumption and binge drinking. These reductions were significant and persisted over 3 years. Further, decreases in blood pressure readings, levels of gamma-glutamyl transferase, psychosocial problems, hospital days, and hospital readmissions for alcohol-related trauma were all significantly reduced. The evidence clearly supports the efficacy and sustainability of brief interventions. Every clinician can provide a brief intervention and the data suggests that the more frequently the brief intervention is reinforced, the better the outcome. It does not take a physician's order or a definitive diagnosis to treat alcohol abuse; it is health behavior counseling that decreases the morbidity and mortality of the disease.

If the client is assessed to have an alcohol use disorder based on the *DSM-5* criteria, the safest recommendation is for the client to abstain from drinking (see Figure 7-7). If a client has an alcohol use disorder and is willing to abstain from alcohol, it is important to provide additional resources. These resources include: 1) referral to an addiction specialist who can evaluate the severity of the clients addiction, provide the resources needed in terms of inpatient detoxification or outpatient management, and determine whether the client needs to be medically managed for withdrawal symptoms; 2) referral to a mutual help group such as AA; and 3) a defined follow-up plan. Table 7-4 provides a listing of all medications generally prescribed for alcohol dependence.

Research demonstrates that, if the client is alcohol dependent or abuses alcohol and is unwilling to abstain, repeated brief interventions result in significant decreases in the amount of alcohol consumed and in cessation of alcohol consumption. For an alcoholic client who is repeatedly hospitalized or who seeks assistance and is in regular contact with a clinician, a brief 2-minute intervention should be done at each visit or hospitalization. The NIAAA (2007) recommends that the clinician take the following steps:

- Acknowledge that change is difficult.
- Support efforts to cut down or abstain, with abstinence as the goal.
- Relate alcohol use to the client's physical, emotional and social problems.
- Address coexisting disorders.
- Consider additional resources such as:
  - an addiction specialist
  - mutual self help group
  - help from significant others
  - referral to a health care provider for medication management.

text continues on page 118

FIGURE 7-7: HOW TO CONDUCT A BRIEF INTERVENTION FOR ALCOHOL USE DISORDERS (ABUSE OR DEPENDENCE)

STEP 3: Advise and Assist.

- **State your conclusion and recommendation clearly:**
  - "I believe that you have an alcohol use disorder and I strongly recommend that you quit drinking and I'm willing to help."
  - Relate to the patient's concerns and medical findings if present.
- **Negotiate a drinking goal:**
  - Abstaining is the safest course for most patients with alcohol use disorders.
  - Patients who have milder forms of abuse or dependence and are unwilling to abstain may be successful at cutting down. (See Step 3 for At-Risk Drinking.)
- **Consider** referring for additional **evaluation by an addiction specialist,** especially if the patient is dependent.
- **Consider** recommending a **mutual help group.**
- For patients who have dependence, **consider**
  - the need for **medically managed withdrawal** (detoxification) and treat accordingly.
  - prescribing a **medication** for alcohol dependence for patients who endorse abstinence as a goal.
- **Arrange follow-up** appointments, including medication management support if needed.

STEP 4: At Follow-up: Continue Support.

REMINDER: Document alcohol use and review goals at each visit. If the patient is receiving a medication for alcohol dependence, medication management support should be provided.

Was the patient able to meet and sustain the drinking goal?

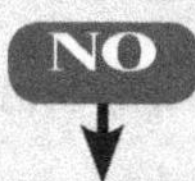

- **Acknowledge that change is difficult.**
- **Support efforts** to cut down or abstain, while making it clear that your recommendation is abstainance.
- **Relate drinking to problems** (medical, psychological, and social) as appropriate.
- If these measures are not already being taken, **consider**
  - referring to an **addiction specialist** or consulting with one.
  - recommending a **mutual help group.**
  - engaging **significant others.**
  - prescribing a **medication** for alcohol-dependent patients who endorse abstinence as a goal.
- **Address coexisting disorders** (medical and psychiatric) as needed.

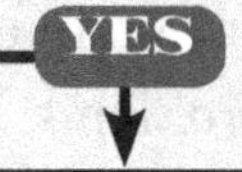

- **Reinforce and support continued adherence** to recommendations.
- **Coordinate care** with a specialist if the patient has accepted referral.
- **Maintain medications** for alcohol dependence for at least 3 months and as clinically indicated thereafter.
- **Treat coexisting nicotine dependence** for 6 to 12 months after reaching the drinking goal.
- **Address coexisting disorders** (medical and psychiatric) as needed.

Note. From *Helping Patients Who Drink Too Much: A Clinician's Guide, Updated 2005 Edition* by National Institute on Alcohol Abuse and Alcoholism, NIH Publication No. 07-3769, 2007. Accessed March 15, 2013, from http://pubs.niaaa.nih.gov/publications/Practitioner/CliniciansGuide2005/guide.pdf

TABLE 7-4: MEDICATIONS FOR TREATING ALCOHOL USE DISORDER

	Naltrexone (Depade,® ReVia®)	**Extended-Release Injectable Naltrexone** (Vivitrol®)	**Acamprosate** (Campral®)	**Disulfiram** (Antabuse®)
Action	Blocks opioid receptors, resulting in reduced craving and reduced reward in response to drinking.	Same as oral naltrexone; 30-day duration.	Affects glutamate and GABA neurotransmitter systems, but its alcohol-related action is unclear.	Inhibits intermediate metabolism of alcohol, causing a buildup of acetaldehyde and a reaction of flushing, sweating, nausea, and tachycardia if a patient drinks alcohol.
Contraindications	Currently using opioids or in acute opioid withdrawal; anticipated need for opioid analgesics; acute hepatitis or liver failure.	Same as oral naltrexone, plus inadequate muscle mass for deep intramuscular injection; rash or infection at the injection site.	Severe renal impairment (CrCl ≤ 30 mL/min).	Concomitant use of alcohol or alcohol-containing preparations or metronidazole; coronary artery disease; severe myocardial disease; hypersensitivity to rubber (thiuram) derivatives.
Precautions	Other hepatic disease; renal impairment; history of suicide attempts or depression. If opioid analgesia is needed, larger doses may be required and respiratory depression may be deeper and more prolonged. Pregnancy Category C. Advise patients to carry a wallet card to alert medical personnel in the event of an emergency. For wallet card information, see *www.niaaa.nih.gov/guide*.	Same as oral naltrexone, plus hemophilia or other bleeding problems.	Moderate renal impairment (dose adjustment for CrCl between 30 and 50 mL/min); depression or suicidal ideation and behavior. Pregnancy Category C.	Hepatic cirrhosis or insufficiency; cerebrovascular disease or cerebral damage; psychoses (current or history); diabetes mellitus; epilepsy; hypothyroidism; renal impairment. Pregnancy Category C. Advise patients to carry a wallet card to alert medical personnel in the event of an emergency. For wallet card information, see *www.niaaa.nih.gov/guide*.
Serious adverse reactions	Will precipitate severe withdrawal if the patient is dependent on opioids; hepatotoxicity (although does not appear to be a hepatotoxin at the recommended doses).	Same as oral naltrexone, plus infection at the injection site; depression; and rare events including allergic pneumonia and suicidal ideation and behavior.	Rare events include suicidal ideation and behavior.	Disulfiram-alcohol reaction, hepatotoxicity, optic neuritis, peripheral neuropathy, psychotic reactions.
Common side effects	Nausea, vomiting, decreased appetite, headache, dizziness, fatigue, somnolence,	Same as oral naltrexone, plus a reaction at the injection site; joint pain; muscle aches or cramps.	Diarrhea, somnolence.	Metallic after-taste, dermatitis, transient mild drowsiness. anxiety.
Examples of drug interactions	Opioid medications (blocks action).	Same as oral naltrexone.	No clinically relevant interactions known.	Anticoagulants such as warfarin; isoniazid; metronidazole; phenytoin; any nonprescription drug containing alcohol.
Usual adult dosage	*Oral dose:* 50 mg daily. *Before prescribing:* Patients must be opioid-free for a minimum of 7 to 10 days before starting. If you feel that there's a risk of precipitating an opioid withdrawal reaction, administer a naloxone challenge test. Evaluate liver function. *Laboratory followup:* Monitor liver function.	*IM dose:* 380 mg given as a deep intramuscular gluteal injection, once monthly. *Before prescribing:* Same as oral naltrexone, plus examine the injection site for adequate muscle mass and skin condition. *Laboratory followup:* Monitor liver function.	*Oral dose:* 666 mg (two 333-mg tablets) three times daily; or for patients with moderate renal impairment (CrCl 30 to 50 mL/min), reduce to 333 mg (one tablet) three times daily. *Before prescribing:* Evaluate renal function. Establish abstinence.	*Oral dose:* 250 mg daily (range 125 mg to 500 mg). *Before prescribing:* Evaluate liver function. Warn the patient (1) not to take disulfiram for at least 12 hours after drinking and that a disulfiram-alcohol reaction can occur up to 2 weeks after the last dose and (2) to avoid alcohol in the diet (e.g., sauces and vinegars), over-the-counter medications (e.g., cough syrups), and toiletries (e.g., cologne, mouthwash). *Laboratory followup:* Monitor liver function.

Note: This chart highlights some of the properties of each medication. It does ***not*** provide complete information and is ***not*** meant to be a substitute for the package inserts or other drug reference sources used by clinicians. For patient information about these and other drugs, the National Library of Medicine provides MedlinePlus (http://medlineplus.gov). Whether or not a medication should be prescribed and in what amount is a matter between individuals and their healthcare providers. The prescribing information provided here is ***not*** a substitute for a provider's judgment in an individual circumstance, and the NIH accepts no liability or responsibility for use of the information with regard to particular patients.

Note. From *Helping Patients Who Drink Too Much: A Clinician's Guide, Updated 2005 Edition* by National Institute on Alcohol Abuse and Alcoholism, NIH Publication No. 07-3769, 2007. Accessed March 15, 2013, from http://pubs.niaaa.nih.gov/publications/Practitioner/CliniciansGuide2005/guide.pdf

LONG-TERM APPROACHES

There are several types of behavioral therapy used to facilitate change and treat alcohol use disorders, including cognitive-behavioral therapies (CBTs), motivational enhancement therapy, the 12-step facilitation treatments (most common is Alcoholics Anonymous [AA]), family-involved treatment, or a combination of these therapies. The two approaches to family-based treatments are alcohol-focused behavioral couple's therapy (ABCT) and family systems approaches. Because the consequences of alcohol use disorders affect the entire family, either one of these approaches has been found to be effective in marriage and family therapies. The major components of ABCT include:

- cognitive-behavioral strategies to help the alcoholic stop drinking and acquire coping skills
- strategies that teach family members to support the drinker's efforts to change, reduce protection for negative consequences, and develop communication skills around alcohol topics and problem solving
- behavioral contract between intimate partners to support the use of medication

(Roberts & McCrady, 2003).

Evidence suggests that ABCT increases marital happiness after treatment, decreases marital separation, and decreases incidents of domestic violence (Roberts & McCrady, 2003). Family systems therapy views drinking as one part of the marital/family relationship and attempts to change family actions that sustain drinking and family members' views of the meaning of drinking. In family systems therapy, the couple will commonly negotiate a drinking goal instead of abstinence. One empiric study has found that this approach is particularly effective in alcoholics who are ambivalent or resistant about changing their drinking behaviors. Both ABCT and family systems therapy are provided by trained therapists and are part of the treatment plan for alcohol use disorders.

The other approach for long-term treatment of alcohol use disorders is referral to community-based services. Alcohol treatment services are available at different levels of care and are often dependent on insurance type. They include inpatient, residential, intensive outpatient, outpatient, or self-help rehabilitation. According to the NIAAA, there are two different approaches to selecting the level of care. "The first approach is stepped care, in which treatment is initiated at the least restrictive level. It is usually a brief outpatient intervention and the intensity of treatment is increased only if the client does not respond to the initial intervention. The second approach, described as client-treatment matching is to select more intensive treatment as the initial approach. Client-treatment matching is recommended by American Society of Addiction Medicine (ASAM), which suggests that the clinician consider the following criteria when selecting an initial level of care" (Roberts & McCrady, 2003). These criteria are:

- severity of alcohol dependence and likelihood of withdrawal syndrome
- medical conditions and complications
- emotional, behavioral, and cognitive conditions or complications
- motivation to change
- relapse or continued use potential
- nature of the recovery environment.

The literature and research is mixed when evaluating the effectiveness of the least restrictive and the more intensive treatment as the initial approach. This decision is often made based on the referring clinician and/or the insurance reimbursement available for treatment.

There are three treatment models that have been extensively studied and supported by the literature – CBT, motivational enhancement therapy (MET), and the twelve-step facilitation (TSF) treatment. CBT focuses on identifying high-risk drinking situations, developing coping strategies, and preventing relapse. CBT is particularly effective for clients who have less severe alcohol dependence (Hester & Miller, 2003; Tonigan, 2003).

MET is a brief, 2- to 4-hour session that combines assessment, feedback, and principles of motivational interviewing. MET is particularly effective for clients who are angry and resistant.

Lastly, TSF is based on the principles of AA. This program or similar treatment programs are the most widely available and seem to be particularly effective with clients who have more severe drinking problems; who socialize with individuals or who are in communities that encourage them to drink; and who have few mental health problems (Tonigan, 2003). AA is free and requires no commitment other than a willingness to stop drinking. For more information about AA, refer to its Web site www.aa.org. The National Clearinghouse for Alcohol and Drug Information provides additional information about other self-help groups and support organizations at http://ncadistore.samhsa.gov/catalog/referrals.aspx?topic=85&h=resources/.

Clinicians should take the time to educate themselves about the available treatment programs in their community and to become familiar with the program, staff, and facility. Treatment facilities and programs may be found through SAMHSA at (800) 622-HELP or located on the internet at http://dasis3.samhsa.gov/.

Behavioral change is difficult and relapse is common. In a review of several large studies of alcoholism treatment, Miller, Walters & Bennett (2001) found that about one-third of alcohol-dependent clients were able to either abstain or drink at moderate levels without negative consequences. Two-thirds of clients had some periods of heavy drinking, but overall they reduced consumption and alcohol-related problems by more than one-half (NIAAA, 2007). The first 12 months are particularly challenging, and relapse is most common during this time. Alcoholism is a chronic disease similar to hypertension and diabetes and recurrence of symptoms is common. If relapse occurs, the client should be encouraged to recommit to abstinence. When a client struggles to abstain, the NIAAA (2007) recommends that the clinician consider the following questions:

- Does the client have a coexisting depression or anxiety disorder?
- What are the triggers for relapse?
- Is the client a candidate for medication for alcohol dependence?
- Is the client attending a mutual help group or therapy?
- Is the client receiving structured follow-up care?

ALCOHOL WITHDRAWAL

A person with an alcohol use disorder who suddenly stops drinking may experience alcohol withdrawal. The severity of these withdrawal symptoms range from feeling anxious and "craving" the substance to severe and generalized seizures. Withdrawal symptoms usually begin within a few hours of abstinence and consist of mild to moderate tremors, irritability, sweating, elevated pulse and blood pressure, nausea, insomnia, and anxiety (Saitz, 1998). Mild withdrawal is the most common form of withdrawal and can be managed successfully in the outpatient setting. A more severe syndrome – alcohol withdrawal delirium – occasionally follows. This generally begins between 24 to 72 hours after alcohol cessation and results in disorientation, poor short-term memory, altered sleep-wake cycle, hallucinations, delirium tremors, and/or seizures.

It is important to identify the client who is at-risk for alcohol withdrawal symptoms, particularly alcohol delirium. Clients who have higher levels of alcohol intake, who have had a longer duration of alcoholism, or who have developed alcohol withdrawal in the past are at increased risk. Clients who are older, have a comorbid acute illness, have elevated liver function tests, or present with intense craving for alcohol are also considered at-risk (Saitz, 1998). The Clinical Institute Withdrawal Assessment for Alcohol, revised (CIWA-Ar) (Sullivan, Sykora, Schneiderman, Haranjo, & Sellers, 1989; Foy et al., 1988) is an instrument that rates 10 withdrawal features and has been found to identify the client at-risk for severe withdrawal symptoms.

The healthcare provider assessing a client for alcohol withdrawal must also consider other associated alcohol problems, including gastritis, gastrointestinal bleeding, liver disease, pancreatitis, electrolyte imbalances, folate and thiamine deficiency, and cardiomyopathy (Saitz, 1998). Managing patients with severe withdrawal should include pharmacotherapy to reduce the risk of associated complications. Benzodiazepines are considered the medications of choice because they improve symptoms and also reduce the incidence of delirium tremens. All benzodiazepines appear to be equally effective; however, such long-acting agents as diazepam, chlordiazepoxide, and lorazepam are generally preferred over short-acting agents because of the decrease risk of rebound (Hoffman & Weinhouse, 2012).

Other agents, such as oral or intravenous anticonvulsants, antipsychotics, and beta-adrenergic blockers are also commonly used for managing severe alcohol withdrawal. Specifically, clonidine, an antihypertensive medication, and the anticonvulsant medication carbamazepine are used in conjunction with benzodiazepines (Myrick & Anton, 1998; Saitz, 1998).

SUMMARY

Alcohol problems are common and healthcare clinicians are in a unique position to identify clients with potential problems and intervene when appropriate. Every client should be screened annually for alcohol use. Alcohol problems are related to the amount consumed and the frequency of consumption (see Figure 7-8). Clients who drink at moderate levels should be encouraged to continue to drink at safe levels. Clients who drink heavily or who

FIGURE 7-8: RELATIONSHIP BETWEEN ALCOHOL USE AND ALCOHOL PROBLEMS

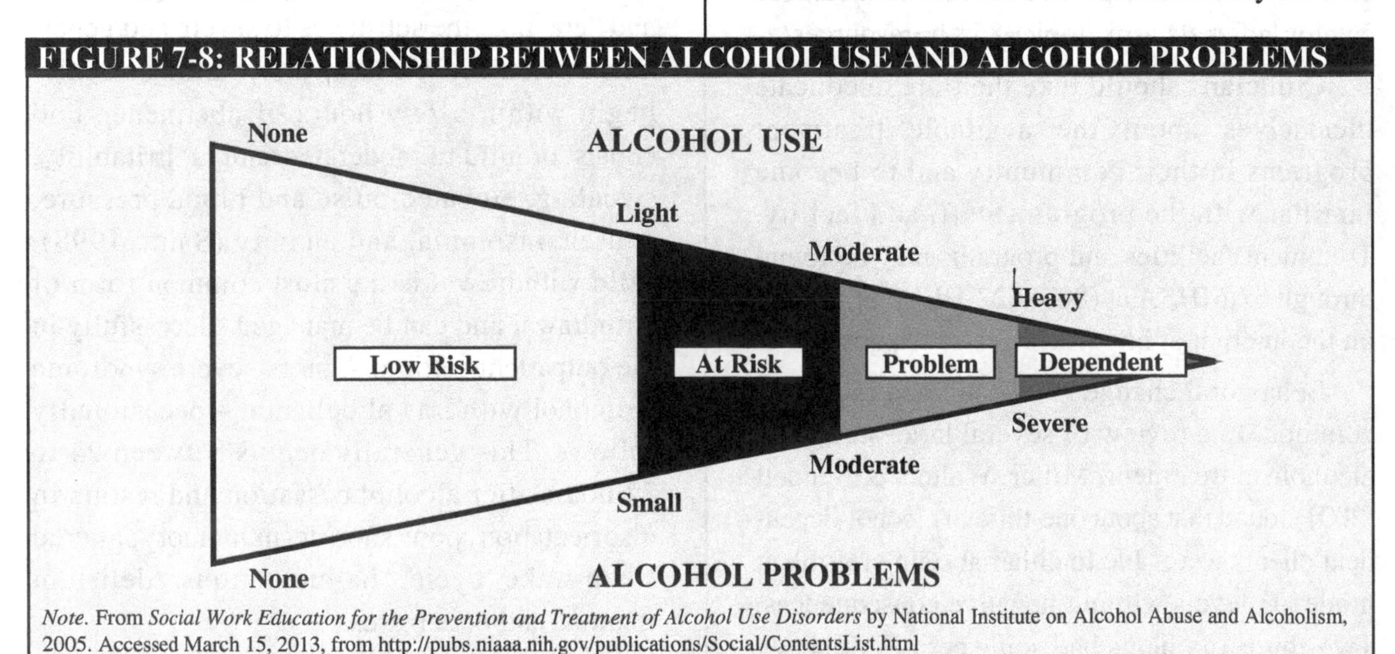

Note. From *Social Work Education for the Prevention and Treatment of Alcohol Use Disorders* by National Institute on Alcohol Abuse and Alcoholism, 2005. Accessed March 15, 2013, from http://pubs.niaaa.nih.gov/publications/Social/ContentsList.html

are at-risk should be counseled to cut down on their alcohol consumption to moderate levels or abstain altogether.

Brief interventions are effective; reliable counseling techniques result in a 30% reduction in alcohol consumption and binge drinking. Brief interventions should be factual and nonconfrontational. Clinicians should state their conclusion and recommendation clearly, focusing on moderate drinking limits and relating these to the clients' concerns and medical findings. Timely follow-up care should be arranged to reinforce these recommendations.

Clients who meet the criteria for alcohol abuse and dependence should be counseled to abstain. The clinician should consider referring the client for evaluation by an addiction specialist and recommend a mutual self-help group. Medically managed withdrawal and pharmacological options should be considered. The client should be followed closely and arrangements should be made for follow-up care.

EXAM QUESTIONS

CHAPTER 7

Questions 34-38

Note: Choose the one option that BEST answers each question.

34. The most common type of alcohol consumed in the United States is

    a. beer.
    b. wine.
    c. spirits.
    d. mixed drinks.

35. A standard drink is any drink that contains 14 grams of pure alcohol. A standard drink equivalent would be

    a. 3 ounces (2 jiggers) of brandy.
    b. an 8-ounce glass of wine.
    c. a 12-ounce can of beer.
    d. a mixed drink with 2 shots of liquor.

36. The National Institute on Alcohol Abuse and Alcoholism defines moderate drinking for healthy men as no more than a daily alcohol consumption of

    a. 1 drink.
    b. 2 drinks.
    c. 3 drinks.
    d. 4 drinks.

37. The most serious signs and symptoms of alcohol withdrawal are

    a. irritability and cravings.
    b. delirium and seizures.
    c. insomnia and mild tremors.
    d. sweating and anxiety.

38. Research studies suggest that brief counseling interventions for patients who drink alcohol at at-risk levels result in approximately

    a. no reduction in alcohol consumption or binge drinking.
    b. a 15% reduction in alcohol consumption and binge drinking.
    c. a 30% reduction in alcohol consumption and binge drinking.
    d. a 50% reduction in alcohol consumption and binge drinking.

REFERENCES

American Psychiatric Association. (2013). *Diagnostic and statistical manual of mental disorders* (5th ed.). Washington, DC: American Psychiatric Association.

Babor, T.F., Higgins-Biddle, J.C., Saunders, J.B., & Monteiro, M.G. (2001). *The Alcohol Use Disorders Identification Test: Guidelines for use in primary care.* World Health Organization. Accessed March 15, 2013, from http://whqlibdoc.who.int/hq/2001/who_msd_msb_01.6a.pdf

Foy, A., March, S. & Drinkwater, V. (1988). Use of an objective clinical scale in the assessment and management of alcohol withdrawal in a large general hospital. *Alcoholism: Clinical and Experimental Research, 12*, 360-364.

Hanson, D. (n.d.). *History of alcohol and drinking around the world.* Accessed March 15, 2013 from http://www2.potsdam.edu/hansondj/Controversies/1114796842.html

Hester, R.K. & Miller, W.R. (Eds.) (2003). *Handbook of alcoholism treatment approaches: Effective alternatives* (3rd ed.). Boston: Allyn & Bacon.

Hoffman, R.S. & Weinhouse, G.L. (2012). *Management of moderate and severe alcohol withdrawal syndromes*. Accessed March 15, 2013 from http://www.uptodate.com/contents/management-of-moderate-and-severe-alcohol-withdrawal-syndromes

Greenfeld, L.A. & Henneberg, M.A. (n.d.). *Victim and offender self-reports of alcohol involvement in crime*. Accessed March 15, 2013 from http://pubs.niaaa.nih.gov/publications/arh25-1/20-31.htm

Knight, J., Sherrit, L., Shrier, A., Harris, S., & Chang, G. (2002). Validity of the CRAFFT substance abuse screening test among adolescent clinic patients. *Archives of Pediatrics and Adolescent Medicine, 156*(6), 607-614.

LaVallee, R., Williams, G.D., & Hsiao-ye, Y. (2009). *Surveillance Report #87: Apparent per capita alcohol consumption: National, state, and regional trends, 1977–2007.* National Institute on Alcohol Abuse and Alcoholism Division of Epidemiology and Prevention Research Alcohol Epidemiologic Data System. Retrieved March 15, 2013 from http://pubs.niaaa.nih.gov/publications/survelliance87/CONS07.htm#fig2

Miller, W.R., Walters, S.T., & Bennett, M.D. (2001). How effective is alcohol treatment in the United States? *Journal of the Study of Alcohol, 62,* 211-220.

McGrew, J. (n.d.). *History of alcohol prohibition.* Shaffer Library of Drug Policy. Accessed March 15, 2013 from http://www.druglibrary.org/schaffer/LIBRARY/studies/nc/nc2a.htm

Muthusamy, R. (2008). *Alcohol metabolism: Interesting facts*. Retrieved March 15, 2013, from http://healthmad.com/health/alcohol-metabolism-interesting-facts/

Myrick, H. & Anton, R. (1998). Treatment of alcohol withdrawal. *Alcohol Health & Research World, 22*(1), 38-43.

National Institute on Alcohol Abuse and Alcoholism. (2004). *Alcohol alert: Alcohol an important women's health issue.* Accessed March 15, 2013, from http://pubs.niaaa.nih.gov/publications/aa62/aa62.htm

National Institute on Alcohol Abuse and Alcoholism. (2005). *Social work education for the prevention and treatment of alcohol use disorders.* Accessed March 15, 2013, from http://pubs.niaaa.nih.gov/publications/Social/ContentsList.html

National Institute on Alcohol Abuse and Alcoholism. (2006). *Alcohol alert: Underage drinking.* Accessed March 15, 2013, from http://pubs.niaaa.nih.gov/publications/AA67/AA67.htm

National Institute on Alcohol Abuse and Alcoholism. (2007). *Helping patients who drink too much: A clinician's guide, updated 2005 edition.* NIH Publication No. 07-3769. Accessed March 15, 2013, from http://pubs.niaaa.nih.gov/publications/Practitioner/CliniciansGuide2005/guide.pdf

Randall, C., Roberts, J., DelBoca, F., Carrol, K., Connors, G., & Mattson, M. (1999). Telescoping of landmark events associated with drinking: A gender comparison. *Journal of the Study of Alcohol, 60*(2), 252-260.

Roberts, L.J. & McCrady, B.S. (2003). *Alcohol problems in intimate relationships: Identification and intervention. A guide for marriage and family therapists.* Accessed March 15, 2013, from http://pubs.niaaa.nih.gov/publications/niaaa-guide/index.htm

Saitz, R. (1998). Introduction to alcohol withdrawal. *Alcohol Health and Research World, 22,* 5-12.

Substance Abuse and Mental Health Services Administration. (2012). *Results from the 2011 National survey on drug use and health: Summary of national findings* (NSDUH Series H-44, HHS Publication No. (SMA) 12-4713). Rockville, MD. Accessed March 10, 2013 from http://www.samhsa.gov/data/NSDUH/2k11Results/NSDUHresults2011.htm

Sullivan, J.T., Sykora, K., Schneiderman, J., Naranjo, C.A., and Sellers, E.M. (1989). Assessment of alcohol withdrawal: The revised Clinical Institute Withdrawal Assessment for Alcohol scale (CIWA-Ar). *British Journal of Addiction, 84,* 1353-1357.

Taj, N., Devera-Sales, A., & Vinson, D. (1998). Screening for problem drinking: Does a single question work. *Journal of Family Practice, 46*(4), 328-335.

Tonigan, J.S. (2003). Applied issues in treatment outcome assessment. In J.P. Allen & V.B. Wilson, *Assessing alcohol problems as a guide for clinicians and researchers* (2nd ed.). NIH Publication No. 03-3745.

World Health Organization. (2004). *Global Status Report on Alcohol 2004.* Department of Mental Health and Substance Abuse. Accessed March 15, 2013, from http://www.who.int/substance_abuse/publications/alcohol/en

World Health Organization. (2009). *Alcohol and injuries: Emergency department studies in an international perspective.* Accessed March 15, 2013 from http://www.who.int/substance_abuse/msbalcinuries.pdf

CHAPTER 8

MARIJUANA/CANNABIS

CHAPTER OBJECTIVE

After completing this chapter, the learner will be able to describe characteristics of marijuana (or cannabis), its health effects, and screening and treatment considerations.

LEARNING OBJECTIVES

After studying this chapter, the learner will be able to:

1. Describe characteristics, common names, and forms of marijuana.
2. Describe the trends and patterns of marijuana use, abuse, and dependence among people in the United States.
3. Describe the biochemical actions and health effects of using marijuana.
4. Describe approaches to screening and treating marijuana abusers.
5. Discuss medicinal uses of marijuana or cannabis and controversies surrounding the legalization of the drug.

OVERVIEW

Marijuana is a mind-altering drug composed of a dry shredded mix of flowers, stems, seeds, and leaves from the hemp plant (Cannabis sativa). The term that is used to refer to marijuana and other drugs made from this plant is called cannabis.

Other forms of cannabis include sinsemilla (high grade marijuana "without seeds"), hashish, and hash oil. The hemp plant varies in quality and potency, which is often dependent on climate, soil, cultivation, and method of preparation (Grinspoon, Bakalar, & Russo, 2005). Preparation of the plant comes in three grades: the cheapest is called bhang and it has the lowest resin; ganja is mid-grade and is obtained from the unfertilized flowering tops and leaves; and the highest grade is called charas (properly called hashish) and is made of the resin itself from the tops of mature plants.

Street names include *pot, gange, reefer, herb, weed, grass, bud, Mary Jane, indo,* and *hydro* (National Institute on Drug Abuse [NIDA], 2011). Most users smoke marijuana in hand-rolled cigarettes called *joints,* while others use pipes or water pipes called *bongs.* Blunts, also popular, are cigars that have been opened and the tobacco is replaced with marijuana alone or marijuana and another drug such as crack cocaine.

Marijuana was most likely first used as an intoxicant in India around 1000 B.C. (National Commission on Marijuana and Drug Abuse, 2002). Another source notes that the drug was recorded in a Chinese compendium of medicines dating back to 2737 B.C. (Grinspoon et al., 2005).

The most famous users were ancient Hindus and the drug was called ganjika in Sanskrit or ganja in modern languages. Cannabis was often used for spiritual purposes.

Even in ancient times, the drug was a subject of controversy, eventually leading to a gradual recognition of its intoxicating properties in the 19th century. In 1857, Fitz Hugh Ludlow influenced members of the French romantic literary movement by publishing a book about the euphoriant properties of cannabis (Grinspoon et al., 2005). In the United States, the U.S. Federal Bureau of Narcotics portrayed marijuana as a powerful addicting substance in the 1930s and, in 1970, the Controlled Substances Act classified marijuana as a Schedule I drug, with high potential of abuse and no accepted medical use.

EPIDEMIOLOGY OF MARIJUANA USE

Marijuana is the most commonly used illicit drug. According to the 2011 National Survey on Drug Use and Health (NSDUH), 18.1 million people in the U.S. aged 12 and older were current marijuana users (Substance Abuse and Mental Health Services Administration [SAMHSA], 2012). This represents 7% of the population.

In the 2011 Monitoring the Future (MTF) study, 16.4% of eighth graders, 34.5% of tenth graders, and 45.5% of twelfth graders reported using marijuana at least once in their lifetime (Johnston, O'Malley, Bachman, & Schulenberg, 2012a). In this same study, 12.5% of eighth graders, 28.8% of tenth graders, and 36.4% of twelfth graders reported using marijuana in the past year.

The overall trends of marijuana use show that annual marijuana use peaked amongst twelfth graders, at 51%, in 1979. Since then, it has fluctuated. A decline was noted for 13 years, evidenced by 22% of twelfth graders reporting marijuana use in 1992. Beginning in 1993, a resurgence of use occurred amongst eighth, tenth and twelfth graders. A peak was reached in 1996 for eighth graders (18.3%) and 1997 for tenth and twelfth graders (34.8% and 38.5%, respectively). From 1998 through 2008, there had been a gradual decline. An upturn that lasted 3 years in the lower grades (and longer in grade 12) was then noted, and in 2011 and 2012, there was some decline in use among 8th graders, with use leveling off among 10th and 12th graders (Johnston, O'Malley, Bachman, & Schulenberg, 2013).

The extent of marijuana use can be seen in the findings from at least two other monitoring systems. The Drug Abuse Warning Network (DAWN), which monitors the health impact of drugs, estimated that marijuana was a contributing factor in more than 461,028 emergency department visits in the United States in 2010 (DAWN, 2012). According to the 2011 Arrestee Drug Abuse Monitoring Program (ADAM II), which surveys drug use among male arrestees in 10 major metropolitan areas across the United States, marijuana is the most common drug detected in arrestees. In 9 of the 10 areas, more than 45% of arrestees tested positive for marijuana (ONDCP, 2012a).

Marijuana use continues to be of concern especially for those who use it more regularly. In 2011, an estimated 5.0 million persons (16.7% of past year marijuana users) were daily marijuana users (i.e., they used marijuana on 300 or more days in the past 12 months) (SAMHSA, 2013). Among young adults ages 19 to 30, approximately 5.1% reported daily marijuana use compared with 1.3%, 3.6% and 6.6% in eighth, tenth and twelfth graders respectively (Johnston et al., 2012a, 2012b).

Marijuana is not only the most commonly used illicit drug but also the most consistently available illicit drug. Marijuana appears to be available to almost all high school seniors; 81.6% reported that they think it would be 'very easy' or 'fairly easy' for them to get marijuana – almost twice the number who reported ever having used it (45.2%). There has been little change in perceived availability from 1975 to 2012, though 81.6% is close to the lowest recorded rate for that timeframe (81.1% in 2009; Johnston et al., 2013).

BIOCHEMISTRY

Although marijuana consists of more than 400 chemicals, the most active chemical in marijuana is delta-9-tetrahydrocannabinol (THC). The amount of THC determines the drug's potency. According to the Office of National Drug Control Policy (ONDCP), the average potency of marijuana available in the United States has more than doubled since 1998 (ONDCP, 2012b). Over the past two decades, the average amount of THC found in marijuana available in the United States has increased from 2.83% in 1985 to 5.81% in 2008. Sinsemilla THC levels have increased from 7.28% to 11.46%. Of the 65,247 marijuana samples analyzed in 2008, marijuana (including sinsemilla) THC concentrations ranged from 0.11% THC to 27.30% THC. Sinsemilla THC levels ranged from 0.82% to 27.3%, while lower grade marijuana ranged from 0.24% THC to 19.48% THC (National Center for Natural Products Research, 2009).

THC is a chemical that is very similar to natural chemicals in the brain called *endogenous cannabinoids*, which help control a wide array of mental and physical processes in the brain and throughout the body, including memory and perception, fine motor coordination, pain sensations, immunity to disease, and reproduction.

When marijuana is smoked, THC travels to many parts of the body, including the brain where its effects begin immediately and last for 1 to 3 hours. The psychological and cardiovascular effects occur within 5 to 10 minutes. At first, the user may feel pleasant sensations but this leads to feelings of sleepiness and depression. Individuals may also feel increased anxiety, fear, distrust, or panic. Heavy use can impair the memory and the ability to recall events and may disrupt coordination and balance.

How Does it Work?

THC attaches to cannabinoid receptors on nerve cells in the brain, leading to a disruption of the endogenous cannabinoids' normal function. The regions of the brain in which cannabinoid receptors are abundant are the cerebellum (body movement), hippocampus (learning and memory), cerebral cortex (higher cognitive functions), nucleus accumbens (reward), and basal ganglia (movement control). This overstimulation of the cannabinoid receptors produces the intoxication experienced by marijuana smokers. THC activates the reward system by stimulating the brain cells to release dopamine, causing the user to feel euphoric or high. With time, the function of cannabinoid receptors may be altered which, along with other changes in the brain, can lead to withdrawal symptoms and addiction (NIDA, 2010).

There is some controversy about whether marijuana is addictive or whether it produces dependency. Tolerance and withdrawal symptoms are signs of addiction and some claim that these are rarely a serious problem for marijuana users (Grinspoon et al., 2005) while others suggest that for chronic users, consequences include behavioral tolerance and withdrawal symptoms upon drug cessation (Lichtman & Martin, 2005).

Long-term use can lead to addiction for some people, resulting in compulsive use that often interferes with life activities. For example, it was found that daily marijuana users were more likely to be unemployed compared to those who reported less-than-daily use (SAMHSA, 2012a). According to the 2011 NSDUH, an estimated 20.6 million people in the U.S. age 12 or older were classified with substance dependence or abuse (8.0% of the total population). Of the estimated 6.5 million people in the U.S. classified with dependence on or abuse of illicit drugs, 4.2 million were dependent on or abused marijuana (SAMHSA, 2012a). MTF findings on youth, marijuana abuse is more prevalent among males than females in the 8th, 10th, and 12th grades (Johnston et al., 2012a).

RELATED MEDICAL PROBLEMS AND CO-OCCURRING DISORDERS

Marijuana abuse is associated with many health effects (NIDA, 2012), including physical, psychological, and behavioral effects that can be divided into acute, persistent, and long-term effects (Table 8-1).

Physical Effects: Respiratory, Neurological, Cardiac, and Immune Systems

The danger of long-term respiratory problems is well confirmed. Smoking marijuana regularly may produce the same health problems as smoking cigarettes on a regular basis, including daily cough, phlegm production, chest illnesses, increased lung infections, and a greater tendency to obstructed airways. There can be a burning and stinging of the mouth and throat with use. There is also evidence that cancer of the respiratory tract and lungs is also a problem because marijuana smoke contains 50% to 70% more carcinogenic hydrocarbons than tobacco smoke (NIDA, 2012).

TABLE 8-1: HEALTH CONSEQUENCES OF MARIJUANA USE

Acute (present during intoxication)

- Impairs short-term memory
- Impairs attention, judgment, and other cognitive functions
- Impairs coordination and balance
- Increases heart rate

Persistent (lasting longer than intoxication, but may not be permanent)

- Impairs memory and learning skills

Long-term (cumulative, potentially permanent effects of chronic abuse)

- Can lead to addiction
- Increases risk of chronic cough, bronchitis, and emphysema
- Increases risk of cancer of the head, neck, and lungs

Note. From *Marijuana abuse.* (Research report series. NIH Publication No. 10-3859), 2010, by National Institute on Drug Abuse. Accessed on March 15, 2013 from http://www.drugabuse.gov/publications/marijuana-abuse/how-does-marijuana-use-affect-your-brain-body

The short-term effects on brain functioning include problems with memory and learning, distorted perceptions, and difficulty in thinking and problem solving. THC alters the way in which information is processed by the hippocampus – the part of the brain responsible for memory formation. There is some evidence that cognitive impairments can last for days, weeks, or even longer depending on the amount smoked. A recent large prospective study that followed individuals over time revealed that those who began smoking marijuana heavily in their teens lost as much as 8 points in IQ between ages 13 and 38, and that their lost cognitive abilities were not restored as adults, even among those who had quit smoking marijuana (NIDA, 2012). Marijuana also disrupts coordination by binding to the receptors in the cerebellum and basal ganglia, the parts of the brain that control balance, posture, coordination, and reaction time. Accidents, including impaired driving performance, are associated with use, especially when used in combination with alcohol.

There is additional evidence that marijuana affects the heart and immune system (NIDA, 2010, 2012). There is evidence that use of marijuana increases heart rate within 5 to 10 minutes of use. One study has indicated a user's risk of heart attack more than quadruples during the first hour after smoking marijuana. There is some indication that THC impairs the immune system's ability to fight disease. This is most likely due to the inhibition of the cells.

Psychological Effects

The *Diagnostic and Statistical Manual of Mental Disorders,* 5th Edition, (*DSM-5*) and the International Classification of Diseases (ICD-10) identifies a cannabis use disorder (American Psychiatric Association, 2013; World Health Organization, 2010). However, there is often difficulty in making a diagnosis because the full criteria are difficult to quantify (Raphael, Wooding, Stevens, & Connor, 2005).

Cannabis withdrawal is included in the *DSM-5* and also included in the ICD-10. Although there is some controversy, heavy use of cannabis results in what has often been described as a cannabis withdrawal syndrome. A recent review found that there is converging evidence from basic laboratory and clinical studies that suggests discontinuation of chronic, heavy use of cannabis results in emotional and behavioral symptoms, appetite change, weight loss, and physical discomfort (Budney, Hughes, Moore, & Vandrey, 2004). However, Budney found that in a sample of adults, the severity of withdrawal was greater for those with psychiatric symptomatology (Budney, Novy, & Hughes, 1999). Haney (2005) describes this less known consequence of daily use as a constellation of symptoms, including irritability, anxiety, marijuana craving, decreased quality and quantity of sleep, and decreased food intake. In an outpatient clinic, nearly two-thirds of the sample of adolescents indicated four or more symptoms. The magnitude of withdrawal severity correlated with current emotional and behavioral symptoms and self-reported problems with cannabis use (Vandrey, Budney, Kamon, & Stanger, 2005).

It has also been suggested that cannabis can produce a "cannabis psychosis," which is another area of disagreement among many researchers. A recent study found that after reviewing studies for a meta-analysis between 1966 and 2004, early use of cannabis did appear to increase the risk for psychosis (Semple, McIntosh, & Lawrie, 2005). Grinspoon and colleagues (2005) summarized the findings, suggesting that the drug may precipitate a toxic psychosis in susceptible people when exposed to a large ingested dose of cannabis. Raphael and colleagues (2005) also summarized the literature, indicating that there appears to be a strong association whereby cannabis precipitates or exacerbates psychosis and schizophrenia.

The relationship between cannabis use disorders and psychiatric conditions has received increasing attention. Co-morbidity is seen with Axis I and II disorders (Stinson, Ruan, Pickering, & Grant, 2006; Bovasso, 2001; Patton et al., 2002). There is evidence for the link between cannabis use and the risk of major depression (Raphael et al., 2005). There is evidence that some cannabis users suffer from an acute anxiety state that may reach a state of panic (Grinspoon et al., 2005). Although these panic reactions are relatively uncommon, the more frequent adverse reaction to moderate use of cannabis is anxiety and paranoid thoughts, which "are more likely in someone who is taking the drug for the first time or in an unpleasant or unfamiliar setting" (Grinspoon et al., 2005, p. 269).

Behavioral Effects

The behavioral effects of marijuana use can impact job performance, including increased absences, tardiness, accidents, worker's compensation claims, and job turnover. From a school performance perspective, students who smoke marijuana get lower grades and are less likely to graduate from high school. There is some indication of a motivational syndrome.

Depression, anxiety, and personality disturbances are associated with marijuana use (NIDA, 2012; Hubbard, Franco, & Onaivi, 1999). Users trying to quit commonly report irritability, anxiety, and difficulty sleeping. On psychological tests, they often display increased aggression (ONDCP, n.d.-b).

SPECIAL POPULATIONS AND RISK IDENTIFICATION

High-risk groups include youth and young adults. In the 2011 NSDUH, young adults ages 18 to 25 had the highest rates for use of illicit drugs, and 19.0% reported using marijuana in the past month. Among youths ages 12 to 17, the statistics vary by age: 1.3% of 12 or 13-year-olds reported current past month use, 6.7% among 14- or 15-year-olds, and 15.1% of 16- or 17-year-olds reported current use (SAMHSA, 2012a). In the 2008 MTF study, 46.6% of college students and 56.3% of young adults (ages 19 to 28) reported lifetime use of marijuana (Johnston et al., 2012b). These statistics clearly indicate that youth and young adults are at particular risk. A recent analysis of 13,718 middle school and high school students found that the student's own and peer involvement with substances, delinquency, and school problems were the three risk factors that predicted marijuana use at all stages of marijuana involvement (initiation of experimental use, initiation of regular use, progression to regular use, failure to discontinue experimental use, and failure to discontinue regular use (van den Bree & Pickworth, 2005). Additional risk factors include less time spent with parents (Best, Gross, Manning, Gossop, & Strang, 2005), positive expectations of use (Chabrol et al., 2006), and male gender (SAMHSA, 2012a).

Cannabis use should be systematically assessed by health care providers through a clinical evaluation of use, frequency and quantity of consumption, and complications from use. Warning signs include a deterioration in school or work performance and a change in recreational activities (giving up activities that were once pleasurable) (Hubbard et al., 1999). All adolescents should be asked about use of drugs – including cigarettes, alcohol, and marijuana – at routine health maintenance visits (Fournier & Levy, 2006). Tools that can be used to do the initial screening include the HEADS (Heyman & Adger, 1997) or the CRAFFT (Knight et al., 1999). The HEADS is used to identify medical, social, and psychological issues in adolescents overall, while the CRAFFT is a series of six questions that are designed to address drug and alcohol misuse or disorders.

Since the 1980s, urine tests have been used to detect 11-nor-delta-9-tetrahydroncannabinol-9-carboxylic acid, a metabolite of delta-9-THC. This is detectable in the urine from 5 to 30 days. In addition, other screening tests may include saliva, sweat patch, and hair tests, although there are limitations associated with these methods.

Drug testing in occupational settings and, more recently, in schools is one of the recommended strategies of the ONDCP. The school recommendation is based on the assumption that drug testing can be a means of preventing and treating youth drug use. The goal is not to punish students who use drugs but rather to prevent drug dependence. There is some evidence that schools that have been doing such testing are seeing a reduction in drug use (ONDCP, 2002).

TREATMENT

There has been a noted increase in marijuana admissions for treatment. From 1992 to 2010, the number of admissions to treatment where the primary substance of abuse was marijuana increased from 93,000 to 353,000 (ONDCP, n.d.-a). The average age at treatment admission for primary marijuana abuse was 25. Approximately 68% of those admitted to treatment were male and 47% were White (SAMHSA, 2012b). However, it should be noted that admissions for marijuana alone is rare because other drugs are also commonly used. These patients reported raised levels of depression, personality disorders, and previous admission to psychiatric hospitals for disorders unrelated to psychoactive substance abuse (Arendt & Munk-Jorgensen, 2004).

In 1997, the U.S. federal government sponsored the Cannabis Youth Treatment (CYT) study, which resulted in innovative and effective treatment methodologies. Various approaches included the following:

- Motivational enhancement therapy (MET) plus cognitive behavioral therapy (CBT) – consisting of two individual MET sessions and three group CBT sessions lasting 6 to 7 weeks. The MET component focused on assisting adolescents to resolve their ambivalence about whether they had a problem with cannabis or substances and increasing their motivation to stop using. The CBT component focused on teaching such skills as refusing offers of cannabis, establishing a social network support of recovery, developing a plan for pleasant activities to replace cannabis activities, and coping with high-risk situations
- Another more in-depth MET/CBT consisting of 12 sessions
- Family support network, which used the MET/CBT of 12 sessions with six parent education group meetings, four home visits, referral to a self-help group, and case management
- Adolescent community reinforcement, which consisted of 10 individual sessions with adolescents, four with caregivers, and limited case management
- Multidimensional family therapy, which consisted of 12 to 15 sessions with adolescents and their family and case management over 12 to 14 weeks.

These were studied for effectiveness in 600 cannabis users (predominately White males, ages 15 to 16) (Dennis et al., 2004). Overall, the CYT study found that all of these interventions demonstrated significant pre- and post-treatment improvements during the 12 months in two main outcomes – days of abstinence and percent of adolescents in recovery.

In a study of adult users, comparable benefits were found from a 14-session cognitive behavioral group treatment and a two-session individual treatment that included motivational interviewing and advice on ways to reduce marijuana use. Use, dependence symptoms, and psychosocial problems decreased for at least 1 year after these treatments. In addition, giving vouchers for abstaining from marijuana also helped to improve outcomes (Budney, Higgins, Radonivich, & Novy, 2000).

Retention of clients is always an issue in treatment. In the CYT study, there were high rates of treatment completion (81%) and high rates of follow-up (Dennis et al., 2002). In another study of 173 youth, factors positively associated with treatment duration included use of drugs in addition to alcohol and marijuana, having less deviant peers, absence of substance-caused emotional problems, and viewing counselor's skills more positively (Battjes, Gordan, O'Grady, & Kinlock, 2004).

Although no medications are available to treat marijuana abuse, work is underway to develop a medication that will block THC's intoxicating effects. This type of medication may be used to prevent relapse to marijuana abuse (NIDA, 2010).

MEDICINAL USE OF CANNABIS AND LEGALIZATION ISSUES

The history of cannabis as a medicinal plant is extensive. The oldest known therapeutic description was by an Emperor in China who used it for beri-beri, constipation, gout, malaria, and absent-mindedness. It has also been used throughout the world for various ailments. For many years, it was listed as a drug of treatment in the United States; however, in 1937, it was outlawed in medical care. Because cannabis is associated with appetite stimulation and pain relief for such illnesses as cancer or AIDS, there is controversy over legalizing cannabis. It has also been used to treat glaucoma and neurological illnesses, such as epilepsy, migraines, nausea in chemotherapy patients, and loss of appetite in patients with AIDS and bipolar disorder (National Commission on Marijuana and Drug Abuse, 2002).

The controversy of legalizing marijuana will most likely continue. Although THC is recognized as an ingredient that can be used to treat some medical problems, marijuana as a smoked product is not proven to be beneficial. There are currently many clinical trials to further study the potential uses of marijuana; in the meantime, the conclusion is that marijuana smoke creates adverse events that do not outweigh the benefits (Drug Enforcement Administration [DEA], 2011). The DEA posits that marijuana "has no accepted medicinal value in treatment in the United States, and evidence that there is a general lack of accepted safety for its use even under medical supervision [exists]" (DEA, 2011).

The federal government has maintained a strong stand against legalizing the medicinal use of marijuana in the United States. Under federal law, marijuana is regulated as a Schedule I controlled substance and its use is prohibited. In 2005, the Supreme Court in Gonzales v Raich declared that the federal government can ban possession of marijuana even in those states that have eliminated sanctions for its use in treating symptoms of illness.

As of February, 2013, there are eighteen states and DC that maintain laws that permit marijuana use for medical purposes (Alaska, Arizona, California, Colorado, Connecticut, DC, Delaware, Hawaii, Maine, Massachusetts, Michigan, Montana, Nevada, New Jersey, New Mexico, Oregon, Rhode Island, Vermont, and Washington). Additionally, as of March 2013, 11 more states had pending legislation to legalize medical marijuana. Maryland currently has a law that protects seriously ill patients from being sentenced to prison for possessing marijuana if they can prove a "medical necessity." However, the law does not protect them from arrest, and it does not provide them with safe access to their medicine (ProCon.org, 2013).

Until the Supreme Court rules directly on the constitutionality of state medical marijuana laws, a conflict remains between federal law which outlaws marijuana use and state laws which may permit its limited medical use. However, those who try to use marijuana as a medical treatment risk legal action by the U.S. Drug Enforcement Administration or other federal agencies, and state medical marijuana laws provide no defense.

SUMMARY

Cannabis has an interesting history relating to recreational and medicinal use. It continues to be a drug with controversial underpinnings.

The use of cannabis as a recreational drug continues to be a concern in our society for several reasons: After several years of decline, marijuana use is once again increasing among high school students; children seem to be initiating use of marijuana at a younger age; the potency of the drug seems to be higher in many cases; and evidence of harmful health effects is present and continues to be studied.

Although drug treatment is effective and is continually studied, it seems that prevention is a critical approach in the future, especially because it is the most common illicit drug used among our youth.

EXAM QUESTIONS

CHAPTER 8

Questions 39-44

Note: Choose the one option that BEST answers each question.

39. The intoxication effect of cannabis is due to

    a. an overstimulation of the cannabinoid receptors in the brain.
    b. an increased need for an increased dose of marijuana.
    c. a stimulation of primarily one area of the brain.
    d. the lack of marijuana brain receptors.

40. Daily marijuana use is greatest among which population?

    a. 8th graders
    b. 10th graders
    c. 12th graders
    d. young adults

41. One of the medical effects of using marijuana is problems with memory. This is most likely due to

    a. delta-9-tetrahydrocannabinol (THC) effects on the cerebellum.
    b. THC effects on the hippocampus.
    c. a psychic dependence in the nucleus accumbens.
    d. the release of dopamine in the brain.

42. Which statement regarding the health effects of marijuana use is true?

    a. Smoking marijuana regularly may produce the same health problems as smoking cigarettes.
    b. Behavioral effects related to job performance from marijuana use are rare.
    c. Coordination, balance, and reaction time is improved with marijuana use.
    d. The heart rate of a person smoking marijuana decreases within the first 5 to 10 minutes.

43. Which statement regarding the treatment of marijuana abusers is true?

    a. There is limited evidence that any type of treatment is effective over a short or long period of follow-up.
    b. Comparable benefits have been found for cognitive behavioral group treatment and individual treatment in adults, including motivational interviewing.
    c. There is no evidence that any type of medication should be developed for marijuana dependence.
    d. Vouchers are an ineffective treatment approach in promoting abstinence from marijuana.

44. Legalizing marijuana for medicinal use is controversial. The Drug Enforcement Agency concludes
    a. marijuana smoke creates adverse events that do not outweigh the benefits.
    b. marijuana use for medicinal purposes should be regulated exclusively by state law.
    c. scientific evidence shows that the positive health effects outweigh the adverse effects.
    d. there is no cause to further study the medicinal value of marijuana.

REFERENCES

American Psychiatric Association. (2013). *Diagnostic and statistical manual of mental disorders* (5th ed.). Washington, DC: American Psychiatric Association.

Arendt, M. & Munk-Jorgensen, P. (2004). Heavy cannabis users seeking treatment-prevalence of psychiatric disorders. *Soc Psychiatry Psychiatric Epidemiology, 39*(2), 97-105.

Battjes, R.J., Gordon, M.S., O'Grady, K.E., & Kinlock, T.W. (2004). Predicting retention of adolescents in substance abuse treatment. *Addictive Behaviors, 29*(5), 1021-1027.

Best, D., Gross, S., Manning,V., Gossop, M., & Strang, J. (2005). Cannabis use in adolescents: the impact of risk and protective factors and social functioning. *Drug and Alcohol Review, 24*(6), 483-488.

Bovasso, G.B. (2001). Cannabis use as a risk factor for depressive symptoms. *American Journal of Psychiatry, 158*(12), 2033-2037.

Budney, A.J., Higgins, S.T., Radonovich, K.J., & Novy, P.L. (2000). Adding voucher-based incentives to coping skills and motivational enhancement improves outcomes during treatment for marijuana dependence. *Journal of Consulting Clinical Psychology, 68*(6), 1051-1061.

Budney, A.J., Hughes, J.R., Moore, B.A., & Vandrey, R. (2004). Review of the validity and significance of cannabis withdrawal syndrome. *American Journal of Psychiatry, 161*(11), 1967-77.

Budney, A.J., Novy, P., & Hughes, J. (1999). Marijuana withdrawal among adults seeking treatment for marijuana dependence. *Addiction, 94*(9), 1311-1321.

Chabrol, H., Chauchard, E., Mabila, J., Mantoulan, R., Adele, A., & Rousseau, A. (2006). Contri-butions of social influences and expectations of use to cannabis use in high-school students. *Addictive Behaviors, 31*(11), 2116-2119.

Dennis, M., Godley, S.H., Diamond, G., Tims, F.M., Babor, T., Donaldson, J., et al. (2004). The Cannabis Youth Treatment (CYT) Study: Main findings from two randomized trials. *Journal of Substance Abuse Treatment, 27*(3), 195-196.

Dennis, M., Titus, J.C., Diamond, G., Donaldson, J., Godley, S.H., Tims, F.M., et al.; C.Y.T. Steering Committee. (2002). The Cannabis Youth Treatment (CYT) experiment: rationale, study design, and analysis plans. *Addiction, 97*(Supplement 1), 16-34.

Drug Abuse Warning Network. (2012). *Highlights of the 2010 Drug Abuse Warning Network (DAWN) findings on drug-related emergency department visits.* Accessed March 15, 2013 from http://www.samhsa.gov/data/2k12/DAWN096/SR096EDHighlights2010.htm

Drug Enforcement Administration. (2011). *The DEA position on marijuana.* Retrieved March 15, 2013 from http://www.justice.gov/dea/docs/marijuana_position_2011.pdf

Fournier, M.E. & Levy, S. (2006). Recent trends in adolescent substance use, primary care screening, and updates in treatment options. *Current Opinion in Pediatrics, 18*(4), 352-358.

Grinspoon, L., Bakalar, J.B., & Russo, E. (2005). Marijuana: Clinical aspects. In J. Lowinson, P. Ruiz, R. Millman, & J.G. Langrod (Eds.), *Substance abuse: A comprehensive textbook.* Philadelphia: Lippincott Williams & Wilkins.

Haney, M. (2005). The marijuana withdrawal syndrome: Diagnosis and treatment. *Current Psychiatry, 7*(5), 360-6.

Heyman, R.B. & Adger, H. (1997). Office approach to substance abuse prevention. *Pediatric Clinics of North America, 44*(6), 1447-1455.

Hubbard, J.R., Franco, S.E., & Onaivi, E.S. (1999). Marijuana: Medical implications. *American Family Physician, 60*(9), 2583-2593.

Johnston, L. D., O'Malley, P. M., Bachman, J. G., & Schulenberg, J. E. (2012a). *Monitoring the Future national survey results on drug use, 1975-2011. Volume I: Secondary school students.* Ann Arbor: Institute for Social Research, The University of Michigan.

Johnston, L. D., O'Malley, P. M., Bachman, J. G., & Schulenberg, J. E. (2012b). *Monitoring the Future national survey results on drug use, 1975-2011. Volume II: College students and adults ages 19-50.* Ann Arbor: Institute for Social Research, The University of Michigan.

Johnston, L. D., O'Malley, P. M., Bachman, J. G., & Schulenberg, J. E. (2013). *Monitoring the Future national results on adolescent drug use: Overview of key findings, 2012.* Ann Arbor: Institute for Social Research, The University of Michigan.

Knight, J.R., Shrier, L.A., Bravender, T.D., Farrell, M., VanderBilt, J. & Shaffer, H.J. (1999). A new brief screen for adolescent substance abuse. *Arch Pediatrics Adolescent Medicine, 153*(6), 591-596.

Lichtman, A.H. & Martin, B.R. (2005). Cannabinoid tolerance and dependence. *Handbook of Experimental Pharmacology, 168,* 691-717.

National Center for Natural Products Research. (2009). *Quarterly Report Potency Monitoring Project.* Report 104, December 16, 2008 through March 15, 2009. Accessed March 15, 2013, from https://www.ncjrs.gov/pdffiles1/ondcp/mpmp_report_104.pdf

National Commission on Marijuana and Drug Abuse. (2002). *History of the medical use of marijuana.* Accessed March 15, 2013, from http://www.skunked.co.uk/articles/history-medicinal-02.htm

National Institute of Drug Abuse. (2010). *Marijuana abuse.* Research report series. (NIH Publication No. 10-3859). Accessed March 15, 2013, from http://www.drugabuse.gov/publications/research-reports/marijuana-abuse

National Institute on Drug Abuse. (2011). *Commonly abused drugs chart.* Retrieved March 15, 2013 from http://www.drugabuse.gov/drugs-abuse/commonly-abused-drugs/commonly-abused-drugs-chart

National Institute on Drug Abuse. (2012). *DrugFacts: Marijuana.* Accessed March 15, 2013, from http://www.drugabuse.gov/publications/drugfacts/marijuana

Office of National Drug Control Policy. (n.d.-a). *Facts and answers to the frequently asked questions about marijuana.* Accessed March 15, 2013, from http://www.whitehouse.gov/ondcp/frequently-asked-questions-and-facts-about-marijuana#treatment

Office of National Drug Control Policy. (n.d.-b). *Marijuana myths and facts.* Accessed March 15, 2013, from https://www.ncjrs.gov/ondcppubs/publications/pdf/marijuana_myths_facts.pdf

Office of National Drug Control Policy. (2002). *What you need to know about drug testing in schools.* Accessed March 15, 2013, from http://www.ncjrs.gov/ondcppubs/publications/pdf/drug_testing.pdf

Office of the National Drug Control Policy. (2012a). *Arrestee Drug Abuse Monitoring Program II 2011 Annual Report.* Accessed March 15, 2013, from http://www.whitehouse.gov//sites/default/files/email-files/adam_ii_2011_annual_rpt_web_version_corrected.pdf

Office of the National Drug Control Policy. (2012b). *Marijuana: Know the facts.* Retrieved March 15, 2013 from http://www.whitehouse.gov/sites/default/files/page/files/marijuana_fact_sheet_3-28-12.pdf

Patton, G.C., Coffey, C., Carlin, J.B., Degenhardt, L., Lynskey, M. & Hall, W. (2002). Cannabis use and mental health in young people: A cohort study. *BMJ, 325*(7374), 1195-1198.

ProCon.org. Medical Marijuana. (2013). *18 Legal medical marijuana states.* Accessed March 15, 2013, from http://medicalmarijuana.procon.org/view.resource.php?resourceID=000881

Raphael, B., Wooding, S., Stevens, G., & Connor, J. (2005). Comorbidity: Cannabis and complexity. *Journal of Psychiatric Practice, 11*(3), 161-176.

Semple, D.M., McIntosh, A.M., & Lawrie, S.M. (2005). Cannabis as a risk factor for psychosis: Systematic review. *Journal of Psychopharmacology, 19*(2), 187-94.

Stinson, F.S., Ruan, W.J., Pickering, R., & Grant, B.F. (2006). Cannabis use disorders in the USA: Prevalence, correlates, and co-morbidity. *Psychological Medicine, 36*(10), 1447-60.

Substance Abuse and Mental Health Services Administration. (2004). *NSDUH report: Daily marijuana users* (Office of Applied Studies). Accessed March 15, 2013, from http://www.oas.samhsa.gov/2k4/dailyMJ/dailyMJ.pdf

Substance Abuse and Mental Health Services Administration. (2012a). *Results from the 2011 National survey on drug use and health: Summary of national findings* (NSDUH Series H-44, HHS Publication No. (SMA) 12-4713). Rockville, MD. Accessed March 15, 2013 from http://www.samhsa.gov/data/NSDUH/2k11Results/NSDUHresults2011.htm

Substance Abuse and Mental Health Services Administration. (2012b). *Treatment Episode Data Set (TEDS) 2000-2010: National admissions to substance abuse treatment services.* Retrieved March 15, 2013 from http://www.samhsa.gov/data/2k12/TEDS2010N/TEDS2010NWeb.pdf

van den Bree, M.B. & Pickworth, W.B. (2005). Risk factors predicting changes in marijuana involvement in teenagers. *Archives of General Psychiatry, 62*(3), 311-319.

Vandrey, R., Budney, A.J., Kamon, JL., & Stanger, C. (2005). Cannabis withdrawal in adolescent treatment seekers. *Drug and Alcohol Dependence, 78*(2), 205-210.

World Health Organization. (2010). *International statistical classification of diseases and related health problems,* 10th revision (ICD-10). Geneva: World Health Organization.

CHAPTER 9

STIMULANTS

CHAPTER OBJECTIVE

After completing this chapter, the learner will be able to describe the effects of stimulant dependence on the body and the current treatment approaches.

LEARNING OBJECTIVES

After studying this chapter, the learner will be able to:

1. Describe the basic effects of cocaine.
2. Describe the differences in the routes of administration of cocaine.
3. Compare and contrast the effects of cocaine and other amphetamines.
4. Discuss current treatment approaches for stimulant dependence.

OVERVIEW

The class of drugs known as *stimulants* is commonly used because of the increased energy individuals experience beyond what would normally be expected. Stimulants may be taken to facilitate weight loss or boost sexual performance. Mild stimulants include nicotine and caffeine, while stronger ones include cocaine and amphetamines. At relatively low doses, use may be equated with perceptions of being more alert, intelligent, energetic, or stronger. At higher doses, euphoria is experienced followed or accompanied by toxic effects.

This chapter will discuss cocaine and amphetamines and their similarities and differences. Methamphetamines – although a stimulant structurally similar to amphetamines – differ in their mechanisms of action and effects on the body (National Institute on Drug Abuse [NIDA], 2006). Methamphetamines will be discussed in Chapter 10.

COCAINE

Overview

Cocaine is found naturally in the leaves of Erythroxylon coca, a shrub native to western South America. It was used frequently in the Inca civilization, primarily in religious ceremonies but also by farmers to lessen fatigue. By the latter half of the 19th century, coca extract was used in multiple products, including soft drinks (such as Coca-Cola) and lozenges. With the development of hypodermic syringes, cocaine was also extracted for use as the first local anesthetic and briefly recommended as treatment for such diverse illnesses as asthma and depression.

As cocaine's use became widespread, its associated problems led most states to regulate its consumption and distribution. In 1914, the federal government instituted the Harrison Act that legally permitted cocaine use by prescription only. Cocaine became less popular by the 1930s, when amphetamines were cheap, legal, and readily available. However, by the 1960s, amphetamines were restricted by law – precipitating the resurgence of cocaine. In 1970, the Controlled Substances Act prohibited cocaine possession in the United States with few medical exceptions. It is classified in the United States as a Schedule II drug, meaning that medical indications exist but there is a very high abuse liability. Despite these restrictions, cocaine use continued unabated, and peaked in 1985 with 5.8 million people in the United States who had used cocaine at least once in the past month (Gold & Jacobs, 2005). Since the mid-1980s, this number substantially decreased to 1.4 million in 2011 (Substance Abuse and Mental Health Services Administration [SAMHSA], 2012a). This decline is attributed to the massive public education about the dangers of cocaine that preceded the marked reductions in experimentation and recreational use, rather than the abuse or dependence that remains a daunting problem (Gold & Jacobs, 2005).

Epidemiology

According to the 2011 National Survey on Drug Use and Health, 670,000 Americans ages 12 and older used cocaine for the first time within the previous year (SAMHSA, 2012a). This number is over 30% lower than the 1.0 million who reported first-time use in 2002. However, current cocaine users, defined as those who used at least once in the past month, totaled 1.4 million or 0.5% of the U.S. population. These numbers represent a decline from 2007 (2.1 million or 0.8%) and 2002 (2 million or 0.9%). The number of first-time users of crack cocaine is smaller at 76,000 in 2011 compared to 337,000 in 2002 (SAMHSA, 2012a).

Since 2006, cocaine has been the third most commonly used illicit drug (SAMHSA, 2012a). According to the Drug Abuse Warning Network (DAWN, 2012), cocaine is the most frequently mentioned illicit drug for emergency department admissions. Of the 488,101 cocaine admissions in 2010, 88.7% were over 21 years of age (DAWN, 2012). Annual prevalence of cocaine use is highest among 23-26 year olds (Johnston, O'Malley, Bachman & Schulenberg, 2012b), . The absolute number of current users are more likely to be of mixed race, employed, and have some college education; however, larger percentages of the unemployed reported current use as well as non-high school graduates (SAMHSA, 2012a; Acosta, Haller, & Schnoll, 2005).

Though rates of use are declining, parallel to the general population there was no significant change in past month use of cocaine by youth ages 12 to 17 over the past decade, remaining at 0.3% in 2011 (SAMHSA, 2012a). In 1999, cocaine use "at least once in their life" peaked at 4.7%, 7.7%, and 9.8% for 8th, 10th, and 12th graders, respectively (Johnston, O'Malley, Bachman, & Schulenberg, 2012a). Use subsequently decreased and, in 2011 was reported as 2.2%, 3.3%, and 5.2% for eighth, tenth, and twelfth graders, respectively (Johnston et al., 2012a). For youth between ages 12 and 21 years, cocaine was involved in 11.3% of the total emergency department drug-related visits (DAWN, 2012) in 2010.

Biochemistry

Cocaine affects the body in three ways. It acts

1. as a vasoconstrictor.
2. to prevent reuptake of neurotransmitters in the brain
3. as a modifier of gene expression.

Cocaine exerts direct effects on the blood vessels and gene expression and indirect effects through excessive neurotransmitter activity. Vasoconstriction means that upon cocaine exposure, blood vessel diameter gets smaller. Neurotransmitters affected by cocaine include dopamine, norepinephrine, and serotonin. Dopamine is involved in the brain's "reward" system and is the key transmitter responsible for cocaine's effects. Norepinephrine is integral to the body's regulation of arousal, and serotonin has a central role in the regulation of hunger. To maintain the body's equilibrium, cells must be able to recycle (i.e., reuptake) excess neurotransmitters, a task accomplished by special transporting proteins. It is the buildup of excess neurotransmitters that results in the receptor cells' overactivity that is responsible for cocaine's effects. Although it does not change the basic function of genes, cocaine, like other psychoactive drugs, can change the *level* of a cell's activity, meaning that cocaine can change gene *expression*. Although a separate and specific gene has not been identified, researchers believe that about one-half of an individual's risk for cocaine addiction is attributed to their genetic makeup (Nestler, 2005).

Areas of the brain with high concentrations of dopaminergic cells include the nucleus accumbens, hippocampus, amygdala, and frontal cortex – all parts of the limbic system. Together, these areas, when exposed to cocaine, are responsible for the intense feelings of pleasure, drug cravings, and compulsive drug-seeking behaviors. The greater number of areas in the brain where dopamine is active may be central to the strong feelings of euphoria compared to the effects of the other neurotransmitters. The location and function of each neurotransmitter and the basic effects of cocaine are summarized in Table 9-1.

Health Effects

Short-term effects

The short-term effects of cocaine that users frequently seek include euphoria, heightened alertness and libido, and a decreased need for food and sleep. Undesirable effects that may occur include pain, headaches, anxiety, and increased blood pressure. See Table 9-2 for a more detailed list of effects organized by body system.

TABLE 9-1: NEUROTRANSMITTER LOCATION AND FUNCTION

Neurotransmitter	Location in Brain	Function	Cocaine Effects
Dopamine	Limbic system: • Hippocampus • Amygdala • Frontal cortex	Reward system	Euphoria Increased feelings of pleasure
Norepinephrine	Brain stem: • Locus ceruleus	Level of arousal and attentiveness	Increased wakefulness Increased alertness
Serotonin	Brain stem: • Raphe nuclei	Hunger control	Decreased food intake and weight loss

TABLE 9-2: COCAINE'S EFFECTS BY BODY SYSTEM

General	Respiratory	Nervous	Gastrointestinal
Decreased appetite and weight loss Insomnia Fever, chills, and sweating	Nasal congestion Hoarseness Shortness of breath Productive cough with black sputum	Euphoria Increased alertness Headache Dizziness Tremor Dilated pupils Restlessness Irritability Anxiety	Nausea and vomiting Abdominal pain
Cardiovascular	**Musculoskeletal**		**Genitourinary**
Palpitations Increased heart rate Increased blood pressure	Weakness Back pain Muscle pain		Increased libido

Influences on cocaine's effects

Cocaine's effects can be influenced by body status, preparation, and route of administration as well as the purity of the cocaine. The body's state can influence the intensity of effects. Cocaine's effects seem to be greater when the user is hungry or not exhausted from sexual activity (Repetto & Gold, 2005). Furthermore, the presence of anxiety, fear, or stress may also potentiate cocaine's euphoric effects.

Forms of cocaine

A paste is made from coca leaves, which is the basis for commonly used preparations. Cocaine hydrochloride in powdered form is readily water soluble and is used intranasally or intravenously (I.V.). Street names for the powdered form include *snow* and *coke*. The powdered form can be inhaled (i.e., smoked) if it is extracted into a volatile organic solvent (such as ether) and heated, a process called *freebasing*. Freebasing became less common when it was discovered that a mixture of cocaine, baking soda (or ammonia), and water hardens and the subsequent rock, known as *crack,* can be heated and the resulting vapors inhaled. See Table 9-3 for other street names for powdered and crack cocaine.

TABLE 9-3: SELECTED STREET NAMES FOR COCAINE

Powder Cocaine	Crack Cocaine
Coke	Rock
Snow	Kryptonite
Snowbirds	Apple jacks
White	Sugar block
Flake	Hard rock
Blow	

Routes of administration

Cocaine can be administered through oral, intranasal, intravenous (I.V.), or inhalation routes, referred to as *chewing, snorting* or *sniffing, mainlining,* and *smoking,* respectively. Although there is some controversy about whether one form of cocaine is more addictive than another (Repetto & Gold, 2005), it is difficult to separate the cocaine form used from its route of administration. Routes with the quickest and highest absorption provide the most potent effects. But, regardless of how cocaine is used, it is possible to absorb sufficient amounts to cause toxicity.

The oral route has the slowest rate of absorption with peak effects taking up to 60 minutes. Furthermore, the bioavailability (the amount of drug available for the body to use) is only 20% to 30% because the liver metabolizes 70% to 80% of the cocaine dose. The slower rate of absorption and lower bioavailability are thought to be the reasons the oral route is associated with lower rates of addiction (Repetto & Gold, 2005).

Cocaine is also poorly absorbed by the nasal mucosa. Because cocaine is a potent vasoconstrictor, the blood vessels rapidly become less able to absorb cocaine through the nasal mucosa; this is compounded by the relatively small area available. Bioavailability for intranasal cocaine use is equal to the oral route at 20% to 30%. However, unlike with oral use, the effects from cocaine through the nasal mucosa are much quicker, with effects felt in 3 to 5 minutes and then disappearing in 60 minutes, when peak effects from the oral route occur.

In contrast, after I.V. injection, the entire dose of cocaine directly enters the bloodstream. With a bioavailability of 100%, effects are felt within 30 seconds and last for 10 to 20 minutes. But the intense high delivered by this route is accompanied by the risks of needle use.

Cocaine through inhalation, whether in freebase or rock form, enters the circulation quicker than with I.V. use, perhaps due to the large surface area available in the pulmonary bed (Ray & Ksir, 2002). Cocaine access to the brain is faster via the pulmonary bed compared to the I.V. route where cocaine must travel through the venous system. Cocaine access to the brain via the pulmonary bed is higher despite the low bioavailability of 6% to 32% that occurs when cocaine is heated in preparation for smoking (Repetto & Gold, 2005).

Purity

Cocaine effects are also influenced by its purity. Purity is lower for oral consumption of the coca leaf at 0.5% vs. the intranasal use of powdered form at 20% to 80%. Purity for I.V. and inhalation forms may range as low as 7% and 40% respectively, to 100% for both preparations. Purity is also affected by what drug dealers use to mix with the cocaine. These additions range from inactive substances, such as sugar or talcum powder to active drugs such as other amphetamines. When cocaine is used with alcohol, another set of problems emerge.

Cocaine and alcohol

Although individuals frequently use other drugs in addition to cocaine, simultaneous alcohol use is particularly common. Initially, alcohol may be used to address the anxiety and insomnia caused by cocaine use. Yet when individuals use alcohol and cocaine simultaneously, the body produces a third product, cocaethylene. Effects observed include those from cocaethylene and the independent effects from each drug – the largest impact may be on the cardiovascular system. For example, chest pain is the presenting complaint for 16% of emergency department drug-related visits (Pozner, Levine, & Zane, 2005). Individually, cocaine and alcohol are vasoconstrictors and impair cardiac function. However, use of both drugs simultaneously appears to have additive effects (Repetto & Gold, 2005). Additionally, cocaethylene has a longer half-life – about 2 hours – compared to about 30 minutes for cocaine. Consequently, the effects on the heart, such as cocaine-precipitated increases in blood pressure, are prolonged with increased chances for lethal heart attacks and strokes. Further complicating this scenario is that alcohol magnifies cocaine's pleasurable effects, increasing cocaine use, and thereby creating a vicious cycle in which abstaining from cocaine is more difficult. See Table 9-4 for a summary of absorption rates and bioavailability by route of administration.

Long-term effects

Long-term effects of cocaine exposure involve physical changes on the nerve cells in the nucleus accumbens. New offshoots from the cell's dendrites occur with cocaine exposure, postulated to permit the collection of more nerve signals from other parts of the brain, such as the hippocampus and amygdala. Tolerance to cocaine, a withdrawal syndrome, and cocaine abuse and dependence are likely outcomes of long-term use.

Tolerance occurs when increasing cocaine doses are needed to obtain the same level of euphoria. This occurs when the brain adapts to cocaine's effect, a process that can develop after a single I.V. dose (Repetto & Gold, 2005). The user then increases the amount of cocaine by

TABLE 9-4: ABSORPTION RATES, BIOAVAILABILITY, AND PURITY

Route	Onset of effects	Duration of effects (min)	Bioavailability (%)	Purity (%)
Oral: coca leaf	5 to 10 min	45 to 90	20 to 30	0.5 to 1
Oral: powder	10 to 30 min	45 to 60	20 to 30	20 to 80
Intranasal	2 to 3 min	30 to 45	20 to 30	20 to 80
Intravenous	30 to 45 sec	10 to 20	100	7 to 100
Inhalation	8 to 10 sec	5 to 10	6 to 32	40 to 100

(Gold & Jacobs, 2005; Repetto & Gold, 2005)

increasing the dose or frequency or changing the route of administration in attempts to recapture the euphoria experienced with the first use. Meanwhile, there is an increased likelihood for adverse effects, acute toxicity, and death.

Until the 1980s, it was commonly believed that there were no consistent signs or symptoms when chronic use of cocaine was discontinued. This may have contributed to the myth that cocaine use was safer than drugs such as heroin that have a definite abstinence syndrome. Although it is true that cocaine does not have a classic abstinence syndrome, there is a definite withdrawal syndrome that occurs a few hours to a few days from the last cocaine use. Such symptoms persist for a minimum of 24 hours. This syndrome is characterized by dysphoric mood (such as irritability, depression, or anxiety) and at least two of the following symptoms:

- insomnia or hypersomnia
- unpleasant dreams
- fatigue
- increased appetite
- psychomotor retardation or agitation.

What distinguishes this withdrawal syndrome from a classic abstinence syndrome is that the cocaine withdrawal symptoms are subjective. There are no objective signs that can be reliably measured; these signs are required to establish the standard abstinence syndrome. Normalization of mood may return within days but it occasionally takes weeks. Similarly, drug craving may continue for weeks after the last cocaine use.

Toxicity

Cocaine intoxication may be observed with any use of cocaine – whether or not it is the first use. Intoxication implies either substantial dose or sensitivity to cocaine and can be differentiated from smaller doses by the associated problems with social or occupational functioning. In addition to recent cocaine use and associated euphoria, affected individuals also may display anxiety and hypervigilance accompanied by a rapid heart rate, perspiration, pupillary dilation, or muscular weakness. These symptoms cannot be attributed to another medical condition.

Medical complications

Most toxicities attributed to cocaine involve the central nervous and cardiovascular systems. Seizures are the most common significant complication of the central nervous system (CNS). Seizures occur as a direct result of cocaine reducing the seizure threshold. Cardiac complications include heart failure, irregular heart rhythm, and heart attack. Chronic use of cocaine is also linked with a more rapid progression of high blood pressure and coronary atherosclerosis (Pozner et al., 2005).

Cocaine toxicity can also cause hallucinations and delusions contributing to psychosis that is commonly accompanied by paranoia. Paradoxically, the body may become more sensitive to the adverse effects of continued cocaine use despite tolerance to its euphoric effects. Death has been documented in the context of seemingly low cocaine doses (NIDA, 2010). See Table 9-5 for a more detailed list of medical complications resulting from cocaine use.

TABLE 9-5: MEDICAL COMPLICATIONS FROM COCAINE USE

Body system	Complication
Central nervous	Seizures Stroke Psychosis Coma
Cardiovascular	Heart attack Heart failure Irregular heart rhythm Aortic dissection Accelerated high blood pressure Coronary atherosclerosis
Genitourinary	Kidney failure
Respiratory	Necrosis of the nasal septum

Treatment

Overall, admission to United States' treatment facilities with cocaine as the primary drug of abuse have decreased in recent years, from 14% in 2004 to 8% in 2010 (SAMHSA, 2012b). The vast majority of admissions were due to the use of smoked cocaine. Specifically, in 2010, smoked cocaine constituted 71% of admissions for cocaine. When considering all treatment admissions for 2010, smoked cocaine constituted 6% of admissions for all substances compared to 2% for other forms of cocaine. Generally, higher rates were reported by the mid-Atlantic and southern-Atlantic states (SAMHSA, 2012b).

General considerations

Treatment begins with a comprehensive assessment that includes whether the individual has cocaine abuse or dependence. This entails an evaluation of data from complete history, physical, and laboratory assessments. If possible, historical data should include information from the client's family or other significant others because the client may not be the most reliable source. The physical examination should target the cardiovascular and neurological systems because they are the systems most frequently affected by cocaine use. Chest X-rays and an electrocardiogram (ECG) should be included.

Laboratory evaluation in the form of testing for the presence of cocaine is vital. In addition to cocaine itself, cocaine metabolites may also be screened for benzoylecgonine (the primary metabolite) and ecgonine methyl ester. Although urine testing is probably the most common approach, the type of testing administered (such as blood testing) is dependent on the rationale for use. For example, if it is most important to determine if cocaine is in the system at the time of the examination, blood testing would be the best choice. If determining history of use beyond one week ago, hair analysis is useful. Specifically, each one-half inch of hair represents about one week of history (Gold & Jacobs, 2005). Saliva testing is increasingly used because of the ease of supervision when compared to urine testing and the difficulty of blood testing. Cocaine levels in saliva have been observed to be similar to cocaine levels observed in plasma.

If urine testing is used, the collection should be witnessed to avoid the client altering the sample (such as diluting with water) to mask the presence of cocaine. With shorter-term cocaine use, urine tests may be positive for cocaine metabolites from 2 to 4 days after use. With longer-term use, positive tests may be noted up to 8 days after use.

The *Diagnostic and Statistical Manual of Mental Disorders*, 5th Edition (*DSM-5*) diagnostic criteria (American Psychiatric Association [APA], 2013) for stimulant use disorder focuses on a maladaptive pattern of use leading to clinically significant impairment or distress observed within a 12-month period. *DSM-5* criteria for stimulant use disorder which includes cocaine (or amphetamine and methamphetamine which are discussed later) are similar to the criteria for the broader diagnosis of substance use disorder.

Essentials of treatment

Phases of treatment can be viewed on a continuum from acute to chronic care. The acute phase addresses the client's life-threatening and severe conditions resulting from cocaine toxicity, and it is conducted in an inpatient setting. After the patient is stabilized, cocaine withdrawal symptoms should be addressed in the subacute phase. If there is not a life-threatening condition, this may be the first phase of treatment. Although intensely uncomfortable, cocaine withdrawal is not life threatening. Even so, unless these symptoms are addressed and treated appropriately, the likelihood of relapse to cocaine use is extremely high.

This phase may occur in an outpatient setting, and should ideally include the support of a 12-step self-help group in the community. From this phase forward, cocaine craving should be addressed. Some form of continuing care (also known as *aftercare)* in the community setting must be in place upon discharge from the formal treatment setting to reduce the likelihood of relapse. Continuing care may be life-long because drug dependence is a chronic condition similar to diabetes or hypertension in that it requires on-going treatment.

Clients with cocaine abuse or dependence can be treated in a full range of settings, including inpatient, outpatient, residential, and community-based care. The correct level of placement considers data obtained from the comprehensive assessment. The American Society of Addiction Medicine (ASAM) developed patient placement criteria for adults and for adolescents that can be used as a guide for appropriate placement.

Six dimensions are considered to determine recommendation for placement in one of five levels of care depending upon the acuity of the client's problems. These dimensions include: 1) acute intoxication and/or withdrawal potential; 2) biomedical conditions and complications; 3) emotional/behavioral/ cognitive conditions and complications; 4) readiness to change; 5) relapse/continued use/continued problem potential; and 6) recovery environment.

The levels of care are early intervention, outpatient treatment, intensive outpatient/partial hospitalization, residential/inpatient, and medically managed intensive inpatient treatment.

Basic principles of treatment include the following:

- It will likely take more than one treatment episode.
- The longer the client can remain in active treatment followed by aftercare, the more likely he or she will achieve successful abstinence.
- Aftercare and active treatment should include a 12-step program.
- A "slip" in drug use does not mean the same as a relapse.
- Treatment at appropriate levels is ongoing and likely life-long

(ASAM, 2001).

Note: At the time of this publication, the ASAM *Patient Placement Criteria* is being revised.

Generally, treatment can be directed towards withdrawal symptoms, reversal of postabstinence craving, and/or prevention or decreasing the likelihood of relapse.

Developing an effective drug for cocaine is under intense research and there are numerous on-going clinical trials testing various drugs. However, the cornerstone of treatment is behavioral therapy because as of yet, there is no specific medication for cocaine abuse approved by the Food and Drug Administration (FDA).

Pharmacologic therapy

Detoxification from cocaine requires no treatment other than stopping its use. However, many clients find the symptoms of withdrawal so intensely dysphoric that they are driven to continue using cocaine to fend off the symptoms. Therefore, any medical treatment that helps relieve withdrawal symptoms improves prospects of recovery. If medications are used, they should not include phenothiazines, especially chlorpromazine or haloperidol, because these drugs may lower the seizure threshold.

The majority of the medications currently under clinical investigation already have an FDA-approved indication for another condition or focus on antibody-based treatments. Due to substantial numbers of cocaine users who are also opioid-dependent, effects of methadone or buprenorphine have also been investigated. For example, although buprenorphine is targeted for opioid abuse, it was noted to reduce cocaine use among a sub-group of depressed clients (Margolin et al., 1995). The approved indications tend to reflect such adverse consequences occurring with cocaine toxicity as seizures and cardiovascular complications. Most of the remaining drug trials target dopamine. In addition to dopaminergic medications, other drugs target gamma aminobutyric acid (GABA), serotonin, 5-hydroxytryptamine2 (5-HT) antagonists, andrenoceptor antagonists, and vasodilators.

Disulfiram (Antabuse) has been well researched and is already approved for alcohol dependence. This drug was initially intended for individuals with coexisting cocaine and alcohol dependence. However, it was observed to work with cocaine use alone and, although the exact mechanism is unknown, it does not appear to promote alcohol prevention. In fact, it may work better for cocaine alone than cocaine and alcohol combined (O'Brien, 2005). Disulfiram increases cocaine plasma concentrations, which increases cocaine's undesirable effects to make cocaine use unpleasant.

GABA drugs, such as topiramate, baclofen, and modafinil, have been observed to be promising drugs for decreasing relapse to cocaine use. This class of drugs is already used as antiepileptics. Specifically, modafinil decreases cocaine's euphoric effects and cravings (O'Brien, 2005).

Serotonergic drugs such as fluoxetine have been observed to decrease cocaine use among methadone-maintained persons; risperidone is believed to block cocaine-induced psychosis while decreasing withdrawal symptoms (Acosta et al., 2005). In another clinical trial, fluoxetine was observed to be significantly more effective than placebo for retaining individuals dependent on crack cocaine in drug treatment (Batki, Washburn, Delucchi & Jones, 1996).

Adrenoceptor antagonists, such as labetolol and carvedilol, have been observed to attenuate blood pressure and heart rate effects from cocaine. The response may be better for individuals with more severe withdrawal symptoms. Similarly, such vasodilators as amiloride and isradipine may improve perfusion in the brain. Currently, findings from this category of drugs have unknown functional or clinical significance.

A rare drug, adrogolide, remains purely experimental and has no approved indication for other disorders. This drug was observed to attenuate some of the subjective effects from cocaine but there was no reduction in use (Sofuoglu & Kosten, 2005).

Antibody-based immunotherapy

Immunotherapy uses antibodies designed to bind with cocaine to block or degrade cocaine so that it is less psychoactive. Due to a short half-life, immunotherapy may be most useful for cocaine overdoses. A disadvantage to their use is that these antibodies do not work directly within the CNS, so successful use is dependent only on peripheral contact between the enzyme (or antibody) and consumed cocaine (Dickerson & Janda, 2005). To combat this disadvantage, continuing research is investigating bacteriophages (viruses that infect bacteria) demonstrated to bind with cocaine when injected intranasally. These bacteriophages, unlike the antibodies, directly enter the CNS to bind with cocaine, without any toxic effects of their own (Dickerson & Janda, 2005). Similarly, a vaccine that prevents cocaine from reaching the brain is currently undergoing clinical testing (Sofuoglu & Kosten, 2005). See Table 9-6 for a summary of pharmacologic therapies being researched.

TABLE 9-6: MEDICATIONS UNDER INVESTIGATION FOR COCAINE TREATMENT

Drug classification	Effect on cocaine treatment	FDA indication	Examples
Blocks alcohol metabolism	Increased undesirable cocaine effects	Alcohol dependence	Disulfiram
Gamma aminobutyric acid	Decreased cocaine craving	Seizures	Baclofen Topiramate Modafinil
Serotonergic	Decreased cocaine use	Depression Schizophrenia	Fluoxetine Risperidone
Adrenoceptor	None	High blood pressure	Labetolol Carvedilol
Vasodilator	Improve brain perfusion	Irregular heart rhythm	Amiloride Isradipine
Experimental	Decreases subjective effects of cocaine	None	Adrogolide
Immunotherapy	Block or degrade cocaine	None	Cocaine vaccine

Behavioral therapy

Because there is no approved drug for cocaine abuse, behavioral therapy is the foundation for treatment. The Matrix Model was developed in the 1980s in response to the lack of effective treatment for stimulant abuse (Obert et al., 2000). The Matrix Model is a structured intensive approach designed to be delivered in the outpatient setting. It includes groups for relapse prevention, education, and social support, in addition to individual counseling, urine toxicology, and breath tests for alcohol. The clinician is supportive of the client and uses a direct (rather than a confrontational) approach. The Matrix Model has been effective in reducing cocaine use (Rawson et al., 2002; Shoptaw, Rawson, McCann, & Obert, 1994).

Specific approaches to behavioral therapy for cocaine abuse include cognitive behavioral, motivational interviewing or enhancement, and contingency management. All treatments may be provided on an individual or group basis, or in combination with one another. Some approaches, such as motivational interviewing and contingency management, are more suited to the individual because these approaches require some degree of tailoring to the individual client. Overall, the strongest evidence-based support has been noted for contingency management and cognitive behavioral therapy (CBT) (Rawson et al., 2002). Unless there is a complication such as cardiac arrest, most treatment is delivered in the outpatient setting.

Contingency management

Much of the research on contingency management (also known as *community reinforcement*) was conducted with clients with cocaine abuse. Contingency management is an approach that emphasizes rewards for positive behavior vs. punishment for negative behavior.

For cocaine-dependence, use of incentives was more effective than standard outpatient behavioral treatment for increasing cocaine abstinence (Higgins et al., 1994). However, incentives alone were most effective when combined with contingency management principles (Higgins et al., 2003). Recently, incentives of higher monetary value were compared to those of lower value. High monetary incentives were observed to be more effective for the short-term only (Higgins et al., 2007).

Cognitive behavioral therapy

CBT is based on the social learning theory and emphasizes modification of the client's thoughts and behaviors. For CBT to be effective for cocaine abusers, clients need to have adequate cognitive functioning; unfortunately, this is usually impaired with extended cocaine use (Aharonovich, Nunes & Hasin, 2003). Aharonovich et al. demonstrated that cognitive functioning was lower among individuals who dropped out of treatment compared with those who completed treatment. Similarly, cocaine abstinence in relation to cognitive functioning followed a similar pattern.

Cocaine Anonymous

Cocaine Anonymous, first adapted from but not affiliated with Alcoholics Anonymous, initially began in Los Angeles in 1982 and is now available in the United States, Canada, and Europe (Cocaine Anonymous, n.d.). As a 12-step self-help group, it does not rely on professional personnel to guide recovery. Twelve-step groups usually follow the same format and guidelines of "working through the steps," commonly encouraging service to others as part of recovery. The goal is to cease using cocaine and other "mind-altering substances" (Cocaine Anonymous, n.d.). Groups involve individuals with similar problems who meet regularly to share their experiences and offer support and encouragement to other group members. Family and friends desiring similar support can contact a Co-Anon Family Group.

Motivational intervention

Motivational interventions have not been a commonly researched approach for cocaine abuse. However, Marsden and colleagues (2006) reported that a brief motivational intervention did not demonstrate significantly better outcomes vs. receiving written information on health risks of stimulants and hazardous alcohol use when they studied a sample of 342 cocaine and crack abusers.

Combination therapy

Combinations of behavioral therapies have been investigated for cocaine dependence. In most studies, cocaine dependence was the key eligibility requirement, regardless of the form (powder and crack) abused. However, occasionally, a treatment study will focus solely on crack cocaine users. While investigators have directly compared combinations of behavioral therapies, there is increasing examination of which therapies work best for specific sub-groups of cocaine abusers.

A five-site randomized clinical trial of four behavioral therapies was sponsored by NIDA; the following therapies were compared:

1. individual counseling plus group counseling
2. CBT plus group counseling
3. supportive-expressive therapy plus group counseling
4. group counseling only

(Crits-Christoph et al., 1999).

Study participants (of whom 79% smoked crack) in the individual plus group counseling treatment group showed the most improvement on cocaine abstinence.

Among a sample of methadone-maintained cocaine-dependent persons, Poling and colleagues (2006) observed that buproprion plus contingency management worked best in combination compared to therapy alone or placebo. Similar results with persons who had co-occuring cocaine and opioid dependence were also observed by Schottenfeld et al. (1997; 2005).

Combination therapy is not always better than either therapy by itself. For example, Rawson et al. (2002) found no significant synergistic effects with combination therapy – specifically, contingency management and CBT. Contingency management was more effective in reducing the number of days of cocaine use in the short-term, while CBT produced comparable results in the long-term.

In a direct comparison of CBT and 12-step self-help groups, CBT was found to be more effective for cocaine abstinence. Notably, study participants all smoked crack and included a higher proportion of participants with other psychiatric problems. Upon further analysis, CBT was noted to work better with individuals who also had depression. It was more effective with individuals demonstrating high abstraction cognitive abilities (supporting Aharonovich et al., 2003) as well. But unexpectedly, individuals in the 12-step self-help group with lower abstraction abilities were more successful than those with higher abstraction abilities in attaining cocaine abstinence.

Carroll, Rounsaville, & Gawin (1991) compared relapse prevention and interpersonal psychotherapy and found differential results that were dependent upon the cocaine user. Relapse prevention was noted to be more effective than interpersonal psychotherapy for abstinence with individuals who had more severe cocaine dependence before study entry (at baseline). However, among individuals with less severe cocaine dependence, both therapies demonstrated equivalent effectiveness.

Special Populations

Women

Female adolescents tend to be more sensitive to cocaine's effects, use greater quantities than male adolescents and are, therefore, more likely to become dependent on cocaine (Repetto & Gold, 2005).

Negative birth outcomes for infants exposed to cocaine in utero include low birth weight, preterm delivery, and small head circumference, and such behavioral abnormalities as developmental difficulties and long-term cognitive problems. These outcomes may not be specific to cocaine because it is almost impossible to distinguish cocaine's affects from those of other drugs, poor nutrition, prenatal care obtained, and other maternal factors known to impact birth outcome.

Psychiatric Comorbidity

The coexistence of cocaine abuse and another psychiatric disorder is substantial. For example, in a community sample of 313 crack users who were not in treatment, the most common comorbid disorders were antisocial personality disorder, depression, and posttraumatic stress disorder, at about 24%, 18%, and 12%, respectively (Falck, Wang, Siegal, & Carlson, 2004). However, it is extremely difficult to differentiate psychiatric disorders that are separate from or preceded cocaine abuse because cocaine use alone can induce psychosis and other psychiatric disorders.

Treatment of comorbid psychiatric disorders first requires abstinence from cocaine use to see what psychiatric symptoms remain. Typically, the comorbid disorder improves with cessation of cocaine use and there is a better response to treatment after abstaining from cocaine. When using antidepressants and antipsychotic medications, it is preferable to avoid those that have significant potential for abuse.

AMPHETAMINES

Overview

Amphetamines have been used for over 5,000 years by physicians in China as Ma-huang, also known as *ephedra*. After initial synthesis in 1887, amphetamines were observed to have both vasoconstricting and bronchodilating properties. In 1932, it was marketed as Benzedrine for treatment of nasal congestion. Amphetamines were also prescribed for narcolepsy and attention deficit hyperactivity disorder (ADHD), then known as *minimal brain dysfunction*. Later, these drugs were widely used to treat weight loss, alleviate fatigue experienced by truck drivers, increase endurance in soldiers during World War II, and enhance athletic performance. However, as early as 1933, reports emerged regarding amphetamine abuse (King & Ellinwood, 2005).

Despite early reports of abuse, legal use continued to increase in the 1960s to epidemic proportions. In 1970, the FDA changed amphetamines with higher abuse liabilities from Schedule III to Schedule II drugs, drastically limiting their availability. Subsequent use peaked in the early 1980s when more than 25% of U.S. adults reported amphetamine use at least once in their lifetime (APA, 2000). Currently in the United States, only two FDA-approved indications for Schedule II amphetamines remain – methylphenidate for ADHD and dextroamphetamine for narcolepsy.

Epidemiology

According to the 2011 National Survey on Drug Use and Health, 970,000 people in the U.S. age 12 or older reported current use of stimulants (excluding methamphetamines and cocaine) and 700,000 reported first-time use. These first-time stimulant users constituted over 10% of all persons reporting first-time nonmedical use of psychotherapeutic drugs (a classification that includes licit narcotics, sedatives, tranquilizers, and stimulants. In 2010, an estimated 31,507 emergency department visits involved the misuse and abuse of CNS stimulants; this represents a 196% increase since 2004 (DAWN, 2012). This number includes methamphetamine visits, but excludes cocaine visits.

Use of amphetamines among 8th and 10th graders has been declining steadily since 1996, with reported lifetime use at 5.2% and 9.0%, respectively, in 2011 (Johnston et al., 2012a). However, the rate of decline has not been so steady among 12th graders. The lifetime use rate for this group of 15.3% in 1996 climbed to 16.8% in 2002, before declining to 12.2% in 2011 (Johnston et al., 2012a).

Categories of Amphetamines

Amphetamines can be divided into three basic categories: methylphenidate and similar drugs licensed for ADHD, anorectic drugs formerly licensed for weight loss, and the natural amphetamines ephedra and khat – a natural amphetamine primarily consumed in East Africa and the Arabian Peninsula. Street names for amphetamines are listed in Table 9-7.

TABLE 9-7: SELECTED STREET NAMES FOR AMPHETAMINES
• Speed
• Uppers
• Black beauties
• Beans
• Pep pills
• A
• Aimies
• Ames
• Amp
• Black birds
• Black bombers
• Blue boy

Methylphenidate

Methylphenidate and similar drugs are Schedule II drugs, which means there are medical indications for their use but they have a high abuse potential. Although principally used to increase concentration and focus in people with ADHD, methylphenidate is also used to treat narcolepsy. Students in particular abuse this drug for its ability to increase concentration and alertness, leading to potential improvements in academic performance.

Methylphenidate tablets can be crushed and used intranasally or mixed with water and injected intravenously. In addition to the well-known adverse effects from needle sharing, a danger of I.V. use is that the fillers in tablets can be insoluble. These insoluble fillers can block small blood vessels, causing potentially lethal damage to the lungs, heart, and brain. Formulations include immediate and sustained release; the latter form is commonly preferred by abusers because crushing the tablet immediately releases the entire dose.

Anorectics

Anorectic drugs are either Schedule III or IV, meaning they have a lower abuse potential compared to methylphenidate. Licensed as appetite suppressants, anorectics include mazindol, benzphetamine, diethylproprion, phendimetrazine and, perhaps the most well-known, phentermine. All have amphetamine-like effects but they are less intense. Phentermine was used with fenfluramine and dexfenfluramine as a widely prescribed combination for weight loss but the latter two were removed from the market because of their tendency to cause heart valve problems.

Khat

Khat is found in the young leaves of the Catha edulis shrub native to East Africa and the Arabian peninsula. Used for hundreds of years and legal in parts of its native region, khat may be smuggled into other countries. Its leaves contain cathine and cathinone and it is used in a manner similar to coffee elsewhere in the world.

Cathine is a Schedule IV substance structurally similar to phenylpropanolamine, which is used in the United States as an over-the-counter appetite suppressant and cold medicine. However, cathinone is a Schedule I substance with no licensed indication in the United States. Cathinone is the component of khat with more potent amphetamine effects. As the leaves dry and age, cathinone is changed to cathine and norephedrine (very similar to phenylpropanolamine), resulting in lessened stimulatory effects. The most intoxicating effects are experienced when the leaves are consumed within 48 hours from the time they are picked. Although fresh leaves are not readily available in the United States, cathinone, used intranasally or orally, may be used in their place.

The leaves are chewed to alleviate fatigue or suppress appetite and, in small to moderate doses, are associated with minimal adverse effects. Dried leaves can also be used to make a tea or paste. Unlike the other amphetamines, khat has some anesthetic effects. Compulsive use is associated with mania, delusions, and paranoia, similar to other types of amphetamines.

Ephedra

Ephedra is a natural herb used in China for asthma, hay fever, and nasal congestion. Its principal active ingredients are ephedrine and pseudoephedrine which, when chemically synthesized, are regulated as drugs by the FDA. It is available in the United States as ephedrine in over-the-counter asthma medications and as pseudoephedrine in nasal decongestants. It was commonly used in appetite suppressants and performance-enhancing drugs. Although pseudoephedrine is still an over-the-counter medication, it is now necessary in the United States to request this product directly from the pharmacist because of its illegal use in making methamphetamines. With chronic use, tolerance can develop; in 2004, the FDA prohibited sale of dietary supplements containing ephedra.

Biochemistry

Amphetamines exert their effects by interfering with dopamine reuptake. In high doses, amphetamines also inhibit the monoamine transporter, further preventing dopamine and norepinephrine reuptake. In addition to the resulting dopamine excess, amphetamines release stores of norepinephrine, epinephrine, and serotonin from nerve endings.

Compared to cocaine, amphetamines have a slower onset of action and a longer half-life; therefore, they produce a longer duration of effects. The half-life of amphetamines is from 4 to 8 hours (vs. about 30 minutes for cocaine), contributing to prolonged stimulatory effects. As previously mentioned, amphetamines can be used orally or intravenously.

Health Effects

Health effects observed with amphetamines are caused by excessive amounts of dopamine, norepinephrine, and epinephrine that stimulate the CNS. Effects may be short- or long-term. Desirable short-term effects include an increased concentration and alertness, increased confidence, and weight loss. These affects may also be accompanied by hurried speech; rapid, irregular heart rate; high blood pressure; hyperactivity; nystagmus; confusion; paranoid delusions; hallucinations; depression; and loss of rapid eye movement (REM) sleep. Additional effects indicative of intoxication include hypervigalance, anxiety, tension, impaired judgement, and stereotypical, repetitive behaviors that may include hand wringing or foot tapping. These effects manifest within minutes to 1 hour after taking the drug.

Typically, after intense use (such as a binge), individuals "crash" and experience withdrawal that includes such symptoms as dysphoria, fatigue, unpleasant dreams, agitation, insomnia or hypersomnia, increased appetite, and consequent craving for more amphetamines. Withdrawal symptoms may last a few hours to a few days. It is not unusual for these persons to use other drugs, such as alcohol, opiates, or benzodiazepines to decrease the nervous feelings from amphetamine use or to combat the withdrawal symptoms.

Long-term effects that represent chronic abuse include tolerance, insomnia, heart failure, psychosis, aggressive behavior, and amphetamine abuse and dependence. Symptoms of amphetamine psychosis include delusions, auditory and visual hallucinations, preoccupation with their own thoughts, and violent, erratic behavior – symptoms not unlike those of schizophrenia. The likelihood of psychosis is greater for those taking amphetamines than for those taking cocaine, perhaps due to the longer drug duration. These neurotoxic symptoms can persist for months or years. Cardiotoxic effects include heart attack and death. Another major cause of death is substantially elevated body temperature that may subsequently lead to stroke, convulsions, and coma.

Treatment

In 2010, treatment for amphetamines has decreased from 0.4% of all admissions compared to 1.1% in 2004 (SAMHSA, 2012b). As with cocaine, treatment begins with a comprehensive health history and physical assessment that includes drug testing to support the diagnosis for amphetamine abuse or dependence. All clients should be explicitly asked about their use of other drugs and medications.

Screening for amphetamines is usually done with urine testing. Amphetamines are typically detected in the urine from 1 to 2 days after last use. Because many of these substances are legal, test results show a greater rate of false positives. This poses a challenge in distinguishing between legal and illegal amphetamine use or abuse.

Any potential treatment previously discussed for cocaine would apply for amphetamine abuse as well. The goal of pharmacotherapy is reversal of the brain changes caused by chronic abuse. Similar to cocaine, there is no FDA-approved drug to treat amphetamine abuse; as with cocaine, behavioral approaches are the primary methods employed. The pharmacologic approach is similar to that of cocaine in that it is targeted to withdrawal symptoms. Tricyclic antidepressants, including imipramine and desipramine were first used to treat amphetamine withdrawal in the 1970s; currently other antidepressanats such as fluoxetine may be used to treat dysphoria. Proposed pharmacologic treatments have included such dopamine agonists as bromocriptine and amantadine to reduce craving for amphetamines.

Special Populations

Unlike with other substances, males and females are almost equally as likely to be treated for amphetamine use. Of the total treatment admissions for amphetamines and methamphetamines in 2010, 46.4% were women (SAMHSA, 2012b).

Use during pregnancy is associated with an increased risk for heart defects, gastrochisis, and cleft lip and palate. Infants are commonly jittery or drowsy, and may experience respiratory distress; however, because many women who use amphetamines use more than one drug, it is difficult to attribute all effects specifically to amphetamine (Moline, 2005).

SUMMARY

Cocaine is the third most commonly used illicit drug but is the most frequently mentioned substance documented in drug-related emergency department admissions. Cocaine acts directly as a vasoconstrictor and prevents the reuptake of dopamine, norepinephrine, and serotonin.

Users experience euphoria and heightened alertness frequently accompanied by irritability and anxiety. Intensity and duration of effects vary with cocaine form and route of administration.

Tolerance develops, requiring the user to increase the dose used to experience the same effects. Adverse effects include seizures and chest pain. Currently, there are no FDA-approved drugs for cocaine but many including immunotherapies are in development. The foundation of effective treatment is behavioral therapy. In the future, the best outcomes will probably be realized with a combination of drug and behavioral therapy.

In 2011, 22% of all Americans reported first-time nonmedical use of psychotherapeutic drugs, with a significant number attributed to amphetamine abuse (SAMHSA, 2012a). Unlike cocaine, amphetamines have licensed medical indications and, with the exception of methylphenidate and similar drugs, several types have less abuse potential. As stimulants, both amphetamines and cocaine interfere with dopamine reuptake and have similar health effects. However, a critical difference is that amphetamines have a much longer half-life; therefore, their effects are prolonged.

Neither amphetamines nor cocaine have an FDA-approved drug to treat abuse. They are both primarily treated with behavioral approaches.

EXAM QUESTIONS

CHAPTER 9

Questions 45-51

Note: Choose the one option that BEST answers each question.

45. The key neurotransmitter responsible for the effects of cocaine is

    a. dopamine.
    b. norepinephrine.
    c. serotonin.
    d. acetylcholine.

46. Bioavailability is the amount of drug available for the body to use. The route of administration of cocaine with the highest bioavailability is

    a. oral.
    b. intravenous.
    c. intranasal.
    d. inhalation.

47. Inhalation of rock cocaine

    a. is associated with a high bioavailability.
    b. is the most common way to use cocaine.
    c. produces fewer toxic effects than intranasal use.
    d. results in the fastest access to the brain.

48. Which statement regarding cocaine withdrawal is correct?

    a. A definite withdrawal syndrome occurs within a few days after the last use.
    b. Drug cravings only last for the first 48 hours after the last use.
    c. Cocaine has a classic abstinence syndrome.
    d. Withdrawal syndrome is characterized by decreased appetite and manic behavior.

49. A basic principle of cocaine treatment is

    a. one treatment episode is all that is required for a permanent cure.
    b. the longer a client remains in active treatment, the more likely he or she will relapse.
    c. a slip in drug use is the same as a relapse.
    d. treatment is ongoing and most likely life-long.

50. The difference between the mechanisms of action of cocaine and those of amphetamines is that amphetamines have a

    a. shortened stimulatory effect.
    b. shorter duration of effect.
    c. slower onset of action.
    d. shorter half-life.

51. Disulfiram is an effective treatment for cocaine dependence by increasing cocaine's undesirable effects. However, the FDA has approved Disulfiram only for the treatment of

    a. opioid dependence.
    b. alcohol dependence.
    c. amphetamine dependence.
    d. nicotine dependence.

REFERENCES

Acosta, M.C., Haller, D.L., & Schnoll, S.H. (2005). *Cocaine and stimulants. In R.J. Frances, S.I. Miller, & A.H. Mack (Eds.), Clinical textbook of addictive disorders* (3rd ed., pp. 184-218). New York: Guilford Press.

Aharonovich, E., Nunes, E., & Hasin, D. (2003). Cognitive impairment, retention and abstinence among cocaine abusers in cognitive-behavioral treatment. *Drug and Alcohol Dependence, 71*(2), 207-11.

American Psychiatric Association. (2013). *Diagnostic and statistical manual of mental disorders* (5th ed.). Washington, DC: American Psychiatric Association.

American Society of Addiction Medicine. (2001). Patient placement criteria for the treatment of substance related disorders (2nd edition, revised). Philadelphia: Lippincott Williams & Wilkins.

Batki, S.L., Washburn, A.M., Delucci, K., & Jones, R.T. (1996). A controlled trial of fluoxetine in crack cocaine dependence. *Drug and Alcohol Dependence, 41*(2), 137-42.

Carroll, K.M., Rounsaville, B.J., & Gawin, F.H. (1991). A comparative trial of psychotherapies for ambulatory cocaine users: Relapse prevention and interpersonal psychotherapy. *American Journal of Drug and Alcohol Abuse, 17*(3), 229-47.

Cocaine Anonymous. (n.d.). *C.A.'s purpose.* Accessed March 15, 2013, from http://www.ca.org/

Crits-Christoph, P., Siqueland, L., Blaine, J., Frank, A., Luborsky, L., Onken, L., et al. (1999). Psychosocial treatments for cocaine dependence. *Arch Gen Psychiatry, 56*:493-502.

Dickerson, T.J. & Janda, K.D. (2005). Recent advances for the treatment of cocaine abuse: Central nervous system immunopharmacotherapy. *American Association Pharm-aceutical Scientists Journal, 7*(3), E579-586.

Drug Abuse Warning Network. (2012). *Highlights of the 2010 Drug Abuse Warning Network (DAWN) findings on drug-related emergency department visits.* Accessed March 15, 2013 from http://www.samhsa.gov/data/2k12/DAWN096/SR096EDHighlights2010.htm

Falck, R.S., Wang, J., Siegal, H.A., & Carlson, H.G. (2004). The prevalence of psychiatric disorders among a community sample of crack cocaine users: An exploratory study with practical implications. *Journal of Nervous Mental Disorders, 192*(7), 503-507.

Gold, M.S. & Jacobs, W.S. (2005). Cocaine and crack: Clinical aspects. In J.H. Lowinson, P. Ruiz, R.B. Millman, & J.G. Langrod (Eds.), *Substance abuse: A comprehensive textbook* (4th ed., pp. 218-251). Philadelphia: Lippincott Williams & Wilkins.

Higgins, S.T., Budney, A.J., Bickel, W.K., Foerg, F.E., Donham, R., & Badger, G.J. (1994). Incentives improve outcome in outpatient behavioral treatment of cocaine dependence. *Archives of General Psychiatry, 51*(7), 568-76.

Higgins, S.T., Heil, S.H., Dantona, R., Donham, R., Matthews, M., & Badger, G.J. (2007). Effects of varying the monetary value of voucher-based incentives on abstinence achieved during and following treatment among cocaine-dependent outpatients. *Addiction, 102*(2), 271-81.

Higgins, S.T., Sigmon, S.C., Wong, C.J., Heil, S.H., Badger, G.J., Donham, R., Dantona, R.L, & Anthony, S. (2003). Community reinforcement therapy for cocaine-dependent outpatients. *Archives of General Psychiatry, 60*(10), 1043-52.

Johnston, L. D., O'Malley, P. M., Bachman, J. G., & Schulenberg, J. E. (2012a). *Monitoring the Future national survey results on drug use, 1975-2011. Volume I: Secondary school students.* Ann Arbor: Institute for Social Research, The University of Michigan.

Johnston, L. D., O'Malley, P. M., Bachman, J. G., & Schulenberg, J. E. (2012b). *Monitoring the Future national survey results on drug use, 1975-2011. Volume II: College students and adults ages 19-50.* Ann Arbor: Institute for Social Research, The University of Michigan.

Johnston, L. D., O'Malley, P. M., Bachman, J. G., & Schulenberg, J. E. (2013). *Monitoring the Future national results on adolescent drug use: Overview of key findings, 2012.* Ann Arbor: Institute for Social Research, The University of Michigan.

King, G.R. & Ellinwood, E.H. (2005). Am-phe-ta-mines and other stimulants. In J.H. Lowinson, P. Ruiz, R.B. Millman, & J.G. Langrod (Eds.), *Substance abuse: A comprehensive textbook (4th ed., pp. 277-302).* Philadelphia: Lippincott Williams & Wilkins.

Margolin, A., Kosten, T.R., Avants, S.K., Wilkins, J., Ling, W., Beckson, M., et al. (1995). A multicenter trial of buproprion for cocaine dependence in methadone-maintained patients. *Drug and Alcohol Dependence, 40*(2), 125-31.

Marsden, J., Stillwell, G., Barlow, H., Boys, A., Taylor, C., Hunt, N., & Farrell, M. (2006). An evaluation of a brief motivational intervention among young ecstasy and cocaine users: No effect on substance abuse and alcohol use outcomes. *Addiction, 101*(7), 1014-26.

Moline, M.L. (2005). *Amphetamine use and pregnancy.* Accessed March 15, 2013, from http://www.obfocus.com/high-risk/amphetamine.htm

National Institute on Drug Abuse. (2006). *Methamphetamine abuse and addiction.* Research report series. (NIH Publication No. 06-4210). Accessed March 15, 2013, from http://www.drugabuse.gov/publications/research-reports/methamphetamine-abuse-addiction

National Institute on Drug Abuse. (2010). *Cocaine abuse and addiction.* Research report series. (NIH Publication No. 10-4166). Accessed March 15, 2013, from http://www.drugabuse.gov/publications/research-reports/cocaine-abuse-addiction

Nestler, E.J. (2005). The neurobiology of cocaine addiction. *NIDA Science & Practice Perspectives, 3*(1), 13-24.

Obert, J.L., McCann, M.J., Marinelli-Casey, P., Weiner, A., Minsky, S., Brethen, P., et al. (2000). The Matrix model of outpatient stimulant abuse treatment: History and description. *Journal of Psychoactive Drugs, 32*(2), 157-164.

O'Brien, C.P. (2005). Anticraving medications for relapse prevention: A possible new class of psychoactive medications. *American Journal of Psychiatry, 162*(8), 1423-1431.

Poling, J., Oliveto, A., Petry, N., Sofuoglu, M., Gonsai, K., Gonzalez, G., et al. (2006). Six-month trial of buproprion with contingency management for cocaine dependence in a methadone-maintained population. *Archives of General Psychiatry, 63*(2), 219-28.

Pozner, C.N., Levine, M., & Zane, R. (2005). The cardiovascular effects of cocaine. *Journal of Emergency Medicine, 29*(2), 173-178.

Rawson, R.A., Huber, A., McCann, M., Shoptaw, S., Farabee, D., Reiber, C., et al. (2002). A comparison of contingency management and cognitive behavioral approaches during methadone maintenance treatment for cocaine dependence. *Archives of General Psychiatry, 59*(9), 817-24.

Ray, O.S. & Ksir, C.L. (2002). *Drugs, society, and human behavior* (9th ed.). Boston: McGraw Hill.

Repetto, M. & Gold, M.S. (2005). Cocaine and crack: Neurobiology. In J.H. Lowinson, P. Ruiz, R.B. Millman, & J.G. Langrod (Eds.), *Substance abuse: A comprehensive textbook* (4th ed., pp. 195-218). Philadelphia: Lippincott Williams & Wilkins.

Schottenfeld, R.S., Chawarski, M.C., Pakes, J.R., Pantalon, M.V., Carroll, K.M., & Kosten, T.R. (2005). Methadone versus buproprion with contingency management or performance feedback for cocaine and opioid dependence. *The American Journal of Psychiatry, 162*(2), 340-9.

Schottenfeld, R.S., Pakes, J.R., Oliveto, A., Ziedonis, D., & Kosten, T.R. (1997). Buprenorphine vs. methadone maintenance treatment for concurrent opioid dependence and cocaine abuse. *Archives of General Psychiatry, 54*(8), 713-20.

Shoptaw, S., Rawson, R.A., McCann, M.J., Obert, J.L. (1994). The Matrix model of outpatient stimulant abuse treatment: Evidence of efficacy. *Journal of Addictive Diseases, 13*(4), 129-141.

Sofuoglu, M. & Kosten, T.R. (2005). Novel approaches to the treatment of cocaine addiction. *CNS Drugs, 19*(1), 13-25.

Substance Abuse and Mental Health Services Administration. (2012a). *Results from the 2011 National survey on drug use and health: Summary of national findings* (NSDUH Series H-44, HHS Publication No. (SMA) 12-4713). Rockville, MD. Accessed March 15, 2013 from http://www.samhsa.gov/data/NSDUH/2k11Results/NSDUHresults2011.htm

Substance Abuse and Mental Health Services Administration. (2012b). *Treatment Episode Data Set (TEDS) 2000-2010: National admissions to substance abuse treatment services*. Retrieved March 15, 2013 from http://www.samhsa.gov/data/2k12/TEDS2010N/TEDS2010NWeb.pdf

CHAPTER 10

METHAMPHETAMINE

CHAPTER OBJECTIVE

After completing this chapter, the learner will be able to describe the history of methamphetamine use in the United States and the profound, long-lasting clinical effects of methamphetamine abuse.

LEARNING OBJECTIVES

After studying this chapter, the learner will be able to:

1. Describe the development of methamphetamine use in the United States.
2. Explain the epidemiology and prevalence of methamphetamine use disorder.
3. Describe the clinical effects of methamphetamine on the brain.
4. Identify common psychological and physical symptoms of methamphetamine use disorders.
5. Describe treatment modalities for methamphetamine use disorder.

OVERVIEW

Methamphetamine is a powerful central nervous stimulant that is highly addictive. The use of methamphetamine has markedly increased in the past decade and research suggests that it is the fastest growing illegal drug in North America (Barr et al., 2006). In many parts of North America and Hawaii, methamphetamine use is at epidemic proportions. Methamphetamine is classified as a psychostimulant and is structurally similar to such other drugs as cocaine and amphetamine. However, unlike cocaine and amphetamine, it has a much longer duration of action and is significantly more neurotoxic. The neurotoxicity of methamphetamine is profound and persists long after its use has discontinued.

HISTORY

Methamphetamine was first synthesized from ephedrine in Japan in the early 1900s and became widely used by Japanese, German, and American soldiers to combat military fatigue during World War II (Meredith, Jaffe, Ang-Lee & Saxon A., 2005). In the 1950s and 1960s several amphetamine products were developed for the purposes of weight loss, energy boosts, and increased alertness. Amphetamine and methamphetamine were also used in over-the-counter inhalers and nasal sprays. Urban legend suggests that Jack Kerouak, under the influence of methamphetamine, wrote *On the Road* in 21 days on a single scroll of paper and that John F. Kennedy relied on injections of methamphetamine during the Cuban Missile Crisis (Case, 2005).

Between 1967 and 1970 more than 31 million prescriptions and 10 billion tablets of legal amphetamine and methamphetamine were dispensed – mostly to women (Case, 2005). As a result of the corresponding increase in methamphetamine and amphetamine addiction; pharmaceutical companies withdrew several of these products and policy makers passed legislation restricting the availability of these drugs.

In response to its decreased availability, underground methamphetamine laboratories emerged in the Bay area of California in the early 1960s and motorcycle gangs developed control of the drug's illegal distribution (Meredith et al., 2005). Hawaii and Western, Northwestern, and Southwestern areas of the United States became hotbeds of illicit methamphetamine activity. In the early 1990s "law enforcement efforts targeting motorcycle gangs, coupled with the development of simpler methods for methamphetamine synthesis, had the effect of shifting control of the U.S. illicit methamphetamine market to Mexican-based traffickers" (Meredith et al., 2005, p. 142).

Most recently, the advent of the ephedrine-pseudophedrine reduction method has resulted in the development of "superlabs" and "mom and pop" laboratories. This method of reduction is quite simple; the processes are available on the internet and the results create a higher yield and a more pure methamphetamine product. Not surprisingly, methamphetamine use disorders have skyrocketed. In addition, the toxic effects of methamphetamine production using the ephedrine-pseudophedrine reduction method have resulted in serious environmental consequences. For every 1 lb of methamphetamine produced, 5 to 6 lb of toxic waste is created (KCI-Anti Meth Site, n.d.), which is dangerous to children, adults, and communities. "Meth cooks often pour leftover chemicals and byproduct sludge down drains in nearby plumbing, storm drains, or directly onto the ground. These byproducts pose long-term hazards because they persist in the soil or groundwater. Clean-up costs are exorbitant because chlorinated solvents and other toxins usually must be incinerated. The cost of cleanup by the EPA ranges from $5000 to $150,000" (KCI Anti-Meth Site, n.d.).

In 2001, Congress passed the Comprehensive Methamphetamine Control Act to increase penalties associated with methamphetamine production and trafficking (KCI-Anti Meth Site, n.d.). In 2006, The Combat Meth Act was signed into law. This law limits the amount of product (ephedrine or pseudoephedrine) that may be sold per day and/or per month, and requires that purchasers provide identification and sign a sales log. Drugs containing pseudoephedrine or ephedrine now must be kept behind the counter or in a locked case. The Food and Drug Administration (FDA) has approved methamphetamine for narcolepsy, attention deficit hyperactivity disorder (ADHD), HIV/AIDS, severe depression, mood disorders, and tardive dyskinesia. However, it is rarely prescribed because of its abuse potential; if it is prescribed, it is generally for narcolepsy and ADHD.

PREVALENCE

The World Health Organization (WHO) estimates that 35 million people worldwide abuse methamphetamine or amphetamine as compared to 15 million cocaine abusers and 10 million opiate users (Meredith et al., 2005). The Community Epidemiology Work Group (CEWG) reported that in 2006 methamphetamine abuse continued to be a problem in the West, with rates indicating high levels of abuse in Honolulu, San Diego, Seattle, San Francisco and Los Angeles. Methamphetamine abuse continued to spread throughout other areas of the country, including rural and urban areas in the South and Midwest. It was reported to be the fastest growing problem in metropolitan Atlanta (NIDA, 2006). In the United States, methamphetamine is second only to marijuana in frequency of abuse (Substance Abuse and Health Services Administration (SAMHSA), 2012b).

In 2011, the number and percentage of persons aged 12 or older who were current users of methamphetamine (439,000 or 0.2 percent) were similar to those from 2007 through 2010, but lower than those from 2002 through 2006. (SAMHSA, 2012a). The Monitoring the Future survey, which assesses the extent of drug use among adolescents, found that in 2011, 2.1% of high school seniors, 2.1% of tenth graders, and 1.3% of eighth graders had reported lifetime use of methamphetamine (Johnston, O'Malley, Bachman, & Schulenberg, 2012).

Methamphetamine use is 5 to 10 times more prevalent in urban gay and bisexual men than it is in the general population because of its stimulant effects, which result in an increase in confidence and libido (Shoptaw, 2006). Evidence suggests that use of methamphetamine during a sexual encounter in gay and bisexual men results in an increased incidence of sexually-transmitted infections and HIV-risk behaviors (Menza et al., 2007).

BIOCHEMISTRY AND HEALTH EFFECTS

Methamphetamine is a major central nervous system (CNS) stimulant that is considered a Schedule II drug with a high abuse potential. Methamphetamine is similar in size, shape, and chemical structure to dopamine and, as a result, triggers the release of large amounts of dopamine and lesser amounts of serotonin and norepinephrine. Dopamine is one of the neurotransmitters involved in reward behavior. All stimulants and most drugs of addiction increase the release of dopamine. The release of dopamine results in a rush of euphoria and a feeling of great pleasure. Cocaine causes the release of 400% more dopamine than occurs naturally. However, crystal methamphetamine releases almost 1500% more dopamine, which is one of the reasons it is so addictive and dangerous. The user pursues drug use in an attempt to continue this reward/pleasure cycle (McVinney, 2005). Although both methamphetamine and cocaine are psychostimulants, there are differences between them. (See Table 10-1).

Animal research shows that high doses of methamphetamine damage neuron cell endings (NIDA, 2006), making it neurotoxic. It appears that the massive release of dopamine and the unusually long duration of action of methamphetamine (12-hour half-life) damages the nerve terminals and interferes with the dopamine and serotonin transmitter systems. Recently, neuroimaging studies of methamphetamine abuse clients confirmed this significant and extensive neural damage (Barr et al., 2006). "Numerous studies have confirmed that methamphetamine abuse is associated with cognitive impairment, the most consistent and severe changes include specific impairments in working memory, attention, and executive function" (Barr et al., 2006, p. 309).

TABLE 10-1: METHAMPHETAMINE VS. COCAINE

Methamphetamine	Cocaine
Stimulant	Stimulant and local anesthetic
Man-made	Plant-derived
Smoking produces a long-lasting high	Smoking produces a brief high
50% of the drug is removed from the body in 12 hours	50% of the drug is removed from the body in 1 hour
Increases dopamine release and blocks dopamine re-uptake	Blocks dopamine re-uptake
Limited medical use	Limited use as a local anesthetic in some surgical procedures

(NIDA, 2006)

Common street names for methamphetamine are *meth, speed, crank, chalk, go-fast, zip, cristy, L.A. ice, crystal, glass,* or *quartz.* It is a white, odorless, bitter-tasting crystalline powder that dissolves in water or alcohol (NIDA, 2006). Methamphetamine can be smoked; snorted; ingested orally; injected intravenously (often referred to as *slamming*), intramuscularly, or through skin-popping; or taken rectally (often referred to as *booty bumping*).

Smoking and injection of methamphetamine results in an immediate "rush" with an onset of action occurring in seconds to minutes. The "high" associated with the other methods of administration lasts longer but is less intense. Because methamphetamine is a psychoactive stimulant, the drug stimulates the sympathetic nervous system. Initially, the drug causes euphoria, a heightened sense of awareness, increased energy, hypersexuality, and decreased anxiety. The methamphetamine user experiences a marked increased heart rate, hypertension, dilation of the pupils, diaphoresis (sweating), increased respiratory rate, decreased appetite, and increased body temperature (NIDA, 2006, 2010; Barr et al., 2006; Meredith et al., 2005). As the initial euphoria declines and tolerance develops, the user will repeatedly administer methamphetamine in an attempt to recapture the feeling of euphoria. This is referred to as the "binge and crash" pattern of use (NIDA, 2006). The "crash" is characterized more by psychiatric complaints than physical complaints. Methamphetamine users describe withdrawal feelings of depression, irritability, restlessness, anxiety, extreme exhaustion, insomnia, suicidal ideation, aggression, and paranoia (Meredith et al., 2005).

CLINICAL IMPLICATIONS

Evidence suggests that methamphetamine abuse clearly damages the neurocognitive ability of the user and that the severity of the damage is related to the duration and amount of use. What is most troubling is that these neurocognitive deficits persist well in to abstinence. Human data suggests that deficits in memory, learning, psychomotor speed, and information processing persist after 3 years of abstinence (Meredith et al., 2005).

Clinical indicators of methamphetamine abuse include anorexia; substantial weight loss; itching and tickling under the skin that clients often describe as "bugs in my skin" ("meth bugs"); scratching and picking at the skin; severe dental problems ("meth mouth"); paranoia and hallucinations; jerky, rapid body movement; and sexual dysfunction ("crystal dick"). Renal failure, dehydration, seizures, hyperthermia, heart attack, and stroke also occur in methamphetamine users. Table 10-2 lists some of the effects of methamphetamine abuse.

Use of methamphetamine places the client at high risk for sexually-transmitted infections and HIV. Intravenous use of methamphetamine increases the risk of transmission of hepatitis B and C and HIV. High-risk sexual practices, men having sex with women, men having sex with men, and trading drugs for sex increases the risk of transmission of HIV, hepatitis B, and other sexually-transmitted infections (NIDA, 2006; Meredith et al., 2005; Barr et al., 2006).

The fetal effects of methamphetamine are a significant problem in the United States. Data suggests that methamphetamine abuse during pregnancy may result in prenatal complications, low birth weight, premature delivery, birth defects, altered behavioral patterns, abnormal reflexes, and extreme irritability of the infant (Smith et al., 2006; Gilbert, 2004). Long-term implications include such learning disabilities

TABLE 10-2: EFFECTS OF METHAMPHETAMINE ABUSE
Short-term effects can include: • increased attention and decreased fatigue • increased activity and wakefulness • decreased appetite • euphoria and rush • increased respiration • rapid/irregular heartbeat • hyperthermia. **Long-term effects can include:** • addiction • psychosis, including – paranoia – hallucinations – repetitive motor activity • changes in brain structure and function • memory loss • aggressive or violent behavior • mood disturbances • severe dental problems • weight loss. (NIDA, 2006)

as ADHD and poor reading and math skills and such aggressive behaviors as oppositional development disorder (Gilbert, 2004).

Maternal red flags for a methamphetamine substance use disorder are similar to those of other drugs and include history of drug use during pregnancy and poor prenatal care; multiple skin lesions and scratching; poor dentition; and the onset of rapid labor and delivery (Gilbert, 2004). Infant red flags include maternal drug use, maternal refusal for drug screening, extreme irritability and jitteriness, poor feeding, and physical features that suggest alcohol or drug use (Gilbert, 2004).

TREATMENT

Treatment outcomes for methamphetamine users appear to be similar to those of cocaine abusers. While the pharmacology and effects of methamphetamine and cocaine differ, these drugs have common elements. Studies suggest that methamphetamine and cocaine users have similar outcomes when exposed to the same treatments (UCLA, n.d.). Currently, there are two treatment approaches that have evidence to support their efficacy in the treatment of methamphetamine abuse – the Matrix Model and the Contingency Management Model (UCLA, n.d.). The Matrix Model incorporates cognitive behavioral therapy (CBT) (which helps clients change their thinking, expectations, and behaviors associated with their drug use), positive reinforcement, components of motivational interviewing, family involvement, a 12-step approach, and regular urine testing.

Counseling is done via group and individual sessions approximately three times per week for 16 weeks; the client then participates in group work for an additional 36 weeks. Methamphetamine users who participated in Matrix Model treatment programs were found to remain in treatment longer, gave more methamphetamine-negative urine samples, and completed treatment at higher rates than those methamphetamine users who received other treatment (UCLA, n.d.). An interesting finding in this study was that methamphetamine users who were ordered to treatment via the court system demonstrated superior results, suggesting that drug-ordered court treatment programs were beneficial (UCLA, n.d.). Additional information about the Matrix Model may be found at www.Hazelden.org or www.SAMHSA.gov.

Contingency management is a model that uses positive reinforcement to produce behavioral change. Positive reinforcement may be verbal and incorporate a reward system that results in greater privileges, higher status, and/or vouchers (dinners, movies, gasoline, etc.) that reward abstinence. "Contingency management techniques have been implemented with meth users in Southern California by the group at UCLA and by researchers in the NIDA Clinical

Trials Network. The results of these investigations have provided powerful support to the efficacy of this behavioral strategy as treatment for meth abuse" (UCLA, n.d.).

One of the challenges of treating methamphetamine users is that the altered neurocognitive abilities associated with methamphetamine use (deficits in memory, learning, psychomotor speed, and information processing) affect the client's ability to adhere and benefit from behavioral treatments. Antidepressant medications are helpful in combating the depressive symptoms that occur in methamphetamine users. Currently, there are no pharmacological treatments for methamphetamine dependence but this remains an active area of pharmaceutical research.

Acute treatment of methamphetamine toxicity should occur in an emergency department and focus on the immediate physical symptoms (NIDA, 2006). Managing the hyperthermia by cooling the client and managing the risk of convulsions with anticonvulsant drugs decreases morbidity and mortality (NIDA, 2006). If the client is not at risk for hyperthermia or convulsions, he or she may be monitored in a quiet area with decreased stimulation. In the presence of extreme agitation, antianxiety agents such as benzodiazepines are helpful (NIDA, 2006). In the presence of methamphetamine psychosis, short-term neuroleptics are effective.

SUMMARY

The use of methamphetamine, a highly additive psychostimulant, is a serious problem in the United States and Canada. The ease of chemically distilling methamphetamine from ephedrine-pseudoephredrine has greatly contributed to the increased prevalence of methamphetamine use disorder.

The long-lasting neurotoxic effects of this drug demonstrate that chronic methamphetamine users exhibit deficits in memory, learning, psychomotor speed, and information processing. These deficits persist at up to 3 years after abstinence occurs and impair the user's cognitive ability.

The effects of methamphetamine on adolescents and fetal growth and development are profound. Treatment options are currently limited and CBT is the mainstay of treatment. Drug companies are aggressively pursuing pharmaceutical treatment options; however, none are currently FDA-approved.

EXAM QUESTIONS

CHAPTER 10

Questions 52-59

Note: Choose the one option that BEST answers each question.

52. Methamphetamine use in the United States has skyrocketed because of the
    a. Comprehensive Methamphetamine Control Act.
    b. over-prescribing of amphetamines by health care providers.
    c. simplified ephedrine-pseudophedrine reduction method.
    d. illegal prescribing of methamphetamine.

53. When ranking illegal drugs abused in the United States, methamphetamine ranks
    a. first.
    b. second.
    c. third.
    d. fourth.

54. Methamphetamine is classified as a(n)
    a. opiate.
    b. stimulant.
    c. hallucinogen.
    d. depressant.

55. Methamphetamine primarily effects the neurotransmitter
    a. dopamine.
    b. serotonin.
    c. norepinephrine.
    d. epinephrine.

56. A common street name for methamphetamine is
    a. baggy.
    b. jack.
    c. L.A. ice.
    d. booty.

57. Methamphetamine abuse primarily affects
    a. liver function.
    b. respiratory function.
    c. immunologic function.
    d. neurocognitive function.

58. Which statement is suggestive of methamphetamine abuse?
    a. "I keep seeing lights all around me."
    b. "I feel like I have bugs under my skin."
    c. "My heart hurts because it's beating so hard."
    d. "I keep hearing voices talking to me all the time."

59. The mainstay of treatment for methamphetamine abuse is
    a. cognitive behavioral therapy.
    b. electroshock therapy.
    c. pharmaceutical therapy.
    d. acupuncture therapy.

REFERENCES

Barr, A.M., Panenka, W., MacEwan, T., Thornton, A., Lang, D., Honer, W., et al. (2006). The need for speed: an update on methamphetamine addiction. *Journal of Psychiatry Neuro-science, 31*(5): 301-313.

Case, P. (August, 2005). *The History of Methamphetamine: An epidemic in context.* Presentation. 1st National Conference on Methamphetamine, HIV and Hepatitis. Salt Lake City, UT.

Gilbert, J. (September, 2004). *Medical effects of methamphetamine on children.* Presentation. Idaho's Second Annual Drug Endangered Children Conference.

Johnston, L. D., O'Malley, P. M., Bachman, J. G., & Schulenberg, J. E. (2012). *Monitoring the Future national survey results on drug use, 1975-2011. Volume I: Secondary school students.* Ann Arbor: Institute for Social Research, The University of Michigan.

KCI: The Anti-Meth Site. (n.d.). *Methamphetamine frequently asked questions.* Retrieved March 15, 2013, from http://www.kci.org/meth_info/faq_meth.htm

McVinney, D. (2005). *The pharmacology of crystal methamphetamine.* Presentation. 1st National Conference on Methamphetamine, HIV and Hepatitis. Retrieved March 15, 2013, from http://www.kci.org/meth_info/PowerPoint/index.html

Menza, T.W., Colfax, G., Shoptaw, S., Fleming, M., Guzman, R., Klausner, J., et al. (2007). Interest in a methamphetamine intervention among men who have sex with men. *Journal of Sexually Transmitted Diseases, 34*(4), 209-214.

Meredith, C.W., Jaffe, C., Ang-Lee, K., & Saxon, A. (2005). Implications of chronic methamphetamine use: A literature review. *Harvard Review of Psychiatry, 13*(3), 141-154.

National Institutes on Drug Abuse. (2006). *Methamphetamine abuse and addiction.* Research report series (NIH Publication No. 06-4210). Retrieved March 15, 2013, from http://www.nida.nih.gov/PDF/RRMetham.pdf

National Institute on Drug Abuse. (2010). *NIDA Info Facts: Methamphetamine.* Retrieved March 15, 2013, from http://www.drugabuse.gov/infofacts/Methamphetamine.html

Shoptaw, S. (2006). Methamphetamine use in urban gay and bisexual populations. *Perspective - Methamphetamine Use, 14*(2), 84-87. Accessed March 15, 2013 from https://iasusa.org/sites/default/files/tam/14-2-84.pdf

Smith, L.M., LaGrasse, L.L., Derauf, C., Grant, P., Shah, R., Arria, A., et al. (2006). The infant development, environment, and lifestyle study: Effects of prenatal methamphetamine exposure, polydrug exposure, and poverty on intrauterine growth. *Pediatrics,118*(3), 1149-56.

Substance Abuse and Mental Health Services Administration. (2012a). *Results from the 2011 National survey on drug use and health: Summary of national findings* (NSDUH Series H-44, HHS Publication No. (SMA) 12-4713). Rockville, MD. Accessed March 15, 2013 from http://www.samhsa.gov/data/NSDUH/2k11Results/NSDUHresults2011.htm

Substance Abuse and Mental Health Services Administration. (2012b). *Treatment Episode Data Set (TEDS) 2000 – 2010: National admissions to substance abuse treatment services*. Retrieved March 15, 2013 from http://www.samhsa.gov/data/2k12/TEDS2010N/TEDS2010NWeb.pdf

UCLA Integrated Substance Abuse Programs. (n.d.). *Methamphetamine treatment*. Retrieved March 15, 2013, from http://www.methamphetamine.org/html/treatment.html

CHAPTER 11

OPIOIDS

CHAPTER OBJECTIVE

After completing this chapter, the learner will be able to describe the effects of opioid use disorder on the body and current treatment approaches.

LEARNING OBJECTIVES

After studying this chapter, the learner will be able to:

1. Identify the major opioid classifications.
2. Describe the effects of the mu, delta, and kappa opioid receptors.
3. Distinguish between an opioid agonist and antagonist.
4. Discuss the short- and long-term effects of heroin.
5. Compare and contrast appropriate prescription opioid use and opioid use disorder.
6. Discuss approaches to treating opioid dependence.

OVERVIEW

Opioids are a class of drugs that include drugs naturally derived from opium and those morphine-like drugs synthesized in the laboratory. All drugs in this class either stimulate or inhibit the activity of specialized receptors in the brain. Morphine is the primary active ingredient in the vast majority of these drugs. Opioids are also referred to as *narcotics* and are defined as drugs with morphine-like properties. Opioids are used medically for anesthetic purposes, to relieve pain and diarrhea, and as cough suppressants. In accordance with the U.S. Controlled Substance Act, most opioids are classified as Schedule II drugs, meaning there are medical indications but that they have a very high potential for abuse.

HISTORY

Morphine occurs naturally in opium, which is found in the seed pod of Asian poppy plants native to the Mediterranean region. Opium has been consumed since 5000 B.C. and is the source of the natural opioids: morphine, codeine, and thebaine. Opium, as well as other opioids, was a common ingredient in numerous medications, including laudanum. Until 1906, ingredients were not required on labels leaving consumers unaware of potential problems. Persons with opium habits, developed from medications or other means, were viewed as more capable of functioning in society than persons with alcohol problems. The problems resulting from compulsive opium use became clearly apparent after the invention of the hypodermic needle and ensuing intravenous (I.V.) drug use. Consequently, in 1909, opium's importation into the United States was restricted.

Morphine, first separated from opium in 1804, preceded heroin as one of the most commonly abused drugs. In 1874, heroin was first synthesized from morphine and it was commercialized in 1898 as a morphine or codeine substitute without addictive properties. But it was soon discovered that all heroin was converted into morphine in the body and heroin's use, along with other opioids under the Harrison Narcotics Act of 1914, was restricted to medicinal purposes. As a result of additional legal measures in the 1920s, unless they were hospitalized, persons who were heroin-dependent were no longer permitted to secure prescriptions, so continued supplies of heroin had to be obtained illegally. With its new illegal status, the cost of heroin – formerly less expensive than alcohol – skyrocketed, and users often committed crimes to obtain the money to purchase it.

To address heroin's problems, synthetic opioids, such as meperidine and fentanyl, were made with the goal of creating a drug with substantial analgesic properties but without the corresponding potential for abuse. Unfortunately, this goal has been less than successful. Drugs representing natural, semi-synthetic, and totally synthetic narcotics are listed in Table 11-1. Of all the opioids, heroin may be the most abused and addictive, largely because it is the most rapid-acting drug.

TABLE 11-1: CLASSIFICATION OF NARCOTICS (OPIOIDS)
Natural
Opium
Morphine
Codeine
Thebaine
Semi-synthetic
Heroin
Hydromorphone
Oxycodone
Hydrocodone
Synthetic
Meperidine
Dextropropoxyphene
Fentanyl
Pentazocine
Butorphanol

EPIDEMIOLOGY

In the United States in 2011, an estimated 620,000 persons ages 12 or older reported heroin use within the past year (Substance Abuse and Mental Health Services Administration [SAMHSA], 2012a). This represents a significant increase from 2007, when only 373,000 had reported past year use. Current users (use in the past 30 days), numbered 281,000 (0.1%). These numbers are not significantly different from those from 2006 to 2010, but do indicate an increase from 2003 (119,000). Individuals between 18 and 25 years of age had the highest rate of past-month use (0.2%) in 2011 (SAMHSA, 2012a).

In contrast, many more individuals reported lifetime nonmedical use of pain relievers with an estimated 34.9 million reporting such use in 2011, a statistically significant increase since the 29.6 million in 2002. The number and percentage of persons aged 12 or older who were current nonmedical users of pain relievers in 2011 (4.5 million or 1.7%) were lower than those in 2010 (5.1 million or 2.0%) and 2009 (5.3 million or 2.1%) (SAMHSA, 2012a).

Among adolescents, lifetime use of heroin in 2011 was about 1.2% for high school students (Johnston, O'Malley, Bachman, & Schulenberg, 2012). The proportions of all youth between ages 12 and 17 reporting current heroin use was no different (0.1%) from the general population. Also similar to the general population, higher percentages of adolescents reported nonmedical use of pain relievers, with 2.1% reporting use in the past month. Unlike the general population, this proportion represented a significant decrease from the 3.2% reported in 2002

(SAMHSA, 2012a). Among emergency department visits in which heroin was the primary drug mentioned, young adults between the ages of 21 and 24 constituted the highest rates (203.1 per 100,000) of drug-related visits (Drug Abuse Warning Network [DAWN], 2011).

FORMS OF OPIOIDS

Biochemistry

To understand opioid's mechanism of action, it is necessary to know two of its basic properties:

1. which type of receptor the opioid has an affinity for – the mu (μ), delta (δ), or kappa (κ) opioid receptor
2. whether the opioid is an agonist, antagonist, or mixed agonist-antagonist.

When activated, the mu receptor is responsible for most of the effects associated with opioids. Activation of the mu receptors affects mood (including reinforcing effects), respiration, pain, blood pressure, gastrointestinal (GI) motility, and endocrine effects. The delta and kappa receptors influence pain in the spinal area. Additionally, stimulation of the kappa receptor may be associated with dysphoria (anxiety, irritability, and depression). Reinforcing effects can be positive or negative. Positive reinforcing effects are observed when the user repeatedly self-administers drugs to experience euphoria. Negative reinforcing effects are observed when the user repeatedly self-administers drugs to alleviate physical pain or painful emotions.

Agonist opioids attach to and activate their specific receptors (for example the mu receptor), while antagonist opioids attach to those same receptors but do not activate them. Further, agonist opioids can completely or partially activate receptors referred to as *full* or *partial* agonists. Partial agonists demonstrate ceiling effects, which means that as the dose of the partial agonist increases, effects at that receptor site also increase to a limit, beyond which further drug increases do not yield increased effects. In contrast, full agonists continue to respond to an escalation in dose beyond those of partial agonists. Opioids of abuse are usually full agonists with preferential binding at the mu receptor.

Mu-opioid receptors are most predominant and are located throughout the brain, spinal cord, and GI system. Opioids are agonists to four endogenous (naturally produced by the body) neurotransmitters: beta endorphins, dynorphins, leu-enkaphalins, and met-enkephalins. In normal conditions, these transmitters are released in the brain and nerve endings to ease pain. When the body is exposed to external opioids, the endogenous opioids are decreased. With continued external exposure, fewer endogenous neurotransmitters are produced and the body becomes dependent on that opioid. This partly explains why users experience pain without a clearly discernable cause when opioids are withdrawn.

Opioids can cause both neurochemical and molecular changes in the brain with chronic use. Typically, their elimination half-life (how long it takes for the body to eliminate half of the drug from the bloodstream) is relatively short, ranging from 2 to 5 hours, with duration of effects of 4 to 5 hours. Bioavailability (amount of drug available for the body to use) for uses other than I.V., can range from 30% to 92%. Bioavailability for I.V. routes is 100% because all of the opioid is immediately available to the body. Oral administration means the opioid is unevenly absorbed in the GI tract, making it more variable because it passes through the liver before it reaches the brain. Morphine and hydromorphone are among the effective analgesics because they are rapidly absorbed into the central nervous system (CNS) while they simultaneously have high thresholds for adverse effects. Codeine is reliably absorbed orally but morphine and meperidine are not.

OPIOID CLASSIFICATIONS

Natural Opioids

Opium

Most of the legally imported opium is used to derive morphine, codeine, and thebaine. The only country permitted to legally harvest opium is India. Concentration of morphine and codeine in opium ranges from 4% to 21% and 0.7% to 2.5%, respectively (Drug Enforcement Agency [DEA], 2011). The half-life for morphine and codeine is relatively short at 2 to 3 hours.

Morphine

Morphine is the standard drug against which all opioids are measured. It is an agonist for the mu-opioid and kappa receptors. When acting as a kappa receptor agonist, morphine produces spinal anesthesia and pupillary constriction. Its bioavailability is about 30%. It is marketed in a high number of preparations and is commonly the drug of choice for treating chronic pain.

Codeine

Codeine is the most widely used opioid prescribed for moderate pain relief and cough suppression. The majority of codeine is now produced from morphine although codeine's effects are less potent. Codeine is also the origin for the semi-synthetic opioid hydrocodone.

Thebaine

Thebaine, a very small component of opium, is not used therapeutically by itself but it is used to make several opioids, including oxycodone, oxymorphone, nalbuphine, naloxone, naltrexone, and buprenorphine. But unlike morphine and codeine, thebaine produces only slight opioid effects.

Semi-synthetic Opioids

Heroin

Heroin is a mu-opioid agonist classified as a Schedule I drug, meaning there is very high potential for abuse with no licensed medical indications for use in the United States. Most of the heroin illegally imported into the United States comes from Mexico and South America (DEA, 2011). Heroin from South America, known to be very pure, is primarily distributed along the East Coast; heroin from Mexico is primarily found on the West Coast. Heroin's origin is differentiated by its color, in which the color of heroin from Mexico is brown to black (known as *black tar*) and heroin from South America can vary from white to brown, depending on the additives incorporated into the drug (DEA, 2011). These additives may range from such substances as sugar to procaine and may include poisons such as strychnine. In the past, heroin was commonly injected; however, with the relatively recent increase in purity, the intranasal and inhalation routes correspondingly deliver increased euphoric effects. Use of these routes became more acceptable and popular because the risks of needle use can be avoided.

The sole difference between heroin and morphine is the addition of two acetyl groups to the morphine molecule (thus the chemical name for heroin, *diacetylmorphine*). This change makes heroin more lipid soluble than morphine. The more lipid soluble a substance is, the faster it crosses the blood-brain barrier. This difference is also responsible for heroin being two to three times more potent than morphine. Once ingested, heroin is converted in the brain to morphine, making heroin a prodrug, which means that heroin is inactive until metabolized (in this case into morphine) in the body. In the brain, it is the morphine molecule that attaches to the opioid receptors to produce its effects. Heroin has a bioavailability of about 35% (for the intranasal and inhalation routes) and a very short half-life of about 30 minutes.

Hydromorphone and oxycodone

Hydromorphone and oxycodone are mu-opioid agonists. Hydromorphone has the same half-life as morphine but is two to eight times more potent. Tablets may be dissolved and injected like heroin. Oxycodone has a bioavailability of about 87% and a half-life of 3 to 4.5 hours. Its sustained release forms are particularly desirable because they contain large amounts of drug that can be released immediately.

Hydrocodone

Hydrocodone is a mu-opioid agonist derived from codeine and thebaine. Compared to hydromorpone and oxycodone, hydrocodone has a longer half-life – 4 to 8 hours. It used to be a Schedule III drug (Schedule V when used as a cough suppressant), meaning that licensed medical indications exist and, although a potential for abuse exists, it is less likely to occur. However, it was recently reclassified as a Schedule II drug, meaning that it has a high potential for abuse, and that abuse of the drug may lead to severe psychological or physical dependence. Hydrocodone is a frequently mentioned drug in emergency department visits and related deaths (DEA, 2011).

Synthetic Opioids

Meperidine

Meperidine is a mu-opioid agonist primarily prescribed for moderate to severe pain relief and used for pre-anesthesia. Its bioavailability is variable and has a half-life of 3 to 5 hours. Because it is more lipid soluble than morphine, it has a more rapid onset of action. Severe adverse effects from meperidine are principally due to its metabolite norpethidine that is associated with convulsions and hallucinations. Unfortunately, unlike those for other opioids, these adverse effects cannot be reversed with the antagonists naloxone or naltrexone.

Dextropropoxyphene

Dextropropoxyphene is a mixed agonist-antagonist used for mild to moderate pain. It is similar to methadone and is one-third to one-half as potent as codeine. At low doses, dextropropoxyphene activates opioid receptors to produce pain relief but, at higher doses, it inhibits these receptors to create a ceiling analgesic effect. Used with other opioids, the overall analgesic effect decreases rather than increases. Depending on its preparation, dextroproproxyphene is a Schedule II or IV drug. It is particularly useful for individuals who cannot metabolize codeine. Its bioavailability ranges from 20% to 50%.

Fentanyl

Fentanyl is a mu-opioid agonist used as an I.V. anesthetic. For chronic pain management, it is available as a patch, lozenge, and an effervescent tablet for absorption through the buccal mucosa. Compared to heroin, there is less euphoria but greater analgesia because it is about 80 times more potent than morphine. Fentanyl has been responsible for an increasing number of deaths because users have started combining it with heroin to augment its potency (Volkow, 2007). The transdermal form has a bioavailability of 92% and the oral form has a bioavailability of 50%. Its half-life ranges from 3 to 12 hours.

Pentazocine

Pentazocine is a mixed agonist-antagonist created to treat mild to moderate pain in an attempt to have an effective analgesic with lower abuse potential. It is a partial kappa agonist/weak mu antagonist that produces analgesia for non-dependent persons and an abstinence syndrome (withdrawal symptoms) for opiate-dependent persons. Despite this formulation, pentazocine was commonly abused and naloxone was added to it to counteract the morphine effects created when the tablet was crushed. It remains classified as a Schedule IV drug. Orally, pentazocine's bioavailability is about 20% with a half-life of 2 to 3 hours.

Butorphanol

Butorphanol is a mixed agonist-antagonist commonly used as a nasal spray to treat migraine headaches and also used parenterally for anesthesia. It is both a partial agonist and antagonist at the mu-opioid receptor and an agonist at the kappa receptor. Similar to pentazocine, it also produces an abstinence syndrome when given to an opiate-dependent person. Because there is a preference for the kappa receptor, if withdrawal symptoms are precipitated, a mu receptor drug would not resolve butorphanol or pentazocine as it would for drugs that have a preference for the μ receptor only. It is categorized as a Schedule IV drug and has a bioavailability of 60% to 70% with a half-life of 4 to 7 hours.

Opioid street names are listed in Table 11-2; Table 11-3 details elimination half-life, bioavailability, and duration of effects.

TABLE 11-2: SELECTED STREET NAMES AND PHARMACOLOGY FOR OPIOIDS

Drug name	Street names	Opioid receptor	Drug type
Morphine	M, Murphy, dreamy	μ and κ	Agonist
Codeine	T3, Captain Cody	μ	Agonist
Heroin	Horse, H-bomb, dragon	μ	Agonist
Hydromorphone	Dillies, hillbilly heroin	μ	Agonist
Oxycodone	OC, oxy	μ	Agonist
Hydrocodone	Vikes, Watson-387	μ	Agonist
Meperidine	Dust, juice	μ	Agonist
Dextropropoxyphene	Fizzies, dollies	μ	Agonist
Fentanyl	China white, good fella	μ	Agonist
Pentazocine	Crackers, yellow footballs	μ	Partial agonist and antagonist
		κ	Agonist

TABLE 11-3: OPIOID PHARMACOKINETICS

Drug name	Half-life	Bioavailability	Duration of effects
Morphine	2 to 3 hours	30%	4 to 5 hours
Codeine	2 to 3 hours	50%	4 to 6 hours
Heroin	30 minutes	35%	4 to 5 hours
Hydromorphone	2 to 3 hours	30% to 35%	4 to 5 hours
Oxycodone	3 to 4.5 hours	87%	4 to 6 hours
Hydrocodone	4 to 8 hours	varies	6 to 8 hours
Meperidine	3 to 5 hours	varies	4 to 6 hours
Dextropropoxyphene	6 to 12 hours	20% to 50%	
Fentanyl (buccal)	2 hours	50%	2 to 3 hours
(transdermal)	12 to 18 hours	92%	72 hours
Pentazocine	2 to 3 hours	20%	4 hours
Butorphanol	2 to 3 hours	60% to 70%	4 hours

HEALTH EFFECTS OF HEROIN AND OTHER OPIOIDS

Route of Administration

Heroin is used through the intranasal, inhalation, intramuscular, or I.V. routes. When heroin crosses the blood-brain barrier, a euphoric effect, referred to as a "rush" or "high," is experienced by the user. This effect is noted in 10 to 15 minutes when used intranasally, 5 to 8 minutes when injected intramuscularly, and as quickly as 5 to 10 seconds when inhaled or used intravenously. The rapid effect is the primary reason heroin is so addictive.

Short-term Effects

At first, the user experiences euphoria, which may be accompanied by dry mouth, a feeling of heaviness in the extremities, and nausea and vomiting. With the initial nausea and vomiting, some individuals may report dysphoria rather than euphoria. Heroin causes a histamine release that leads to dilation of the peripheral blood vessels and a warm flushing of the skin with severe itching. Peristalsis is slowed in the GI tract causing constipation. At the same time, the urinary bladder contracts, resulting in perceptions of urinary urgency.

After these initial effects, users are often drowsy for several hours and mental function is clouded. Vomiting, observed initially, ceases so much so that even emetic agents usually do not succeed in inducing vomiting. Blood pressure decreases and the heart and respiratory rates decrease – sometimes fatally.

Long-term Effects

Tolerance

As the body adapts to heroin, the user consumes increasingly greater amounts to achieve that same level of euphoria or analgesia, a process known as *tolerance*. Tolerance is the outcome of the adjustments made at the opioid receptors to the almost continuous binding to external rather than from the body's internal opioid substances. To overcome tolerance, the user must increase the heroin dose. Tolerance to opioids other than heroin occurs, an effect known as *cross-tolerance*. Consequently, the user requires greater than normal doses for other opioids to achieve a substantial analgesic effect.

Tolerance is not limited to euphoria and analgesia because the body also becomes less responsive to heroin's effects on respiratory depression, nausea, and vomiting. There is also a reduced impact on the mental state and the user is less lethargic. But this effect is less marked for blood pressure, which may continue to decrease, along with increased constipation and urinary urgency. There is also very little effect on pupillary constriction.

Tolerance usually refers to the user's physical state but it may be behavioral as well. Behavioral tolerance refers to the user whose body reflexively learns to anticipate heroin's effects after repeated exposure to heroin. The body begins to respond as if the heroin had already been consumed. This is such a strong conditioned response that, given the appropriate stimuli (anything that reminds the user of heroin), physiological changes (such as body temperature or intestinal motility) ensue in anticipation of the drug. Physical tolerance is reversed during periods of abstinence from heroin but the behavioral tolerance is far more persistent and is the basis of drug craving.

Opioid withdrawal

Symptoms of withdrawal result when the opioid is stopped or an antagonist is administered. In both circumstances, a typical abstinence syndrome begins. The prerequisite for withdrawal is the user must be physically dependent on the drug. The degree of physical dependence and tolerance is based on a continuum rather than absolutely present or absent. Severity of withdrawal depends on the degree of physical dependence and tolerance as well as how gradually the external opioid is removed from its receptor site. A more sudden removal results in a more intense abstinence syndrome.

Symptoms of withdrawal are secondary to rebound of the sympathetic nervous system, which results in hyperactivity. Because these symptoms represent sympathetic nervous system hyperactivity, specific symptoms are too many to name in total. These symptoms tend to occur sequentially and typically begin with anxiety and drug craving, progressing to yawning, muscle aches, and runny nose, and then to vomiting and diarrhea. Although acutely uncomfortable, heroin withdrawal is rarely fatal if the person is otherwise healthy (National Institute on Drug Abuse [NIDA], 2005). Signs and symptoms of the abstinence syndrome and their typical timing of appearance for heroin and morphine are detailed in Table 11-4.

The most rapid removal of opioid from its receptor site is accomplished by opioid antagonists, which selectively compete for the site but have no agonist properties. Shorter-acting opioids exit the receptor site more promptly than do opioids with longer half-lives. Thus, heroin and morphine produce intense abstinence syndromes with relatively rapid onset and progression. For such shorter-acting drugs as heroin and morphine, withdrawal usually begins within 6 to 8 hours of the last dose. Major withdrawal symptoms peak between 24 and 72 hours after the last dose of heroin and subside within about 5 to 10 days.

After resolution of the acute abstinence syndrome, a more subtle abstinence syndrome may be present for many months, causing risk of relapse to heroin use to be high during this period. Symptoms include drug craving, anxiety, irritability, difficulty sleeping, increased sensitivity to pain, loss of pleasure (anhedonia), and a reduced ability to endure stress. Additionally, the respiratory system is less responsive to carbon dioxide. Normally, when levels of carbon dioxide get too high, the brain automatically directs the body to breathe to lower these levels. A dampened response to this automatic reflex occurs among heroin users even after use has ceased.

Opioid abuse and dependence

Abuse of opioids is less problematic compared to dependence from a physiologic perspective. Individuals who abuse opioids tend to use them less frequently and, consequently,

TABLE 11-4: ABSTINENCE SYNDROME SYMPTOMS AFTER HEROIN OR MORPHINE

Signs	Approximate hours after last dose
Drug craving, anxiety	6
Yawning, perspiration, runny nose, teary eyes	14
Increase in above symptoms, pupil dilation, piloerection (goose bumps), tremors (muscle twitches), hot and cold flashes, aching bones and muscles, loss of appetite	16
Increased intensity of above symptoms; insomnia; increased blood pressure; fever; increased pulse rate, respiratory rate and depth; restlessness; nausea	24 to 36
Increased intensity of above symptoms, being in a curled-up position, vomiting, diarrhea, weight loss, spontaneous ejaculation or orgasm, high hematocrit, increased blood glucose levels	36 to 48

(Ray & Ksir, 2002)

do not experience significant tolerance or physical dependence. Withdrawal symptoms for this group are essentially absent. When considering persons using opioids for a medical condition, abuse is defined as use in excess of what is needed for the medical problem.

In contrast, users who are opioid dependent have escalated their dose of drug in response to tolerance and are physically dependent on the drug. Among individuals from various clinical settings, opioid withdrawal occurred in 60% of individuals who had used heroin at least once in the prior 12 months (American Psychiatric Association [APA], 2013). These individuals have substantial psychosocial troubles in addition to their physical problems.

Intoxication, overdose, and medical complications

Opioid intoxication is defined as "the presence of clinically significant maladaptive behavioral or psychological changes that develop during, or shortly after, opioid use" (APA, 2013, p. 546). It can occur with the first dose or after chronic use, and the symptoms represent many of the same ones described previously as short-term effects, but are more intense. Opioid intoxication begins with euphoria and progresses to irritability, anxiety, depression, restlessness or decreased activity, and impaired judgment, social, or occupational functioning. These psychological symptoms are accompanied by pupillary constriction and decreased consciousness that varies from lethargy to coma. These symptoms usually last for several hours, a time-frame consistent with the half-life of most opioid drugs.

Opioid's strong depressant effect on the respiratory system is usually the cause of acute overdose and death. Mortality rates as a result of heroin use has been estimated to be nearly 20 times higher than the general population (Dilts & Dilts, 2005). Other common causes of death include drug-related infections (such as from needle use or overall depressed immune function), suicide, homicide, or accidental death.

Endocrine (including thyroid, adrenal, and gonadotropin) activity is all reduced through heroin's effects on the pituitary gland and tends to be evident after chronic heroin use. Examples of pituitary dysfunction include erectile dysfunction and irregular menstrual periods. Other complications may be noted as a result of chronic or short-term use. For example, medical complications include hepatitis and HIV infection that may be direct complications of I.V. use, particularly with shared needles. Risky behaviors such as unprotected sex with multiple partners also contribute to HIV and other sexually transmitted infections. About 70% to 80% of the 35,000 new hepatitis C infections that occur annually in the United States are among I.V. drug users (NIDA, 2005). Further, the likelihood of infections is augmented by the impaired immune function observed among chronic opioid users.

Beyond infections, I.V. heroin users may attempt to block the entry of the contaminants often added to heroin, by injecting the drug through cotton. Although this practice may obstruct contaminants, small particles of cotton can gain entry to the circulatory system potentially leading into pulmonary emboli. Selected medical complications of chronic heroin use are included in Table 11-5.

TREATMENT

In 2010, 14% of the total admissions for substance abuse treatment were opioid related admissions for which heroin was the primary drug of abuse, constituting 62% of all opioid admissions (SAMHSA, 2012b). This represents a decline since 2000, when 15% of total admissions were heroin-related, constituting 91% of all opioid admissions. Of the total admissions for opioids, youth between ages 12 and 19 made up 3.5% of primary heroin admissions, while indi-

TABLE 11-5: COMPLICATIONS OF HEROIN USE
Injection
• Scarred or collapsed veins
• Lymphadenopathy
• Bacterial infections of blood vessels and heart valves
• Abscesses or soft tissue infections/osteomyelitis
• Liver disease or hepatitis B, C
• HIV
• Kidney disease
Nasal inhalation
• Pneumonia
• Tuberculosis
• Hepatitis B, C
• HIV
• Septic emboli to the lungs
Subsequent to overdoses with anoxia or coma
• Partial paralysis
• Parkinsonism
• Intellectual impairment
• Personality changes
• Peripheral neuropathy
• Acute transverse myelitis
• Blindness
(NIDA, 2005; Dilts & Dilts, 2005)

viduals aged 20-24 years made up 51.6%%. The number for the total population is smaller than the numbers reported in 2005; however, heroin constituted a larger percent of the total opioid admissions. In 2005, heroin comprised 81% of total opioid admissions. Treatment admissions for opiates other than heroin increased from 50,520 in 2005 to 155,722 in 2010, representing an increase of more than 300% (SAMHSA, 2012b).

General Considerations

Treatment for opioid dependence can include drug and/or behavioral therapies. Drug therapy may include medications to treat withdrawal, an opioid agonist to substitute for heroin, and/or an opioid antagonist for relapse prevention. A comprehensive history, physical, and laboratory assessment should be completed before making treatment decisions. Historical data should include information from the user's family or significant others because the client may not be the most reliable historian. All individuals should be asked about their use of other drugs. Laboratory evaluation in the form of testing for the presence of opioids is vital and should include routine screening for hepatitis B and C and HIV with informed consent.

Urine tests are usually employed and remain positive for most opioids from 12 to 36 hours after last use. Longer acting opioids such as methadone can be identified in urine for several days. It is important to know which opioids you are screening for because all tests may not detect all opioid use. For example, fentanyl is not detected by standard urine tests although it is possible to do so with more refined procedures (APA, 2013, p. 544).

Phases of treatment can be viewed on a continuum from acute to sub-acute to continuing care. The *acute* phase addresses the client's life-threatening and severe conditions resulting from opioid toxicity, for which supportive care is given in the hospital setting. After a client is stabilized, a *sub-acute* phase can address the client's withdrawal symptoms. If there is not a life-threatening condition present, this can be the first phase of treatment. Although intensely uncomfortable, opioid withdrawal is not life threatening if the client is otherwise healthy. Yet, even if the client is healthy, unless these symptoms are addressed and treated appropriately, the likelihood of relapse to opioid use is extremely high. This phase may occur in an outpatient setting, and should ideally include the support of a 12-step self-help group in the community. Some form of *continuing care* (also known as *aftercare*) in the community setting must be in place upon discharge from the formal treatment setting to reduce the likelihood of relapse to opioid use. Continuing care should include participation in a 12-step self-help group and may include maintenance drug therapy. Continuing care may need to be life-long because drug dependence is a chronic condition, such as that of diabetes or hypertension, which requires on-going treatment.

Although these phases are discussed separately, recovery does not occur in distinct phases. There is substantial overlap for which drug combinations and behavioral therapy can accommodate individual client needs.

Acute Phase: Opioid Overdose

Individuals who have overdosed on opioids usually have severe respiratory depression and may be comatose. The first priority in this situation is to re-establish adequate respiration by immediately giving an opioid antagonist such as naloxone, preferably intravenously. A rapid response should be observed within 1 to 2 minutes; if not, other causes should be considered. After a sufficient improvement is noted, monitoring must continue because the relatively short half-life of naloxone means that additional doses may be required, depending on the half-life of the opioid responsible for the overdose. After the individual has been stabilized, dosing with naloxone may be replaced with oral naltrexone, a longer-acting antagonist. However, this must be done with caution because naltrexone is capable of precipitating severe withdrawal symptoms (Knapp, Ciraulo, & Jaffe, 2005). When life-threatening events have been resolved, users have four basic treatment options: detoxification, drug substitution, behavioral therapy, or a combination of drug and behavioral therapies.

Subacute Phase: Opioid Detoxification

The goal of detoxification is to achieve safe withdrawal from opioids with minimal withdrawal symptoms. How a client is withdrawn from the drug depends in part upon:

- the degree of withdrawal symptoms he is willing to tolerate
- any coexisting medical problems that may complicate the withdrawal process
- the available treatment setting in which withdrawal can occur.

Because withdrawal is not inherently dangerous among healthy users, they may opt to withdraw without the support of medications. Otherwise, withdrawal can be treated by substituting another opioid drug and then slowly tapering its dose. Alternatively, withdrawal can be treated with use of non-opioid medications. Sedatives can help treat the restless sleep and insomnia that often persist for many days or weeks. Sedative use is not recommended as first-line treatment because clients may develop physical dependence to them.

Clonidine, a central acting alpha-2 agonist used to treat high blood pressure can also be used. Clonidine acts by dampening parts of the sympathetic nervous system made hyperactive by opioid withdrawal. It suppresses many of the autonomic signs and symptoms of withdrawal, such as nausea, vomiting, perspiration, intestinal cramps, and diarrhea. However, clonidine does not significantly improve the muscle aches, back pain, insomnia, and craving for opioids. Further, use of clonidine is limited by its own adverse effects of sedation and low blood pressure.

Within the inpatient setting, a standard approach to detoxification is methadone use, which is often substituted for shorter-acting opioids by stabilizing the client on a given dose, usually a total of 40 mg in divided doses. After 1 to 2 days, the dose is reduced by about 20% each day. With this schedule, the user experiences mild withdrawal symptoms beginning about the third or fourth day. These symptoms often continue after hospital discharge when methadone is completely withdrawn.

Alternatively, ultrarapid detoxification approaches have been developed for use in the hospital setting that uses such antagonists as naloxone to precipitate opioid withdrawal while the client is heavily sedated with short-acting benzodiazepines. This approach, which takes 48 hours, has been demonstrated to be successful in the short-term because few or no withdrawal symptoms are observed when the sedation tapers off (Knapp et al., 2005). The client may then be transitioned to naltrexone. However, because some clients continue to have minimal withdrawal symptoms with naltrexone after discharge, many stop taking it. Another approach is to premedicate clients with buprenorphine before they undergo ultrarapid detoxification because it may diminish the occurrence of some adverse effects, such as nausea and vomiting that may otherwise occur after the detoxification procedure (Dilts & Dilts, 2005).

Inpatient programs, especially ultrarapid detoxification, are expensive and the likelihood of rapid relapse to opioid use is substantial, especially given the continued presence of withdrawal symptoms (Knapp et al., 2005). However, an advantage of detoxification over longer-term substitution with methadone is that the duration of the acute abstinence syndrome is shortened.

Subacute Phase: Pharmacotherapy

Drug Substitution

The rationale for drug substitution is that for some individuals, prolonged exposure to opioids induced long-lasting adaptive changes. Continued administration of an opioid is then necessary to maintain normal mood states and responses to stress. Goals of drug substitution include minimizing the abstinence syndrome, blocking the euphoric effects of the abused opioid, and relieving opioid craving.

Methadone and buprenorphine are available for drug substitution.

Methadone

Methadone is the oldest and most commonly used drug in the treatment setting. Methadone is a synthetic mu-opioid agonist that blocks the effects of heroin when given at adequate doses, while simultaneously eliminating withdrawal symptoms and alleviating the craving for heroin. It is absorbed well when given orally and, at appropriate doses, is neither intoxicating nor sedating, so its effects do not interfere with activities of daily living. The effects of methadone can last for 24 hours, permitting once daily dosing while suppressing withdrawal symptoms from heroin for 24 to 36 hours. Methadone has been demonstrated to be safe even when used continuously for 20 years or more. Consequently, in support of the current belief of drug dependence as a chronic disorder, life-long use of methadone is not considered inappropriate (Marion, 2005).

Similar to all opioids, long-term use leads to tolerance and physical dependence; however, withdrawal symptoms from methadone compared to heroin are less severe but longer in duration due to methadone's lengthier half-life. In contrast to heroin in which withdrawal may begin as soon as 6 hours after the last dose, methadone can take 2 to 4 days to manifest with the abstinence syndrome taking from 2 to 3 weeks to resolve.

Buprenorphine

Buprenorphine is a mixed agonist-antagonist that has revolutionized opioid treatment. It is the first medication approved, by the Food and Drug Administration (FDA) in 2002, outside of substance abuse treatment programs for the private physician's office (after 8 hours of approved training), designed to make this option more accessible and common. Buprenorphine is a semi-synthetic opioid derived from thebaine: a partial mu-agonist and a kappa-antagonist. Buprenorphine attaches to the same receptors as morphine, but because it is a partial agonist, it yields similar effects but at a reduced intensity. Because buprenorphine is also an antagonist at the kappa-receptor, it may inhibit some of the dysphoric effects experienced as part of withdrawal.

Similar to methadone, buprenorphine has an analgesic potency 30 to 50 times greater than morphine. It is capable of blocking the reinforcing effects of other opioids and suppressing drug craving while causing far less respiratory depression – a substantial advantage over methadone. Further, buprenorphine generates less physical dependence and, therefore, fewer withdrawal symptoms than methadone. Both buprenorphine and methadone have a long duration of action but unlike methadone, buprenorphine may be used only three times per week for maintenance (Knapp et al., 2005).

Buprenorphine is poorly absorbed when swallowed so it is administered sublingually. Sublingual tablets are available in two forms: those containing only buprenorphine and those that contain buprenorphine and naloxone to minimize its abuse potential through I.V. use. The inclusion of naloxone means that when the tablet is crushed, the naloxone is activated and precipitates withdrawal symptoms. Buprenorphine is particularly useful for detoxification. It is as effective as clonidine in suppressing withdrawal symptoms but has minimal effects on blood pressure (Knapp et al., 2005). Due to buprenorphine's strong affinity for its receptors, larger doses of naloxone are often necessary to reverse its effects if individuals overdose on it.

Subacute Phase: Behavioral Therapy

The most effective approach may be the use of both pharmacotherapies and behavioral treatments. The mainstay approaches to behavioral therapy include cognitive behavioral therapy (CBT), motivational interviewing or enhancement, contingency management, and therapeutic community. All may be provided on an individual or group basis or in combination. Some approaches, such as motivational interviewing and contingency management, are more suited to the individual because these approaches require some degree of tailoring to the individual client. Therapeutic community treatment is designed for implementation in a residential setting, relying on treatment through a group approach.

Contingency Management

Contingency management is an approach that emphasizes rewards for positive behavior vs. punishment for negative behavior. This approach has four principles:

1. rapid and accurate detection of drug use
2. positive reinforcement of abstinence
3. loss of positive reinforcement upon detection of drug use
4. development of positive reinforcers to compete with drug use.

Urine specimens are tested three times weekly with abstinence based on these urine results. Abstinence is reinforced with vouchers that can be redeemed for various desirable services or cash. These vouchers increase in value with each consecutive drug-free specimen. Drug-positive urines result in no receipt of vouchers and a reset of the voucher to the initial baseline value.

Cognitive Behavioral Therapy

CBT is based on the social learning theory and emphasizes modification of the client's thoughts and behaviors. The goal is to encourage abstinence by helping clients learn and master effective coping skills that can help them to believe they can resist returning to substance abuse. The focus is on the exploration of the positive and negative consequences of substance use. This approach is the foundation for relapse prevention because clients are taught the skills needed to prevent a return to substance abuse after treatment.

Motivational Interventions

Motivational interventions (MIs) are based on the Transtheoretical Model of Change (Miller, 1999). The stages are described in Table 11-6. MI strategies adapt to each stage to meet clients at their current state rather than presenting treatment options without considering the client's present readiness to change. Strategies are based on the concept that motivation is the key to changing clients' behavior. This approach can be incorporated into the clinician's interviewing style (then referred to as *motivational interviewing*) used for assessment as well as treatment. MI can be combined with other approaches, such as for brief interventions and contingency management.

Therapeutic Community

Therapeutic community (TC) involves residing in a facility with 24-hour supervision. It uses a structured living environment as an integral part of the client's treatment plan. These settings may be ideal for clients with a substance dependence diagnosis that is accompanied by severe psychosocial impairment who do not meet clinical criteria for hospitalization. Adherence is reinforced with rewards for responsible social behavior and punishments for non-adherence. Traditionally, length of stay in TCs ranged between 18 to 24 months but, with the advent of managed care, typical length of stay is now 12 months or less. Varied individual and group therapy sessions using such approaches as CBT are also implemented within TCs.

12-step Self-help Groups

Self-help or 12-step groups are widely available and most notably include Narcotics Anonymous (NA). They are unique in that they do not rely on professional personnel to guide recovery. Twelve-step groups usually follow the same format and guidelines of "working through the steps." As a rule, the group's philosophy is highly spiritual, but not associated with a specific denomination or religion. New group members are typically sponsored by another person who is further along in recovery and who acts as a guide to the novice. These support groups are free and typically anonymous and confidential. The goal is total abstinence – a drug-free existence where use of any medications (including methadone) is not well supported for the long term. Members focus on staying drug-free "one day at a time" and expect their members to demonstrate a wish to cease substance use.

TABLE 11-6: STAGES OF CHANGE

Stage	Definition
Precontemplation	Individual is in denial about changing his or her substance use behavior and has no plans to change
Contemplation	Individual is thinking about a change in his or her substance use behavior suggesting recognition of a serious problem, but still ambivalent
Preparation	Individual expresses readiness to make a change in his or her substance use behavior
Action	Individual has begun to make changes in his or her substance use behavior and possibly participating in a defined treatment program
Maintenance and relapse prevention	Individual has accomplished his or her initial goals and has made changes in his or her life, but may temporarily return to using substances

Note. From *Enhancing Motivation for Change in Substance Abuse Treatment* by W.R. Miller, 1999, Treatment Improvement Protocol (TIP) Series 35. DHHS Publication No. (SMA) 99-3354. Rockville, MD: Substance Abuse and Mental Health Services Administration, Center for Substance Abuse Treatment.

Continuing Care: Pharmacotherapy

Naltrexone

Naltrexone is a long-acting opioid antagonist that can be used to prevent relapse to opioid use. Unlike methadone and buprenorphine, it is not possible to develop tolerance; therefore, physical dependence and subsequent withdrawal from naltrexone is not possible. Correspondingly, it is not a controlled substance and can be prescribed outside of the drug treatment setting without any additional requirements, such as those required by buprenorphine.

It is similar to methadone and buprenorphine in that it blocks the euphoric effects of heroin. However, because there are no opioid agonist effects, craving for opioids is not alleviated. Importantly, with naltrexone, any opioid use will precipitate withdrawal symptoms. Further, because abstinence from drug use reduces tolerance (and therefore physical dependence), drug use at levels that were previously tolerated can, in this instance, lead to overdose – a fact that clients should be warned about. Knowledge of this fact is the key to naltrexone's use for relapse prevention. It is also the reason that many individuals do not adhere to its regimen.

Evidence-based practice suggests that individuals with the following characteristics are more likely to be successfully maintained on naltrexone:

- less severe opioid dependence
- high motivation
- presence of sanctions if they fail to adhere to the regimen or relapse to drug use
- substantial positive social support

(Sullivan, Comer, & Nunes, 2006).

Initiation of naltrexone requires that clients have not used opioids of any kind in the previous 10 days to avoid withdrawal symptoms. Nonadherence to naltrexone can be addressed through administering it as a long-lasting depot formulation that blocks opioid-induced euphoria for 3 to 5 weeks (Knapp et al., 2005).

PRESCRIPTION OPIATES

Abuse of prescription opiates differs from heroin abuse in that for the majority of cases, abuse begins secondary to ineffective chronic pain management. There has been increased emphasis on appropriate pain management, exemplified by The Joint Commission, which requires pain, respiration, temperature, blood pressure, and pulse assessment. Opioids have since been more frequently prescribed to address effective pain management (Ling, Wesson, & Smith, 2005).

In the chronic pain setting, the term "misuse" is commonly used instead of "abuse." Misuse includes the clinician's behavior – for example, prescribing opiates for an inappropriate health problem, at an excessive dose, or for a longer duration than necessary. As such, it is a very widespread problem among the elderly population.

In contrast, substance abuse and dependence are characterized by explicit behaviors. An individual may be physically dependent on opioids, yet not meet the APA diagnostic behavioral criteria for abuse or dependence. Instead the term "pseudoaddiction" may be used for drug-behaviors consequent to inadequate pain treatment. Ling and colleagues (2005) describe the following phases:

- inadequate prescription of analgesics
- patient's escalation of analgesic demands and behavior changes to convince others of the severity of their pain and need for relief
- mistrust between the clinician and patient.

Although there appears to be more overdose deaths attributed to opiates, it is difficult to determine if the victims are chronic pain clients (Ling et al., 2005). This is complicated by the common use of conversion tables that are based on the setting of acute rather than chronic pain and do not account for possible physical dependence. These conversion tables often presume that methadone and morphine have about equal potency; however, clinical experience suggests that methadone is actually more potent, perhaps due to its better oral absorption (Walsh & Strain, 2006). Clinicians prescribing methadone for chronic pain clients may be prescribing a dose that is too high and these persons may be more likely to experience a lethal overdose (Ling et al., 2005).

Another concern is prescribing opioids to clients with a history of opioid or alcohol abuse. Dunbar and Katz (1996) observed that individuals with substance abuse histories were at no greater risks of relapsing to drug use when prescribed short-term opioids. Interestingly, those who had a history of substance abuse were less likely to misuse the prescription opioid compared to persons without this history. These results can be attributed to the one group that demonstrated continued involvement in such self-help groups as NA, as a result of their prior drug abuse history, in addition to having a more stable support system. The important message from this study is that having a history of substance abuse alone should not preclude adequate pain management.

Further complicating the issue is the evidence that chronic opioid use leads to increased sensitivity to pain when the drug is withdrawn (Ling et al., 2005). Chabal and colleagues (in Ling et al.) use the following behaviors to suggest prescription drug abuse:

- overemphasis on opioid issues during pain clinic visits that persists beyond the third treatment session
- pattern of early refills (three or more) or dose escalation in the absence of acute changes in medical condition
- multiple phone calls or visits to request more opioids or refills or to discuss problems associated with opioid prescription
- pattern of such prescription problems as lost, spilled, or stolen medication
- supplemental sources of opioids obtained from multiple providers, emergency departments, or illegal sources.

Three of these criteria should be met to qualify for abuse. In their study of 403 patients being treated for chronic pain, history of opioid or alcohol abuse did not predict prescription opioid abuse.

SPECIAL POPULATIONS

Chronic Pain

Chronic nonmalignant pain is reported in up to 40% of U.S. adults (Verhaak, Kerssens, Dekker, Sorbi & Bensing, 1998). Both misuse of prescription opioids and illicit drug use are commonly detected among persons presenting for chronic pain management (Manchikanti et al., 2006). Among individuals with chronic pain, identified risk factors for opioid abuse or illicit drug use include age younger than 45 years, pain subsequent to a motor vehicle accident, involvement of more than two areas of the body, and a past history of illicit drug use (Manichikanti et al., 2006).

As part of the routine history and physical (including record request from previous providers) to evaluate chronic pain, all clients should be explicitly asked about a past or current history of illicit substance use or misuse of prescription opioids. Those persons with a recent history of illicit drug use or prescription opioid misuse should be simultaneously enrolled in a substance abuse treatment or comprehensive pain program respectively, based upon the clinician's evaluation. Other guidelines might include the following:

- An agreement or contract clearly detailing expectations from the client and the clinician should be used. Even though there is no consensus on the use, elements, or effectiveness of these agreements (Arnold, Han, & Seltzer, 2006), an agreement might include these requirements:
  - — clients will not obtain opioids from other sources
  - — early refills will not be permitted
  - — clients will adhere to scheduled follow-up visits that may include urine toxicology screening
  - — the understanding that the clinician can terminate opioid prescribing if the agreement is broken (Kahan, Srivastava, Wilson, Mailis-Gagnon, & Midmer, 2006).
- Initiate an appropriate dose for the chronic pain condition after confirming that non-opioid treatments were ineffective.
- Increase the dose gradually and adjust appropriately to achieve satisfactory analgesia with manageable adverse effects.

Most chronic pain clients can be stabilized on a daily dose of less than 300 mg of morphine or its equivalent (Kahan et al., 2006). Although methadone is inexpensive and highly effective in the drug treatment setting, it is less desirable for clients with chronic pain. Methadone's long half-life lends itself to once daily dosing for heroin-dependent clients; however, clients with chronic pain often require more frequent dosing. Furthermore, it is known that methadone's half-life can vary from person to person ranging from 12 to more than 150 hours (Portenoy, Lussier, Kirsh, & Passik, 2005). Therefore, more than once daily dosing leads to subsequent concerns of dangerous accumulation in the body. Similarly, partial agonists or agonist-antagonists are not recommended because they can precipitate an abstinent syndrome (Portenoy et al., 2005). Fentanyl patches should be restricted to clients who are completely tolerant to morphine or other potent opioids (Kahan et al., 2006).

This dose adjustment phase usually takes about eight weeks. If dose escalation does not lead to satisfactory pain relief, the clinician can consider one of the following alternatives:

- Rotate opioids in cases where cross-tolerance is incomplete. When initiated, clients should be started at one-half the dose of the previous opioid.
- Wean off the current opioid and restart it after a period of abstinence during which other pain treatments are used. Not infrequently, clients either have an improved response to the restarted opioid or they find better satisfaction with the other treatment and no longer desire opioid treatment.
- Re-evaluate the underlying condition (if present) believed to be responsible for the pain, considering the possibility of a new problem requiring additional or different treatment.
  - — Address and treat any associated psychological disorders such as depression.
  - — Require that refills be picked up in person on a monthly basis.
- Ideally follow-up every three months

(Ballantyne & Mao, 2003; Kahan et al., 2006).

Pregnant Women

Based on 2010 and 2011 data, 5.0% of pregnant women 15-44 years of age used illicit drugs in the past month (SAMHSA, 2012a). During pregnancy, heroin crosses the placenta into the fetal circulation. Although heroin withdrawal is not fatal to an otherwise healthy pregnant woman, withdrawing from heroin (which commonly occurs because heroin is short acting) can kill the fetus. Additionally, low birth weight is associated with heroin use during pregnancy and, unlike with cocaine, labor is frequently prolonged.

To prevent these outcomes, methadone, a long-acting opioid, is commonly substituted for heroin to prevent withdrawal symptoms. Even though women maintained on methadone will instead be dependent on a longer acting opioid, women's maintenance on methadone ultimately means that withdrawal may occur only once after birth vs. several times in utero from heroin use. Also, methadone helps women care for themselves and their fetus because withdrawal is prevented while the drug craving is targeted. Buprenorphine has been observed to be equally safe and effective during pregnancy, offering an alternative treatment to methadone (NIDA, 2005). Pregnant women can also undergo detoxification from heroin; however, relapse rates to heroin use are high and subsequent withdrawal will continue to be a concern until delivery. After birth, infants exposed to opioids (whether heroin or methadone) in utero, usually display withdrawal syndromes referred to as infant *abstinence syndrome*.

Psychiatric Comorbidity

The presence of another substance use disorder and coexisting psychiatric disorder is extremely common for opioid users. Problems with alcohol and benzodiazepines often coexist because these drugs are commonly used to address the adverse effects from heroin. Alternatively, other drugs may be used to potentiate opioid-induced euphoria. One frequent example is simultaneous cocaine use called a *speedball,* used to produce a more intense euphoria but less intense adverse effects (Knapp et al., 2005).

Among other mental disorders, depression and personality disorder are the most frequently diagnosed (Dilts & Dilts, 2005). Major depression is the most common mood disorder, diagnosed at almost 16%. It occurs more frequently in women than in men, as it does in the general population. Coexisting depression is more strongly associated with a history of concomitant polydrug abuse. The dysphoria evident as part of withdrawal is not responsive to antidepressants, and pharmacologic treatment for depression is only effective after a period of abstinence (Dilts & Dilts, 2005).

Of all the personality disorders, antisocial personality disorder is the most commonly diagnosed (mostly among men) seen in as many as 25% of opioid abusers seeking treatment. Unlike depression, antisocial personality disorder can be reliably diagnosed historically in most individuals because it typically manifests at a young age, before the onset of opioid dependence.

The relationship between opioid abuse and antisocial personality is complicated and appears to be influenced by a genetic factor. When antisocial personality and opioid dependence coexist, the treatment of either problem is challenging. The overall outcome is poor and is associated with inadequate time in treatment, relapse to opioid use, criminal behavior, and difficulty establishing rapport with a therapist. The one exception appears to be the antisocial addict who has both an opioid disorder and depression. Surprisingly, these individuals respond much better to treatment in a manner similar to the average opioid addict without significant psychiatric comorbidity (Dilts & Dilts, 2005). Youth with a history of conduct disorder have been observed to be at particular risk for substance use, especially with opioids (APA, 2000).

Anxiety disorders are observed in about 10% of opioid users (Dilts & Dilts, 2005). Members of this group are typically younger in age and higher in socioeconomic status, with less extensive drug histories than typical opioid users. Other disorders, such as psychosis, schizophrenia, and mania, are rarely seen among opioid users in drug treatment.

SUMMARY

In 2011, approximately 4.5 million people in the U.S. reported current nonmedical use of pain relievers and 281,000 reported current heroin use (SAMHSA, 2012a).

Opioids may be naturally derived or synthetic. Their actions demonstrate agonist or antagonist activity depending on their binding to specific opioid receptors.

Opioid effects of euphoria and analgesia may diminish when tolerance occurs, resulting in physical dependence. Abrupt cessation of the opioid produces a distinct abstinence syndrome.

Unlike other substances of abuse, there are many pharmacologic approaches to treatment including methadone and, most recently, buprenorphine. The introduction of buprenorphine expands access to treatment beyond the drug treatment setting and will hopefully increase the number of individuals accepting treatment for opioid dependence.

EXAM QUESTIONS

CHAPTER 11

Questions 60-69

Note: Choose the one option that BEST answers each question.

60. Morphine is classified as a(n)
    a. artificial opioid.
    b. natural opioid.
    c. semi-synthetic opioid.
    d. synthetic opioid.

61. When activated, the receptor responsible for most of the effects associated with opioids, including mood, is the
    a. delta (δ).
    b. mu (μ).
    c. kappa (κ).
    d. alpha (α).

62. Which statement about the properties of opioids is true?
    a. Full agonist opioids attach to and activate their receptors.
    b. Full agonist opioids attach to but do not activate their receptors.
    c. Antagonist opioid attach to and activate their receptors.
    d. Partial agonist opioids attach to but do not activate their receptors.

63. In observing for signs of heroin withdrawal, the clinician would look for
    a. slow pulse, cough, and paralysis.
    b. constricted pupils and low blood pressure.
    c. dilated pupils, perspiration, and vomiting.
    d. increase in appetite and constipation.

64. Severity of withdrawal symptoms depends on the
    a. amount of drug craving.
    b. extent of attachment to the opioid receptor.
    c. extent of physical dependence.
    d. number of withdrawal symptoms.

65. Cause of death from opioids is usually due to
    a. homicide.
    b. HIV.
    c. profound respiratory depression.
    d. suicide.

66. After ultra-rapid detoxification, one of the problems in using naltrexone post-discharge is that
    a. it competes with heroin for the same receptor site.
    b. it is associated with a severe decrease in blood pressure.
    c. withdrawal symptoms may persist.
    d. it works too quickly.

67. A substantial advantage of using buprenorphine over methadone is that buprenorphine
    a. attaches to a different receptor.
    b. causes far less respiratory depression.
    c. is a more potent drug.
    d. has a long duration of action.

68. According to Dunbar and Katz, individuals with substance abuse histories

    a. are at greater risk for relapsing when prescribed short-term opioids.

    b. are at no greater risk for relapsing when prescribed short-term opioids.

    c. are more likely to misuse prescription opioids than people without substance abuse histories.

    d. should never be prescribed short-term opioids for pain management.

69. When treating opioid dependence in pregnant women, maintenance on methadone

    a. is never recommended due to increased risk to the fetus.

    b. helps the woman take care of herself and her fetus.

    c. is much more effective than buprenorphine.

    d. prevents infant withdrawal syndromes.

REFERENCES

American Psychiatric Association. (2013). *Diagnostic and statistical manual of mental disorders* (5th ed.). Washington, DC: American Psychiatric Association.

Arnold, R.M., Han, P.K., & Seltzer, D. (2006). Opioid contracts in chronic nonmalignant pain management: Objectives and uncertainties. *American Journal of Medicine, 119*(4), 292-6.

Ballantyne, J.C. & Mao, J. (2003). Opioid therapy for chronic pain. *New England Journal of Medicine, 349*(20), 1943-53.

Drug Enforcement Agency. (2011). *Drugs of abuse.* Retrieved March 15, 2013, from http://www.justice.gov/dea/docs/drugs_of_abuse_2011.pdf

Drug Abuse Warning Network. (2011). *2009 National estimates of drug-related emergency department visits.* Retrieved March 15, 2013 from http://www.samhsa.gov/data/2k11/DAWN/2k9DAWNED/HTML/DAWN2k9ED.htm

Drug Abuse Warning Network. (2012). *Highlights of the 2010 Drug Abuse Warning Network (DAWN) findings on drug-related emergency department visits.* Accessed March 15, 2013 from http://www.samhsa.gov/data/2k12/DAWN096/SR096EDHighlights2010.htm

Dilts, S.L. & Dilts, S.L. (2005). Opioids. In R.J. Frances, S.I. Miller, & A.H. Mack (Eds.), *Clinical textbook of addictive disorders* (3rd ed., pp. 138-156). New York: Guilford Press.

Dunbar, S.A. & Katz, N.P. (1996). Chronic opioid therapy for nonmalignant pain in patients with a history of substance abuse: Report of 20 cases. *Journal of Pain and Symptom Management, 11*(3), 163-171.

Johnston, L.D., O'Malley, P.M., Bachman, J.G., & Schulenberg, J.E. (2009). *Teen marijuana tilts up, while some drugs decline in use.* Ann Arbor, MI: University of Michigan News Service. Retrieved July 7, 2010 from http://monitoring thefuture.org

Johnston, L. D., O'Malley, P. M., Bachman, J. G., & Schulenberg, J. E. (2012). *Monitoring the Future national survey results on drug use, 1975-2011. Volume I: Secondary school students.* Ann Arbor: Institute for Social Research, The University of Michigan.

Kahan, M., Srivastava, A., Wilson, L., Mailis-Gagnon, A., & Midmer, D. (2006). Opioids for managing chronic non-malignant pain. Safe and effective prescribing. *Canadian Family Physician, 52*(9), 1091-6.

Knapp, C. M., Ciraulo, D. A., & Jaffe, J. (2005). Opiates: Clinical aspects. In J.H. Lowinson, P. Ruiz, R.B. Millman, & J.G. Langrod (Eds.), *Substance abuse: A comprehensive textbook* (4th ed., pp. 180-195) Philadelphia: Lippincott Williams & Wilkins.

Ling, W., Wesson, D.R., & Smith, D.E. (2005). Prescription opiate abuse. In J.H. Lowinson, P. Ruiz, R.B. Millman, & J.G. Langrod (Eds.), *Substance abuse: A comprehensive textbook* (4th ed., pp. 459-468) Philadelphia: Lippincott Williams & Wilkins.

Manchikanti, L., Cash, K.A., Damron, K.S., Manchukonda, R., Pampati, V. & McManus, C.D. (2006). Controlled substance abuse and illicit drug use in chronic pain patients: An evaluation of multiple variables. *Pain Physician, 9*(3), 215-26.

Marion, I.J. (2005). Methadone treatment. *NIDA Science and Practice Perspectives, 3*(1), 25-33.

Miller, W.R. (1999). Enhancing motivation for change in substance abuse treatment. Treatment Improvement Protocol (TIP) Series 35. DHHS Publication No. (SMA) 99-3354. Rockville, MD: Substance Abuse and Mental Health Services Administration. Retrieved March 15, 2013, from http://www.ncbi.nlm.nih.gov/bookshelf/br.fcgi?book=hssamhsatip&part=A61302

National Institute on Drug Abuse. (2005). *Heroin abuse and addiction.* Research report series (NIH Publication No. 05-4165). Retrieved March 15, 2013, from http://www.nida.nih.gov/PDF/RRHeroin.pdf

Portenoy, R.K., Lussier, D., Kirsh, K.L., & Passik, S.D. (2005). Pain and addiction. In R.J. Frances, S.I. Miller, & A.H. Mack (Eds.), *Clinical textbook of addictive disorders* (3rd ed., pp.367-95). New York: Guilford Press.

Ray, O.S. & Ksir, C.J. (2002). *Drugs, society, and human behavior.* New York: McGraw Hill.

Sullivan, M.A., Comer, S.D., & Nunes, E.V. (2006). Pharmacology and clinical use of naltrexone. In E.C. Strain & M.L. Stitzer (Eds.), *The treatment of opioid dependence* (pp. 295-320). Baltimore: Johns Hopkins University Press.

Substance Abuse and Mental Health Services Administration. (2012a). *Results from the 2011 National survey on drug use and health: Summary of national findings* (NSDUH Series H-44, HHS Publication No. (SMA) 12-4713). Rockville, MD. Accessed March 15, 2013 from http://www.samhsa.gov/data/NSDUH/2k11Results/NSDUHresults2011.htm

Substance Abuse and Mental Health Services Administration. (2012b). *Treatment Episode Data Set (TEDS) 2000 - 2010: National admissions to substance abuse treatment services.* Retrieved March 15, 2013 from http://www.samhsa.gov/data/2k12/TEDS2010N/TEDS2010NWeb.pdf

Verhaak, P.F., Kerssens, J.J., Dekker, J., Sorbi, M.J., & Bensing, J.M. (1998). Prevalence of chronic benign pain disorder among adults: A review of the literature. *Pain, 77*(3), 231-9.

Volkow, N.D. (2007). *Fentanyl use in combination with street drugs leading to death in some cases.* Retrieved March 15, 2013, from http://www.drugabuse.gov/about/welcome/messagefentanyl606.html

Walsh, S.L. & Strain, E.C. (2006). Pharmacology of methadone. In E.C. Strain & M.L. Stitzer (Eds.), *The treatment of opioid dependence* (pp. 59-77). Baltimore: Johns Hopkins University Press.

CHAPTER 12

CENTRAL NERVOUS SYSTEM DEPRESSANTS

CHAPTER OBJECTIVE

After completing this chapter, the learner will be able to discuss the characteristics of and issues related to the abuse of central nervous system (CNS) depressants.

LEARNING OBJECTIVES

After studying this chapter, the learner will be able to:

1. Identify populations at risk for abuse of CNS depressants.
2. Identify CNS depressants most commonly abused.
3. Identify health risks related to the abuse of CNS depressants.
4. Select appropriate strategies to address CNS depressant abuse.

OVERVIEW

CNS depressants are drugs that dampen function of the CNS on a continuum that can range from reducing anxiety to, with the exception of benzodiazepines, coma and fatal respiratory depression. Sedative medications are designed to decrease anxiety while hypnotic medications are designed to encourage sleep. Making a distinction between sedatives and hypnotics is somewhat arbitrary because sedative drugs at higher doses also produce sleep, which is why sedatives and hypnotics are often discussed as a single drug class. CNS depressants are available legally for medical purposes with a prescription, and obtained illegally for recreational or nonmedical purposes. Most people use sedatives and hypnotics responsibly but substantial numbers of people misuse them. These drugs are typically classified as Schedule II or III drugs because of their abuse potential.

One of the oldest and most universally used CNS depressants is alcohol. Over the years, hundreds of substances within this category have been developed. These drugs have been referred to as *downers, sedatives, hypnotics, minor tranquilizers, anxiolytics,* and *anti-anxiety medications*. Most of these medications have been developed for legitimate therapeutic uses but are sometimes used illegally. This chapter will discuss current and common CNS depressants, particularly barbiturates and benzodiazepines.

HISTORY

Historically, most cultures have used substances to reduce stress, relieve anxiety, and produce sleep. Chloral hydrate and paraldehyde are two of the oldest pharmaceutical depressants still used today. Chloral hydrate, known as "knockout drops" or "Mickey Finn" when mixed with alcohol, was first developed in 1832 but not used clinically until 1869 (Drug Enforcement Agency [DEA], 2011). It is an excellent drug for inducing sleep and remains in use today. Paraldehyde was developed in 1829 but not introduced clinically until 1882. It also remains in use today because it is highly effective with minor respiratory depression. In the nineteenth century, bromide salts were widely used to induce sleep but caused serious adverse effects due to a build-up of bromide metabolites in the body. These adverse effects included dermatitis, constipation, motor disturbances, delirium, and psychosis. Consequently, bromides are no longer used in legal medications (Ksir, Hart, & Ray, 2005).

Barbiturates were first developed in the early 1900s. Although many were developed, not all were marketed for human use and about one-half continue to be used in medical settings. One of the major limiting factors with this class of drugs is the rapid development of tolerance, and resultant physical and psychological dependence.

In the 1960s, the development of benzodiazepines represented major progress because they evidenced less addictive potential than barbiturates. Today, about 20% of all prescribed controlled substances are benzodiazepines (DEA, 2011).

In 1954 until 1965, glutethimide and methaqualone were introduced (respectively) as safer barbiturates. But by 1972, they were actively abused by college students and young adults, producing tolerance, dependence, and withdrawal symptoms. Production of methaqualone was stopped in 1984 when it was reclassified as a Schedule I drug. In 1991, glutethimide was changed to a Schedule II drug to minimize the abuse potential (DEA, 2011). From 1972 to 1978, diazepam was the leading seller of prescription drugs (Ksir et al., 2005). Multiple national surveys suggest that the use of medical benzodiazepines peaked by 1976 and decreased by 25% by the late 1980s (Dupont & Dupont, 2005).

In the 1990s, flunitrazepam and gamma hydroxybutyric acid (GHB) emerged as illegal designer or club drugs. These drugs have been implicated in sexual assaults causing them to be referred to as *date rape* drugs (DEA, 2011).

EPIDEMIOLOGY

In 2011, approximately 231,000 people aged 12 or older, reported current nonmedical use of sedatives, and 1.8 million reported current use of tranquilizers (Substance Abuse and Mental Health Service Administration [SAMHSA], 2012). Over 1 million (1.2) people aged 12 and older used tranquilizers for the first time in 2011, and 0.7 million used sedatives for the first time on a nonmedical basis. Tranquilizers representing the second most frequently used category of prescription drugs (SAMHSA, 2012). These figures have not significantly changed in the past few years. Though sedatives and hypnotics are prescribed more often for persons ages 60 and older, misuse is most frequent among individuals between ages 18 and 25 (Suzuki & Sola, 2006).

In 2009, the Drug Abuse Warning Network (DAWN) found that one of the most frequently reported prescription medications was benzodiazepines. The two most frequently abused benzodiazepines were alprazolam (Xanax) and clonazepam (Klonopin) (DAWN, 2011).

BIOCHEMISTRY

CNS depressants slow normal brain function by stimulating gamma-aminobutyric acid (GABA) activity. When stimulated, GABA, the most widely dispersed inhibitory CNS neurotransmitter, inhibits or "depresses" discharge from neurons in the CNS, decreasing brain activity. There are three known GABA receptors: GABA-A, GABA-B, and GABA-C (Dupont & Dupont, 2005). Stimulation of

GABA-A receptors are primarily associated with seizure activity, anxiety, and sleep; GABA-B receptors are chiefly associated with memory and analgesia. Both receptor types are associated with mood changes. The function of GABA-C receptors is uncertain. Benzodiazepines bind to specific receptor sites in the brain causing increased GABA activity. Barbiturates bind to a separate receptor site nearby and also cause increased GABA (Ksir et al., 2005) activity. Elevated GABA activity results in, at minimum, a calming effect.

CLASSIFICATIONS OF SEDATIVE-HYPNOTICS

Depressants used in moderate doses induce a state of intoxication much like that of alcohol. Due to similar drug profiles, they exhibit cross tolerance; that is, effects demonstrated with one drug in this class will also be seen if another drug in the same class is taken.

Barbiturates are normally categorized according to the speed of onset and the duration of the effect. The classifications are ultrashort, short, intermediate, and long-acting. The ultrashort-acting barbiturates are Schedule IV drugs used intravenously to produce anesthesia in about 1 minute. The short-acting and intermediate drugs are usually taken orally and have an onset of action within about 15 to 40 minutes and duration of about 6 hours. The indication for these drugs is normally insomnia and preoperative sedation. The long-acting barbiturates have an onset of action after about 1 hour and last for about 12 hours. The primary purpose for these drugs is the treatment of seizure disorders and daytime sedation. Table 12-1 provides a listing of available barbiturates and their classifications.

Benzodiazepines are also used therapeutically to produce sedation, induce sleep, relieve anxiety, and muscle spasms, and prevent seizures. These drugs are available with both shorter and longer durations of action. The shorter acting preparations are often used with individuals who have difficulty getting to sleep. Some of the shorter-acting benzodiazepines include estazolam, flurazepam, temazepam, triazolam, and midazolam. The longer duration drugs are often used in individuals with daytime anxiety who also experience insomnia and in those who have seizures. Some of the longer-acting benzodiazepines include alprozolam, chlordiazepoxide, clorazepate, diazepam, halazepam, lorazepam, oxazepam, prazepam, quazepam, and clonazepam (DEA, 2005). Table 12-2 provides a listing of some of the commonly used benzodiazepines. Table 12-3 lists selected street names for benzodiazepines.

TABLE 12-1: BARBITURATES

Type	Time of Onset	Duration of Action
Short-acting Pentobarbital (Nembutal) Secobarbital (Seconal)	15 minutes	2 to 3 hours
Intermediate-acting Aprobarbital (Alurate) Amobarbital (Amytal) Butaboarbital (Butisol)	30 minutes	5 to 6 hours
Long-acting Mephobarbital (Merbaral) Phenobarbital (Luminal)	1 hour	6 to 10 hours
(Ray et al., 2005)		

TABLE 12-2: BENZODIAZEPINES

Generic Name	Trade Name	Indication
Alprazolam	Xanax	Antianxiety
Chlordiazepoxide	Librium	Antianxiety
Clonazepam	Klonopin	Anticonvulsant
Clorazepate	Tranxene	Antianxiety
Diazepam	Valium	Antianxiety
Estazolam	ProSom	Hypnotic
Flumazenil	Romazicon	Antagonist
Lorazepam	Ativan	Antianxiety
Midazolam	Versed	Anesthesia
Oxazepam	Serax	Antianxiety
Quazepam	Doral	Hypnotic
Temazepam	Restoril	Hypnotic
Triazolam	Halcion	Hypnotic

(Lowinson, Ruiz, Millman, & Langroud, 2005)

TABLE 12-3: SELECTED STREET NAMES FOR BENZODIAZEPINES

Reds	Barbs
Red devils	Downers
RDs	Busters
Fender benders	Butisol
Yellow	Courage pill
Yellow jackets	Florinal
Blues	G.B.s
Blue heavens	Goof balls
Rainbows	Green dragons
Christmas trees	King Kong pills
Pink ladies	Lotusate
Micky finn	Peanuts
Knockout drops	Ludes

Zolpidem is a hypnotic chemically unrelated to benzodiazepines but with a similar mechanism of action in that it binds to a similar GABA receptor. Zolpidem is absorbed quickly with a short half-life of about 2 hours. To date, few cases of zolpidem abuse have been reported (Wesson, Smith, Ling, & Seymour, 2005).

Comparably, *buspirone* is an anxiolytic that is neither chemically nor pharmacologically related to either the benzodiazepines or barbiturates and for this reason buspirone does not demonstrate cross-tolerance with either benzodiazepines or barbiturates. Consequently, this is not a drug used to treat sedative-hypnotic withdrawal.

Flunitrazepam, also known as the *date rape drug,* is a benzodiazepine that is not legally produced or marketed in the United States. Also known as *rophies, roach,* or *roofies,* flunitrazepam is a popular club or designer drug. This drug is usually added to a victim's drink without their knowledge causing them to be incapacitated and preventing them from resisting sexual assault. GHB is similar to flunitrazepam in that the victim cannot resist sexual assault and experiences amnesia-like effects. The use of this drug in sexual assault crimes is often difficult to prove because the drug is eliminated from the body quickly.

HEALTH EFFECTS OF SEDATIVE-HYPNOTICS

CNS depressants are excellent drugs and provide therapeutic benefits but also have a high abuse potential. The most frequently illegally used drugs are alprazolam (Xanax) and diazepam (Valium). Although they are still readily abused, benzodiazepines are well known for their better safety profiles when compared to barbiturates. Generally, benzodiazepines are much safer than barbiturates and cause significantly less respiratory depression. Compare this to the short- and intermediate-acting barbiturates that are fatal if taken in greater than 10 times the therapeutic dose (Wesson et al., 2005). It is essentially impossible to take a fatal benzodiazepine dose when taken by itself (Wesson et al., 2005). However, given the cross-tolerance among barbiturates, benzodiazepines, and alcohol, any combination of these substances can be fatal. The uses and consequences of commonly used CNS depressants are presented in Table 12-4.

Adverse effects of sedative-hypnotics include disinhibition, slurred speech, loss of motor coordination, impaired judgment, and decreased concentration (DEA, 2011). Various emotional effects include euphoria, depression, suicidal tendencies, and laughing or crying for no apparent reason. One effect of benzodiazepines is anterograde amnesia – loss of new memories during the period of intoxication, while past memory remains intact. This effect is intentionally targeted for surgical procedures requiring conscious sedation.

Adverse effects or toxicities from benzodiazepines can be seen in repeated use of large doses or in some cases daily doses of the substances. Signs and symptoms suggesting intoxication are obvious and include sustained horizontal nystagmus in addition to impaired gait, speech, and judgement (Wesson et al., 2005), observed

TABLE 12-4: CENTRAL NERVOUS SYSTEM DEPRESSANTS

Barbituates

- Mephobarbital (Mebaral)
- Pentobarbital sodium (Nembutaal)

Benzodiazepines

- Diazepam (Valium)
- Chlordiazepoxide hydrochloride (Librium)
- Alprazolam (Xanax)
- Triazolam (Halcion)
- Estazolam (ProSom)
- Clonazepam (Klonopin)
- Lorazepam (Ativan)

Prescription indications

- Anxiety
- Tension
- Panic attacks
- Acute stress reactions
- Sleep disorders
- Anesthesia (at high doses)

Effects on the body

Central nervous system (CNS) depressants slow brain activity through actions on the GABA system, producing a calming effect.

Effects of short-term use

A "sleepy" and uncoordinated feeling during the first few days; as the body becomes accustomed (tolerant) to the effects, these feelings diminish.

Effects of long-term use

Physical dependence and addiction are possible.

Possible negative effects

Seizures may follow a rebound in brain activity after reducing or discontinuing use.

Contraindications

They should not be used with other substances that cause CNS depression, including:

- alcohol
- prescription opioid pain medicines
- some over-the-counter cold and allergy medications.

Note. From *Prescription Drugs: Abuse and Addiction* by National Institute on Drug Abuse, Research report series (NIH Publication No. 11-4881), 2011. Accessed on March 15, 2013, from http://www.drugabuse.gov/PDF/RRPrescription.pdf

when the effects are below that of intoxication. Such symptoms as amnesia, hostility, irritability, and vivid or disturbing dreams have also been reported (DEA, 2011). The impaired judgment and decreased concentration associated with depressant intoxication also increases the risks associated with driving a car or using other mechanical equipment.

Tolerance and Dependence

Tolerance – physical and psychological dependence – can develop quickly and are related to the dose, frequency, and duration of use. Tolerance is thought to occur from the long-term use of sedative-hypnotics that results in down regulation (decreased sensitivity of the GABA receptors) (Sola, 2011). The development of tolerance causes the safety margin between the effective and dangerous doses to narrow, resulting in potential coma or death. Overdose of depressants produces effects that are similar to alcohol overdose. The person becomes very drowsy and unconscious, develops cold and clammy skin and decreased heart rate, and has shallow respirations. Death may occur from respiratory failure.

Psychological dependence or reinforcement is the potential for these medicines to be abused or "liked." Among alcoholics and others with substance use problems, benzodiazepines are relatively weak reinforcers compared to opiates, stimulants, and barbiturates (Dupont & Dupont, 2005). Benzodiazepines are not normally primary drugs of abuse but they are commonly used by addicts to increase the effect of heroin, marijuana, or alcohol. In fact, benzodiazepines are commonly employed to decrease the withdrawal associated with alcohol, cocaine, heroin, or methamphetamines (Dupont & Dupont, 2005).

Physical dependence is seen in this class of drugs as noted by a characteristic withdrawal syndrome. Individuals more prone to dependence include those prescribed higher doses, those who use them in combination with alcohol or other sedative drugs, and those with a family history of alcoholism. The latter group may be more susceptible due to genetic influences. Dependence at higher doses may be evident in as little as one month (Sola, 2011). This syndrome differs from opioid withdrawal in that it lasts longer and is usually perceived as more unpleasant. The sedative or hypnotic withdrawal syndrome includes the potential for seizures so it is essential to withdraw the drug slowly after daily use for more than a few weeks (Dupont & Dupont, 2005).

Withdrawal

Withdrawal from sedative-hypnotics is potentially life-threatening and may require hospitalization; death occurs in as many as 5% of those seeking care (Ksir et al., 2005). Typical signs and symptoms of withdrawal often reflect CNS hyperactivity and include anxiety, tremors, seizures, nightmares, delirium, insomnia, anorexia, nausea, vomiting, elevated pulse and blood pressure, and fever. Short-acting medications, such as pentobarbital and secobarbital, have withdrawal symptoms that usually start 12 to 24 hours after the last dose, peaking in intensity between 1 and 3 days after the last dose. Symptoms are delayed and/or prolonged if the person has liver disease. Such long-acting medications as phenobarbital, diazepam, and clordiazepoxide have a withdrawal syndrome that usually commences between 1 and 2 days after the last dose, peaking in intensity on the fifth to eighth day (APA, 2013; Wesson et al., 2005). Clinically significant withdrawal signs and symptoms can occur when taken at as low as twice the maximum therapeutic range for more than 1 month (Wesson et al., 2005).

When used in lower doses and/or for short periods of time, discontinuing benzodiazepines may not cause withdrawal symptoms but can cause symptom reemergence. Some persons experience symptom rebound during the first week or two after stopping benzodiazepines. A small number of individuals experience severe or extended withdrawal symptoms after discontinuing benzodiazepines, referred to as a *protracted withdrawal syndrome* (Dupont & Dupont, 2005). These symptoms can be mild or severe and present intermittently over many months. Symptoms include mild to moderate anxiety, mood instability, sleep disturbances, increased sensitivity to light and sound, and psychosis. One way to distinguish symptom rebound from protracted withdrawal is that symptoms due to withdrawal slowly decrease with continued benzodiazepine abstinence, whereas symptom reemergence does not. Persons at increased risk for developing a withdrawal syndrome from chronic but low drug doses are those with a family or personal history of alcoholism, those who use alcohol daily, and those who concomitantly use other sedatives (Wesson et al., 2005).

TREATMENT

Treatment for sedative-hypnotic withdrawal is required because the symptoms can be life-threatening. Standard treatment is the gradual withdrawal of the drug of dependence.

Three basic treatment strategies include the use of gradually decreasing doses of the sedative-hypnotic, substitution of a long-acting barbiturate followed by gradual withdrawal of the substituted long-acting sedative-hypnotic, and substitution of an anticonvulsant such as tegretol or depakote (Wesson et al., 2005; Dupont & Dupont, 2005).

Treatment for sedative-hypnotic withdrawal with the substitution of phenobarbital has multiple benefits. As a long-acting drug, any withdrawal symptoms that may occur are mild. It also maintains a relatively stable blood level with appropriate dosing. Its margin for safety is much wider than the shorter acting drugs; therefore, only extremely high doses are lethal. Furthermore, if toxicity occurs with phenobarbital, the signs are easily recognized and include "sustained nystagmus, slurred speech, and ataxia" (Wesson et al., 2005). Finally, even if the individual does become intoxicated, effects of high doses do not include disinhibition, a desired state for many individuals who misuse the drug. The only significant disadvantage is the tedious calculations for conversion from the abused drug. Additionally, 1% to 5% of individuals, so treated, develop a rash (Wesson et al., 2005).

As part of the stabilization process, individuals must be carefully evaluated before administering the next dose. If signs of sedative-hypnotic intoxication occur (slurred speech, sustained nystagmus), the dose is reduced; if symptoms of withdrawal occur (such as intense nightmares, muscle twitching, psychosis), the dose is increased. After stabilization (meaning no signs of intoxication or withdrawal are present), phenobarbital can be gradually withdrawn, typically by 30 mg each day.

The use of an anticonvulsant as a substitute for sedative-hypnotic withdrawal has been clinically successful. Tegretol and depakote are both effective in suppressing withdrawal symptoms because they increase GABA function. Patients with pre-existing seizure disorders readily tolerate the use of tegretol (Dupont & Dupont, 2005). Perhaps most importantly, neither of these drugs has effects sought after by those who misuse sedative-hypnotics.

Benzodiazepine overdose is most dangerous in combination with other sedative-hypnotic drugs. A benzodiazepine antagonist, flumazenil, is available for treating acute benzodiazepine intoxication. This drug must be used with caution because it may not reverse respiratory depression completely and can provoke withdrawal seizures in persons with benzodiazepine dependence. In a barbiturate overdose, the individual is treated with urine alkalinization to increase drug excretion. The goal is to maintain a urine pH of 7.5. Sodium bicarbonate can be given intravenously but severely ill persons may require dialysis. An overdose with these drugs requires not only immediate intervention but also medical observation for several days because they have extremely long half lives and are metabolized slowly.

Although minimal research regarding the treatment of barbiturate and benzodiazepine addiction exists, addicted clients should undergo medically supervised detoxification. Additionally, cognitive behavioral therapy (CBT) can be offered which is based on social learning theory and emphasizes modification of the individual's thoughts and behaviors. CBT has been used to successfully help individuals to adapt to a discontinuation of benzodiazepines. A supportive organization based on the 12-step Alcoholics Anonymous model is Pills Anonymous. A goal for both approaches is to encourage abstinence by helping clients learn and master effective coping skills that can help them believe they can resist relapsing to substance abuse. The focus is on the exploration of positive and negative consequences of substance use. Because clients are taught the skills needed to prevent a return to substance abuse after treatment, this approach is the foundation for relapse prevention.

SCREENING OF SPECIAL POPULATIONS AND RISK IDENTIFICATION

Most people use prescription medications responsibly, taking only the medications prescribed, at the prescribed dose, and for the prescribed time. It is important that individuals be appropriately diagnosed and medically treated as necessary. Most people who abuse benzodiazepines maintain their own supply by getting medication from several different physicians, forging prescriptions or buying illegal pharmaceuticals. Because more than 80% of Americans have contact with a healthcare provider once a year, these providers are in a unique position to potentially identify and address problems with sedative-hypnotics (NIDA, 2011). Prevention strategies include responsible prescribing and monitoring of these substances as well as helping individuals identify actual and potential problems. Health care providers, including primary care providers, pharmacists, and nurses, have a role in preventing prescription drug abuse. It is essential that primary care providers be comfortable and competent in counseling persons in the area of drug abuse. In the research study Missed Opportunity: National Survey of Primary Care Physicians and Patients on Substance Abuse 2000, more than 40% of physicians reported having difficulty discussing substance abuse with their patients (The National Center on Addiction and Substance Abuse at Columbia University, 2000). The Benzodiazepine Checklist for Long-term Use, presented in Table 12-5, is a tool that health care providers can use as they structure the pharmacological therapy for their patients.

Older Adults

For persons older than age 65, symptoms of sedative-hypnotic withdrawal develop slower than the 12- to 24-hour period stated previously. Similarly, duration of withdrawal will be longer. This group is more vulnerable to the cognitive impairment that may arise with these drugs and should be evaluated carefully to determine if the benefits outweigh the risks. Due to the presence of other comorbid medical disorders, distinguishing the symptoms of intoxication and withdrawal are more challenging.

Psychiatric Comorbidity

Benzodiazepines are frequently illicitly used by people with other substance use disorders such as cocaine or by those who are enrolled in methadone maintenance programs for opioid

TABLE 12-5: BENZODIAZEPINE CHECKLIST FOR LONG-TERM USE
1. *Diagnosis.* Is there a current diagnosis that warrants the prolonged use of a prescription medication?
2. *Medical and nonmedical substance use.* Is the dose of the benzodiazepine the client is taking reasonable? Is the clinical response to the benzodiazepine favorable? Is there any use of non-medical drugs, such as cocaine or marijuana? Is there any excessive use of alcohol (such as a total of more than four drinks per week or more than two drinks per day)? Are there other medicines being used that can depress the functioning of the central nervous system?
3. *Toxic behavior.* Is the patient free of evidence of slurred speech, staggering, accidents, memory loss, or other mental deficits or evidence of sedation?
4. *Family monitor.* Does the family confirm that there is a good clinical response and no adverse reactions to the patient's use of a benzodiazepine?
Standard for continued benzodiazepine use: a "yes" to all four questions.
(Frances, Miller, & Mack, 2005)

dependence. They are usually self-administered by persons with cocaine abuse to decrease agitation caused by cocaine use or to augment methadone's effect to produce euphoria. Clonazepam is particularly favored by this group because it is usually not included in urine toxicology screens (Wesson et al., 2005). The depressant effects of tricyclic antidepressants, such as amitriptyline, may also be used to enhance the sedative effects of methadone (Wesson et al., 2005).

It is essential that we accurately differentiate medical and nonmedical use of these medications. First, consider if the substance being prescribed will treat a diagnosed health problem. Secondly, consider the drugs impact on the user's life. For example, individuals misusing a substance often experience deterioration, denial, and negative consequences in their lives. In therapeutic situations, control of the substance use is shared by the provider and the patient; in nonmedical situations, the user is in complete control.

The pattern of use is also important. In most situations, these medications are prescribed for periods that correspond to the health problem. Lastly, consider if the substance is being obtained legally or illegally. As controlled substances, they can be obtained only with a medical prescription (Dupont & Dupont, 2005). Many people who abuse benzodiazepines obtain their drugs by getting prescriptions from various health providers, from people with valid prescriptions, by forging prescriptions, or by buying illegal substances off the street.

SUMMARY

CNS depressants function to substantially slow normal brain function by affecting the neurotransmitter GABA. In lower doses, they act as a sedative; in higher doses, the effect is hypnotic. These are commonly prescribed substances that are useful in treating anxiety and sleep disorders but are also at risk for misuse and abuse.

People need to be appropriately diagnosed and managed (treated, followed, and educated) to be safely treated with these medications at the correct prescription. With appropriate care and consideration, these substances are safe and effective medications.

EXAM QUESTIONS

CHAPTER 12

Questions 70-73

Note: Choose the one option that BEST answers each question.

70. Although sedatives and hypnotics are prescribed more often for persons ages 60 and older, misuse is most frequent among individuals

    a. younger than age 18.
    b. between ages 18 and 25.
    c. between ages 35 and 55.
    d. older than age 55.

71. According to the Drug Abuse Warning Network, in 2009, the most frequently illegally abused benzodiazepines includes

    a. alprazolam and clonazepam.
    b. rohypnol and lorazepam.
    c. lorazepam and methqualone.
    d. midazolam and diazepam.

72. The most serious health risk(s) associated with central nervous system (CNS) abuse include(s)

    a. death from respiratory failure.
    b. HIV and sexually-transmitted infections.
    c. liver failure.
    d. cerebral vascular accident (stroke).

73. An appropriate strategy to address CNS depressant abuse is

    a. relapse prevention only.
    b. medically supervised detoxification and cognitive behavioral therapy.
    c. medically supervised detoxification only.
    d. cognitive behavioral therapy only.

REFERENCES

American Psychiatric Association. (2013). *Diagnostic and statistical manual of mental disorders* (5th ed.). Washington, DC: American Psychiatric Association.

Drug Abuse Warning Network. (2011). *National estimates of drug-related emergency department visits.* Office of Applied Studies, SAMHSA. Retrieved March 15, 2013, from http://www.samhsa.gov/data/2k11/DAWN/2k9DAWNED/HTML/DAWN2k9ED.htm

Drug Enforcement Administration. (2011) *Drugs of abuse – Chapter 7: Depressants.* U.S. Department of Justice. Retrieved March 15, 2013, from http://www.justice.gov/dea/docs/drugs_of_abuse_2011.pdf

Dupont, R.L. & Dupont, C.M. (2005). Sedatives/hypnotics and benzodiazepines. In R.J. Frances, S.I. Miller, & A.H. Mack (Eds.), *Clinical textbook of addictive disorders* (3rd ed., pp. 219-244). New York: Guilford Press.

Frances, R.J., Miller, S.I., & Mack, A.H. (Eds.) 2005. *Clinical textbook of addiction disorders,* (3rd ed.), New York: Guilford Press.

Ksir, C., Hart, C.L., & Ray, O.S. (2005). *Drugs, society, and human behavior,* 11th ed. New York: McGraw-Hill.

National Institute on Drug Abuse. (2011). *Prescription drugs: Abuse and addiction.* Research report series (NIH Publication No. 11-4881). Retrieved March 15, 2013, from http://www.drugabuse.gov/PDF/RRPrescription.pdf

Substance Abuse and Mental Health Services Administration. (2012). *Results from the 2011 National survey on drug use and health: Summary of national findings* (NSDUH Series H-44, HHS Publication No. (SMA) 12-4713). Rockville, MD. Accessed March 15, 2013 from http://www.samhsa.gov/data/NSDUH/2k11Results/NSDUHresults2011.htm

Sola, C.L. (2011). *Sedative, hypnotic, anxiolytic use disorders.* Retrieved March 15, 2013, from http://www.emedicine.com/med/topic3119.htm

The National Center on Addiction and Substance Abuse at Columbia University. (2000). *Missed opportunity: National survey of primary care physicians and oatients on substance abuse.* Retrieved April 3, 2013, from http://www.casacolumbia.org/templates/Publications_Reports.aspx#r41

Voshaar, R.C., Couvee, J.E., Van Balkom, A.J.L., Mulder, P.G., & Zitman, F.G. (2006). Strategies for discontinuing long-term benzodiazepine use. *British Journal of Psychiatry, 189,* 213-220.

Wesson, D.R., Smith, D.E., Ling, W., & Seymour, R.B. (2005). Sedative-hypnotics. In J.H. Lowinson, P. Ruiz, R.B. Millman, & J.G. Langrod (Eds.), *Substance abuse. A comprehensive textbook* (4th ed.). Philadelphia: Lippincott Williams & Wilkins.

CHAPTER 13

INHALANTS

CHAPTER OBJECTIVE

After completing this chapter, the learner will be able to describe the characteristics and health effects of inhalant use in the U.S. population.

LEARNING OBJECTIVES

After studying this chapter, the learner will be able to:

1. Discuss how inhalants are used.
2. Define the four different categories of inhalants.
3. Describe trends and patterns of inhalant use in the U.S. population.
4. Describe the health effects of inhalant use.
5. Discuss the role of screening and treatment in addressing this health issue.

OVERVIEW

Inhalants are volatile solvents and substances that produce chemical vapors, which are inhaled for purposes of producing a mind-altering effect. The term refers to more than a thousand household and commercial products that are generally easily accessible and available at low cost. Inhalants are the third most widely used class of illicit drugs among adolescents (Wu, Pilowsky, & Schlenger, 2004). The substances are inhaled in various ways, including "sniffing," "snorting," "bagging," or "huffing." Sniffing or snorting involves the inhalation directly from containers or a heated pan. Bagging refers to the inhalation of vapors from plastic bags containing the substance. Huffing is the inhalation of vapors by taking a cloth saturated with the substance and placing the cloth over the nose and mouth or stuffing it in the mouth. Inhaling from balloons filled with nitrous oxide is another method of using the substances. Some common street names for inhalants or using inhalants are *laughing gas* (nitrous oxide), *snappers* (amyl nitrite), *poppers* (amyl nitrite and butyl nitrite), *whippets* (fluorinated hydrocarbons, found in whipped cream dispensers), *bold* (nitrites), and *rush* (nitrites) (National Institute on Drug Abuse [NIDA], 2013).

CATEGORIES OF INHALANTS

There are four general categories of inhalants (Table 13-1). Volatile solvents are liquids that vaporize at room temperature. These are found in such common household and industrial goods as paint thinners or removers, dry cleaning fluids, gasoline, correction fluids, and felt tip markers. Some of the chemicals within these products include propane, butane, trichloroethane (TCE), benzene, methylene chloride, and toluene. A street name for toluene is *tolly*.

TABLE 13-1: CATEGORIES OF INHALANTS, SAMPLE PRODUCTS, AND CHEMICALS FOUND IN INHALANTS

Category of Inhalant	Examples of Products	Examples of Chemicals Found in Inhalants
Volatile solvents	Paint thinners, paint removers, dry cleaning fluids, gasoline, glue, correction fluids, felt-tip markers, degreasers	Methylene chloride, Toluene, Benzene, Trichlorethylene
Aerosols	Spray paints, deodorant and hair sprays, vegetable oil sprays, fabric protector sprays	Hydrofluorocarbons
Gases	Medical anesthetics, gases in household products (butane lighters, propane tanks, whipped cream dispensers, and refrigerants)	Ether, Chloroform, Halothane, Nitrous oxide, Butane, Propane, Freon
Nitrites	Video head cleaner, room odorizers, leather cleaner, or liquid aroma	Cyclohexyl nitrite, Isoamyl (amyl) nitrite, Isobutyl (butyl) nitrite

(NIDA, 2012)

Aerosols are the second category and are sprays that contain propellants and solvents that can be found in hair sprays, spray paints, deodorants, and vegetable sprays. The chemicals associated with these selected products include butane and propane.

The third category is gases. Gases include household and commercial products as well as medical anesthetics. Of the medical anesthetic gases, nitrous oxide is the most frequently abused and can be found in whipped cream dispensers and products that increase octane levels in racing cars. Some common street names for nitrous oxide include *whippets, laughing gas,* and *buzz bomb.*

The fourth category, nitrites, includes cyclohexyl nitrite, isoamyl (amyl) nitrite, and isobutyl (butyl) nitrite. Street names include *poppers*, *snappers*, *bullets*, *Amys*, *Ames*, or *pearl*. Although nitrites are prohibited by the Consumer Product Safety Commission, they can still be found in products labeled as "video head cleaner," "room odorizer," "leather cleaner," or "liquid aroma" (NIDA, 2012a; NIDA, 2013).

In an analysis of 12- to 17-year-olds who participated in the National Survey on Drug Use and Health, the most commonly used inhalants by self-report were glue, shoe polish, and/or toluene. Other inhalants used included gasoline or lighter fluid, spray paints, aerosol sprays (other than spray paint) correction fluid or cleaning fluid, locker room odorizers, lacquer thinner, lighter gases (such as butane or propane), and nitrous oxide or "whippits" (NSDUH, 2010). The percentage of youths aged 12 to 17 who currently use inhalants was 0.9% in 2011, indicating a long-term gradual decline in inhalant use. It is interesting to note that inhalant use is more common among youth in the lower end of the 12-17 age range – a trend that lies directly opposite of that for virtually all other drugs. The annual prevalence of use is 6%, 4%, and 3% in grades 8, 10, and 12, respectively (Johnston, O'Malley, Bachman, & Schulenberg 2013). For the three grades combined, the 0.6% drop in inhalant use in 2012 was significant.

EPIDEMIOLOGY OF INHALANT USE

There are approximately 20.5 million people in the U.S. ages 12 and older who reported using inhalants at least once during their lifetime (Substance Abuse and Mental Health Services Administration [SAMHSA], 2012a). This represents 8.0% of the population ages 12 and older. In the same survey, the 2011 National Survey on Drug Use and Health (NSDUH) found that nearly 2 million Americans (0.7%) reported past year inhalant use and 624,000 (0.2%) reported past month inhalant use (SAMHSA, 2012). In the 2009 Monitoring the Future study, 13.1% of eighth graders, 10.1% of tenth graders, and 8.1% of twelfth graders reported lifetime use of inhalants, while the past month use ranged from 1.0% in the twelfth graders to 3.2% in the eighth graders (Johnston, O'Malley, Bachman, & Schulenberg, 2012a). Among students surveyed in the 2009 Youth Risk Behavior Surveillance System, 11.4% reported using inhalants at least one time during their lifetimes (Centers for Disease Control and Prevention [CDC], 2012). In a sample of college students, 3.7% reported lifetime use while 7.2% of young adults (ages 19 to 28) reported lifetime use of inhalants (Johnston, O'Malley, Bachman, & Schulenberg, 2012b).

In looking at the patterns of use over time, inhalant use increased by one-third among eighth and tenth graders from 1991 to 1995 but declined gradually at all grade levels from 1995 to 2002. From this point on, the trends in the three grades have slightly diverged: 8th graders showed a significant increase in use for 2002 and 2004, followed by a decline from 2005 to 2012; 10th graders showed an increase after 2002, but some decline since 2007 (including a significant decrease in 2011); 12th graders showed some increase from 2003 to 2005, but a decline since then (Johnston, O'Malley, Bachman, & Schulenberg, 2013). It is also clear from the NSDUH that new inhalant users are predominately younger than 18; in 2011, 67.1% of new users were under 18 years of age (SAMHSA, 2012a).

Gender differences also exist in inhalant use but vary by age. Among 8th graders, females actually have higher rates of annual inhalant use than males. However, among twelfth graders, males reported using inhalants in the past year more than females (Johnston, O'Malley, Bachman, & Schulenberg, 2012a). In the NSDUH, similar proportions of boys or girls age 12 to 17 abused inhalants but among those age 18 to 25, males were twice as likely to abuse them as females (SAMHSA, 2012a).

Other risk factors for inhalant use include adverse socioeconomic conditions, a history of childhood abuse, poor grades, and dropping out of school. Inhalant use is found in urban and rural settings (NIDA, 2012a). There is also evidence that some Hispanic groups and American Indians on reservations have a higher percentage of inhalant users than the general population (Sharp & Rosenberg, 2005).

In looking at adults, the risk factors associated with inhalant use were being age 18 to 25, Asian, past year alcohol abusers and dependents, lifetime drug users, and White women and men reporting symptoms of mental illness. For inhalant disorders, the adults were primarily age 35 to 49 years, had less education, had a coexisting alcohol disorder, used inhalants weekly, and had received professional treatment for emotional or psychological problems (Wu & Ringwalt, 2006).

BIOCHEMISTRY

The chemicals that are inhaled are rapidly absorbed through the lungs into the bloodstream. They are distributed to the brain and other organs and, within seconds of inhalation, intoxicating feelings similar to the effects of alcohol are experienced. These effects can include slurred speech, an inability to coordinate movements, euphoria, dizziness, lightheadedness, hallucinations, and delusions. Nearly all abused inhalants (except for the nitrites) have neurobehavioral effects similar to central nervous system (CNS) depressants such as alcohol, sedatives, and anesthetics (NIDA, 2012a). Neuroimaging techniques have revealed that various inhalants affect the brain differently by affecting different regions of the brain.

Nitrites are a special class of inhalants in that they, unlike the other inhalant categories, do not act on the CNS but act directly on the blood vessels and muscles. They dilate the vessels, increase heart rate, create a sensation of heat and excitement, and cause such other effects as dizziness and headaches. Nitrites are also used to enhance sex (NIDA, 2012a).

There is evidence of a mild withdrawal with the continued use of inhalants (NIDA, 2012a). Studies have found that the rewarding effects of toluene, for example, are related to levels of brain dopamine (NIDA and Fogarty International Center, 2005).

SCREENING OF SPECIAL POPULATIONS AND RISK IDENTIFICATION

Youth are at particular risk for inhalant use. Early identification and intervention are the best public health measures in addressing this problem. Some potential signs of a serious inhalant problem are chemical odors on breath or clothing; paint or other stains on face, hands, or clothes; hidden empty spray paint or solvent containers and chemical-soaked rags or clothing; drunk or disoriented appearance; slurred speech; nausea or loss of appetite; or inattentiveness, lack of coordination, irritability, and depression (NIDA, 2012a).

It has been suggested that drug screening may be useful in monitoring inhalant abusers of toluene. According to one source, routine urine screens for hippuric acid, a major metabolite of toluene, could be performed two to three times weekly (Sharp & Rosenberg, 2005).

Pregnant women are a special population for consideration. There have been some case reports noting abnormalities in newborns and subsequent developmental impairments. Although there is limited research that links exposure to a specific birth defect or developmental problem, some animal studies have found that toluene or trichloroethylene can result in reduced birth weight and skeletal abnormalities (NIDA, 2012a).

RELATED MEDICAL PROBLEMS AND CO-OCCURRING DISORDERS

The medical consequences of inhalant use can be very severe. The most drastic consequence of use is death. The syndrome "sudden sniffing death," which is usually associated with the abuse of butane, propane, and chemicals in aerosols, occurs after sniffing highly concentrated amounts of chemicals. These chemicals can induce heart failure and death within minutes of repeated inhalations. Death can also occur from suffocation, which may occur when inhaling from a paper or plastic bag in a closed area, convulsions or seizures, coma, choking on vomit after inhalation, or a fatal injury suffered while intoxicated (NIDA, 2012a).

Chronic abuse can cause severe damage to several body systems. The most significant is damage to the brain and other parts of the CNS. Volatile solvents such as toluene can damage the protective sheath around certain nerve fibers in the brain and peripheral nervous system. Major neurotoxic syndromes seen in people exposed to organic solvents include peripheral neuropathy, ototoxicity (damage to the ears, hearing problems), and encephalopathy (affecting the brain). Less common conditions are cerebellar ataxic syndrome, Parkinsonism, or myopathy (muscle weakness) (Sharp & Rosenberg, 2005).

Neurological syndromes will reflect damage to the part of the brain involved in cognition, movement, vision, or hearing. The symptoms can be cognitive impairments (mild to severe dementia), difficulty coordinating movement, spasms of the limbs, or a loss of feeling, hearing, and vision. A study by Mathias (2002) examined the extent of brain damage and neuropsychiatric impairment induced by chronic abuse of inhalants and cocaine. Inhalant abusers performed significantly worse on tests involving working memory and executive cognitive functions. In addition, the inhalant abusers were more likely to have brain abnormalities on magnetic resonance imaging scans.

Other organs of the body can also be affected by exposure to solvents. Toluene and chlorinated hydrocarbons can cause damage to the liver and kidneys. Methylene chloride can cause a reduction of the oxygen carrying capacity of the blood and changes to the heart muscle and heartbeat. Benzene, which is found in gasoline, can cause bone marrow injury, impaired immunologic function, an increased risk of leukemia, and reproductive toxicity (NIDA, 2012a).

Nitrites are a special category. Because nitrites are often used to enhance sexual function, research shows that abuse of these drugs is associated with unsafe sexual practices, increasing the risk of sexually-transmitted infections. In addition, there is also a link to the development of other infectious diseases and tumors because nitrites impair the immune system and cause injury to red blood cells (NIDA, 2012a).

There is some controversy about the reversibility of damage to the body with use of inhalants. In general, acute high- and low-level exposure to organic solvents are associated with full reversibility. Chronic neurotoxic injury related to solvents is slowly and incompletely reversible and usually does not progress upon cessation of exposure (Sharp & Rosenberg, 2005). Other sources have stated that chronic exposure to inhalants can produce significant and sometimes irreversible damage to the heart, lungs, liver, and kidneys (NIDA, 2012a). For example, the irreversible effects of solvents include hearing loss (toluene, trichroethylene), peripheral neuropathies or limb spasms (hexenes, nitrous oxide), CNS or brain damage (toluene), and bone marrow damage (benzene) (NIDA, 2012b).

Besides the medical effects, there are also psychosocial correlates with inhalant use, such as delinquent behavior. In 2011, youths ages 12 to 17 who reported having been in a serious fight at school or work, or in some other form of delinquent behavior, were more than twice as likely than other youths to have used illicit drugs (includes inhalants) in the past month; past month illicit drug use was reported by 18.5% of 12-17 year olds who had been in a serious fight, and 8.0% who had not been in a serious fight (SAMHSA, 2012a).

TREATMENT

The number of admissions to treatment in which an inhalant was the primary drug of abuse decreased from 1994 to 2004; in 1994, there were 2,676 admissions, which gradually dropped to 1,209 in 2004. From 2005 to 2009, the number increased from 1,068 to 1,558, before declining in 2010 to 1,449. And while the numbers have changed, the percentage of admissions to treatment in which an inhalant was the primary drug of abuse has remained constant for the period from 2000 to 2010 at 0.1%, indicating an increase in the number of people seeking treatment for drug abuse (SAMHSA, 2012b). Over 60% of the admissions involved clients younger than age 30 (SAMHSA, 2012b).

Research regarding the prevention of inhalant use and treatment of addiction is limited

(Ridenour, 2005). Treatment is mainly supportive with attention to airway, breathing, and circulation management being paramount when a client presents to a medical setting. No medication is available to reverse the effects of inhalants; neuroleptics and other forms of pharmacotherapy are not useful in treatment (Greene, Ahrendt & Stafford, 2006; Sharp & Rosenberg, 2005).

There are often associated psychosocial problems and the possibility of brain injury, which makes progress difficult. Previous studies have found that inhalant abusers have unique psychiatric symptomatology (Ridenour, 2005). In a group of 847 adolescents being treated for substance addiction to inhalants, the adolescents were more likely to have another disorder related to alcohol, nicotine, cocaine, amphetamine, or halluconogen addiction; major depression; or attempted suicide, underscoring the need to address inhalant use and addiction in treatment settings (Sakai, Hall, Mikulich, & Crowley, 2004).

Overall, treating a person with an inhalant disorder is similar in some ways to treating clients with other substance abuse disorders (Brouette & Anton, 2001). The first step is getting a detailed history (products used, how often they are used, and the medium used) and a physical examination. With chronic inhalant abusers, attention to the neurological examination and laboratory work to assess organ damage (liver, kidney, and heart) is indicated. Attention to the possibility of withdrawal warrants close monitoring. In adults, CBT, 12-step facilitation, or motivational enhancement may be beneficial, although many inhalant users have neurocognitive deficits, which may make cognitive behavioral approaches difficult initially.

Differences from standard substance treatment are also present. Detoxification from poisonous chemicals must be accomplished before planning treatment. This detoxification cannot be accomplished in a 14-, 21-, or 28-day model but will most likely take 90 to 120 days. The client will most likely have a short attention span, poor impulse control, and poor social skills not appropriate for group therapy. Lastly, neurocognitive damage may impair decision-making skills (National Inhalant Prevention Coalition, n.d.). Other treatment suggestions by the National Inhalant Prevention Coalition are found in Table 13-2.

TABLE 13-2: SPECIFIC INHALANT TREATMENT CONSIDERATIONS

- Standard substance abuse treatment is generally ineffective for inhalant abusers.
- Detoxification, medical screening, and neurological screening must be initiated before a treatment plan is constructed.
- Neurocognitive assessments are important to assess impairment.
- Neurocognitive rehabilitation should be provided to those who are "impaired."
- There is a need to consider academic progress for students.
- A peer patient advocate system may be established to assist incoming patients.
- A team approach is imperative and where indicated, occupational and physical therapy must be included in a comprehensive treatment plan.
- Access to inhalable substances must be eliminated or restricted.
- Aftercare planning is critical and must take into consideration easy availability to inhalants, residual cognitive impairments, and poor social functioning.

(National Inhalant Prevention Coalition, n.d.)

SUMMARY

Inhalant use continues to be an important public health issue. The number of eighth graders using inhalants is of particular concern, especially because this number has increased in recent years.

Psychosocial problems are commonly present along with use and there is also evidence that use of inhalants is associated with the use of other illicit drugs, such as injection drug use (Wu & Howard, 2006). All of these issues point to the fact that screening, prevention, and treatment interventions for individuals using inhalants is critical. The international meeting of scientists – *Inhalant Abuse Among Children and Adolescents: Consultation on Building an International Research Agenda* – in November 2005 attests to the significance of this issue. The issues that emerged from that meeting confirm the findings of recent studies. Some of the priority research areas include standardizing and adapting surveillance methods for inhalant abuse; designing, implementing, and evaluating treatment and prevention interventions tailored to inhalant abuse; expanding basic science studies to better understand the mechanisms of action; and investigating the interaction among underlying factors that may contribute to inhalant abuse and consequences (National Institute on Drug Abuse and Fogarty International Center, 2005).

EXAM QUESTIONS

CHAPTER 13

Questions 74-79

Note: Choose the one option that BEST answers each question.

74. The inhalation of vapors by taking a cloth saturated with the substance and placing it over the nose and mouth or stuffing it in the mouth is called

    a. sniffing.
    b. bagging.
    c. huffing.
    d. snorting.

75. The category of inhalants that are used to enhance sexual function is

    a. volatile solvents.
    b. aerosols.
    c. nitrites.
    d. gases.

76. The types of inhalants most frequently used by adolescents ages 12 to 17 are

    a. glue, shoe polish, and/or toluene.
    b. gasoline and lighter fluid.
    c. nitrous oxide inhalants.
    d. spray paints.

77. One of the most serious medical effects of using inhalants is death. This is most likely due to

    a. effects of gases on the cerebellum.
    b. damage to the liver and kidneys.
    c. heart failure or suffocation.
    d. the release of dopamine in the brain.

78. Which statement about the mechanisms of action of nitrites is true?

    a. Nitrites have a neurobehavioral effect similar to other depressants.
    b. Nitrites act as an anesthetic agent on the body.
    c. Nitrites dilate and relax blood vessels.
    d. Nitrites activate the brain's dopamine system.

79. Screening for hippuric acid in urine is used to identify abuse of which inhalant?

    a. Ether
    b. Nitrite
    c. Toluene
    d. Hydroflurocarbon

REFERENCES

Brouette, T. & Anton, R. (2001). Clinical review of inhalants. *The American Journal on Addictions, 10,* 79-94.

Centers for Disease Control and Prevention. (2012). Youth risk behavior surveillance – United States, 2011. *Morbidity & Mortality Weekly Report, 61*(SS-04). Retrieved March 15, 2013 from http://www.cdc.gov/mmwr/preview/mmwrhtml/ss6104a1.htm

Greene, J.P., Ahrendt, D., & Stafford, E.M. (2006). Adolescent abuse of other drugs. *Adolescent Medicine, 17*(2), 283-318.

Johnston, L. D., O'Malley, P. M., Bachman, J. G., & Schulenberg, J. E. (2012a). *Monitoring the Future national survey results on drug use, 1975-2011. Volume I: Secondary school students*. Ann Arbor: Institute for Social Research, The University of Michigan.

Johnston, L. D., O'Malley, P. M., Bachman, J. G., & Schulenberg, J. E. (2012b). *Monitoring the Future national survey results on drug use, 1975-2011. Volume II: College students and adults ages 19-50.* Ann Arbor: Institute for Social Research, The University of Michigan.

Johnston, L. D., O'Malley, P. M., Bachman, J. G., & Schulenberg, J. E. (2013). *Monitoring the Future national results on adolescent drug use: Overview of key findings, 2012.* Ann Arbor: Institute for Social Research, The University of Michigan.

Mathias, R. (2002). *Chronic solvent abusers have more brain abnormalities and cognitive impairments than cocaine abusers.* National Institute on Drug Abuse, Research Findings, Vol 17, No. 4. Retrieved March 15, 2013, from http://archives.drugabuse.gov/NIDA_Notes/NNVol17N4/Chronic.html

National Inhalant Prevention Coalition. (n.d.). *Inhalants: Guidelines.* Accessed March 15, 2013, from www.inhalants.org/guidelines.htm

National Institute of Drug Abuse. (2012a). *Inhalant Abuse.* Research report series (NIH Publication Number 10-3818). U.S. Department of Health and Human Services. Bethesda, MD: National Institutes of Health. Retrieved March 15, 2013, from http://nida.nih.gov/PDF/RRInhalants.pdf

National Institute on Drug Abuse. (2012b). *NIDA Info Facts: Inhalants.* Retrieved March 15, 2013, from http://www.drugabuse.gov/infofacts/inhalants.html

National Institute on Drug Abuse. (2013). *Facts on drugs: Inhalants*. Retrieved March 15, 2013 from http://teens.drugabuse.gov/drug-facts/inhalants

National Institute on Drug Abuse and Fogarty International Center. (2005). *Inhalant abuse among children and adolescents: Consultation on building and international research.* Meeting summary. Rockville, MD. Accessed March 15, 2013, from http://international.drugabuse.gov/sites/default/files/pdf/inhalant_summary.pdf

Ridenour, T.A. (2005). Inhalants: Not to be taken lightly anymore. *Current Opinions in Psychiatry, 18*(3), 243-247.

Sakai, J.T., Hall, S.K., Mikulich, G.S., & Crowley, T.J. (2004). Inhalant use, abuse, and dependence among adolescent patients: Commonly comorbid problems. *Journal of the American Academy of Child and Adolescent Psychiatry, 43*(9), 1080-1088.

Sharp, C.W. & Rosenberg, N.L. (2005). Inhalants. In J. Lowinson, P. Ruiz, R. Millman, & J.G. Langrod, (Eds.). *Substance abuse: A comprehensive textbook.* Philadelphia: Lippincott Williams & Wilkins.

Substance Abuse and Mental Health Services Administration. (2010). *Adolescent inhalant use and selected respiratory conditions.* Retrieved March 15, 2013 from http://www.samhsa.gov/data/2k10/175/175RespiratoryCond.htm

Substance Abuse and Mental Health Services Administration. (2012a). *Results from the 2011 National survey on drug use and health: Summary of national findings* (NSDUH Series H-44, HHS Publication No. (SMA) 12-4713). Rockville, MD. Accessed March 15, 2013 from http://www.samhsa.gov/data/NSDUH/2k11Results/NSDUHresults2011.htm

Substance Abuse and Mental Health Services Administration. (2012b). *Treatment Episode Data Set (TEDS) 2000-2010: National admissions to substance abuse treatment services.* Retrieved March 15, 2013 from http://www.samhsa.gov/data/2k12/TEDS2010N/TEDS2010NWeb.pdf

Wu, L.T., Pilowsky, D.J., & Schlenger, W.E. (2004). Inhalant abuse and dependence among adolescents in the United States. *Journal of the American Academy of Child and Adolescent Psychiatry, 43*(10), 1206-1214.

Wu, L. & Ringwalt, C.L. (2006). Inhalant use and disorders among adults in the United States. *Drug and Alcohol Dependence, 85*(3), 1-11.

Wu, L. & Howard. M. (2006). Is inhalant use a risk factor for heroin and injection drug use among adolescents in the United States? *Addictive Behaviors, 32*(2), 265-281.

CHAPTER 14

HALLUCINOGENS

CHAPTER OBJECTIVE

After completing this chapter, the learner will be able to discuss the characteristics and issues related to the abuse of hallucinogenic substance use.

LEARNING OBJECTIVES

After studying this chapter, the learner will be able to:

1. Discuss the history of hallucinogenic substances and how their use has evolved.
2. Identify the hallucinogenic substances most commonly abused.
3. Describe the physiological and psychological effects of hallucinogens.
4. Identify the health risks associated with abusing hallucinogenic substances.
5. Select appropriate treatment strategies used to combat the abuse of hallucinogens.

OVERVIEW

Hallucinogens are drugs that cause dramatic alterations in mood and perception. People under the influence of hallucinogenic drugs commonly report seeing images, hearing sounds, and feeling sensations that seem real, but do not exist (National Institute on Drug Abuse [NIDA], 2009.). The drug class name hallucinogens is misleading because these substances do not consistently produce hallucinations – defined as false perceptions with no basis in reality – but rather they cause changes in mood and thought (United States Drug Enforcement Agency [DEA], n.d.-a).

Hallucinogens include both naturally occurring substances, such as plants, fungi, and such synthetically-produced substances as lysergic acid diethylamide (LSD). Historically, naturally occurring hallucinogens have been used by many different cultures for thousands of years to create mystical experiences. The Hindu holy book, Rig Veda, mentions soma, thought to be derived from the mushroom Amanita Muscaria, as a sacred substance used to induce higher levels of consciousness. In pre-Columbian Mexico, teotlaqualli, made from the hallucinogenic flower ololiuqui, was used by soldiers during ceremonial times. Hallucinogens are also thought to have been associated with the "immoral" behavior of witches during the Salem, Massachusetts, witch trials (Parish, 2011).

The first synthetic hallucinogen was accidentally discovered in 1938 in a Sandoz laboratory while conducting medical research on lysergic acid compounds. This compound is derived from a fungus ergot, which develops on rye grass. Searching for a therapeutic ergot-derived analeptic agent, dozens of lysergic acid compounds were created. LSD-25 was discovered by a Swiss chemist named Albert Hoffman.

Five years later, in 1943, he accidentally ingested some of the drug and experienced some frightening sensory effects leading to the discovery of the drug's hallucinogenic effects (DEA, n.d.-b).

In 1947, Sandoz Laboratories began marketing the new compound LSD-25 as Delysid. Delysid was used by psychiatrists who believed its use in psychotherapy could help access repressed emotions (Parish, 2011). This compound was also used as a tool to research mental illness. The U.S. Central Intelligence Agency conducted human experiments with LSD, testing its use as an interrogation tool and as a control agent (Parish, 2011).

In the early 1960s, Timothy Leary, a psychology instructor at Harvard University, began experimenting with hallucinogens. Leary claimed that LSD provided instant happiness, enhanced creativity in art and music, facilitated problem-solving ability in school and at work, increased self-awareness, and helped psychotherapy (Pechnick & Ungerleider, 2005). Leary was not reappointed to the faculty of Harvard and became a self-proclaimed martyr for the LSD cause. In the early years, LSD users banned together, organized their lives around the use of the drug and ultimately created a subculture. Initially, users were young adults about 21 years of age, and usually used only LSD.

By the late 1960s, the cultural revolution was actively being influenced by LSD, psychedelics, and such other hallucinogenic compounds as mescaline and psilocybin (Pechnick & Ungerleider, 2005). The media publicized the introduction of LSD and indirectly aided in its growth. Musicians, rock music, the hippie lifestyle, and flower children were loosely associated with the Leary philosophy. Eventually, the use of LSD spread through all socioeconomic groups, particularly the middle-class and affluent youth. Users of LSD became more involved in polydrug abuse. The general population became anxious and concerned about the increasing drug abuse problem until the nation declared a war on drug abuse (Pechnick & Ungerleider, 2005).

As the popularity and use of hallucinogens increased, so did the reporting of adverse affects. The reporting of "bad trips" and resulting accidents and suicides focused attention on the seriousness of the LSD problem. In late 1966, Sandoz Laboratories stopped distributing the drug and all existing supplies of the drug were turned over to the government, which would make the drug available for legitimate concerns. In 1967, the federal government classified LSD as a Schedule I drug and, in 1970, it continued to be classified a Schedule I drug according to the Comprehensive Drug Abuse Prevention and Control Act. Today, LSD is considered to have no acceptable medical use in the United States (Pechnick & Ungerleider, 2005). The use of illegally manufactured hallucinogens declined until the 1990s when its popularity started to grow, presumably because of its low cost (McDowell, 2005).

Hallucinogens are a diverse group of substances that differ in their chemical structures, mechanisms of action, and adverse effects. Most of the naturally occurring hallucinogens can be recreated synthetically and are more potent than in their natural form. The main groups of hallucinogens include lysergamides (LSD, morning glory seeds, or Hawaiian woodrose), indolealkylamines (psilocybin, psilocin, bufotenin, dimethyltrptamine [DMT], 5-MeO-DMT), phenylethylamines (mescaline, methamphetamines, 3,4-methylenedioxy-N-methylamphetamine [MDMA], 3,4-methylenedioxy-N-ethylamphetamine [MDEA], 3-methoxy-4,5-methylenedioxyamphetamine [MMDA], 2,6-dimethoxy-4-methylamphetamine [DOM]), piperidines (ketamine, phencyclidine [PCP]), cannabinols (marijuana, hashish), and dextromethorphan. The best known, most famous, and by far the most potent hallucinogen is LSD.

LYSERGAMIDES

Lysergamides include naturally occurring morning glory seeds and LSD. As mentioned previously, LSD was initially produced from the ergot alkaloids from the fungus *Claviceps purpurea*, a contaminant of wheat and rye flour. LSD is now synthesized from lysergic acid and is a clear or white, odorless, water-soluble material. The crystal can be crushed into a powder and mixed with binding agents to produce tablets known as "microdots" or thin squares of gelatin known as "window panes." It is most commonly diluted and applied to paper known as "blotter acid." Today, the typical dose of LSD is 20 to 80 mcg. The initial effects of LSD begin about 30 to 90 minutes after ingestion and continue for about 12 hours with the peak effect noted at about 4 hours (DEA, n.d.-b). LSD is known by various street names, usually referring to the pattern printed on the blotter paper, such as *'cid*, *acid*, *Bart Simpsons*, and *Sandoz*. Table 14-1 provides a list of LSD street names. LSD is usually taken orally but can also be taken via intranasal, sublingual, parenteral, inhalation, or even conjunctival routes (Parish, 2011).

The precise mechanism of action for LSD remains unclear. It is structurally similar to the neurotransmitter serotonin and disrupts the interaction of nerve cells. The neurotransmitter serotonin modulates mood, pain, sensory perception, personality, sexual activity, and other functions. LSD affects the electrical activity of the neurons in the locus ceruleus, some cortical regions and, at a system level, these effects could change how the brain handles sensory information, as well as alter cognitive and perceptual processing (Petchnick & Ungerleider, 2005). The hallucinogenic activity of LSD is thought to be mediated by LSD's effect on serotonin-2 receptors. LSD acts postsynaptically to inhibit serotonin release and increase retention of serotonin-2 receptors. The net effect is that of a serotonin agonist (Parish, 2011).

TABLE 14-1: SELECTED STREET NAMES FOR LSD

LSD Street or Slang Names
'Cid
Acid
Blotter
Blotter acid
Bart Simpson
Beavis and Buttheads
Dots
Lucy in the Sky with Diamonds
Mellow yellow
Microdot
Pane
Paper acid
Sugar
Sugar cubes
Sorcerer's apprentice
Trip
Window glass
Window pane
Zen

The effects of LSD vary dramatically with the amount of the drug ingested and the user's personality, mood, expectations, and surroundings. The first 4 hours after ingesting the drug are often referred to as a "trip." Initially, users experience dizziness, parethesias, weakness, and tremors. Later, the users experience a marked increase in vision and auditory changes, mood changes, altered time sense, and depersonalization. Sensory input becomes mixed together and users report "hearing" colors or "seeing" smells. Emotions are often labile and intense, shifting rapidly through a range from fear to euphoria. The sense of touch is significantly magnified.

Symptoms of a transient depression may occur after LSD use. The major physiologic effects of the drug include increased blood pressure, heart rate, dizziness, dilated pupils, loss of appetite, dry mouth, sweating, nausea, numbness, and tremors (NIDA, 2009). A list of the effects of LSD is provided in Table 14-2.

TABLE 14-2: EFFECTS OF LSD

Physical
Dilated pupils
Higher body temperature
Increased heart rate
Elevated blood pressure
Increased sweating
Loss of appetite
Sleeplessness
Dry mouth
Tremors
Psychological
Intense sensory experiences
Mixing of senses (hearing colors, seeing sounds)
Distorted sense of time
Distorted body image
Fear of
• Losing control
• Insanity
• Death
Flashbacks, which may cause
• Distress
• Impairment of functioning
Paranoia
Confusion
Acute panic (bad trip)

(NIDA, 2009)

During the peak effects of LSD, the user usually experiences a decrease in the ability to make sensible judgments and avoid common dangers, making them susceptible to personal injury. Occasionally, users experience acute panic reactions referred to as a "bad trip." Some fatal accidents have occurred during states of LSD intoxication, yet no deaths have been reported due to LSD ingestion alone, regardless of the dose (Parish, 2011).

LSD is not considered a physically or psychologically addictive drug because it does not produce compulsive drug-seeking behavior. LSD does produce tolerance, so users who take the drug repeatedly must take progressively higher doses to achieve their desired level of intoxication (NIDA, 2009). LSD use also creates a cross tolerance to other hallucinogenic drugs, such as psilocybin and mescaline. Drug tolerance resolves after several days without substance use. Most LSD users usually limit themselves to taking the drug once or twice per week. There are no withdrawal symptoms experienced with stopping LSD use. One of the most dangerous aspects of LSD is its unpredictable nature, even in experienced users.

Long-term effects of LSD use include the risk of persistent psychosis and hallucination persisting perception disorder (HPPD). The cause of these conditions is unknown. They are most commonly identified in people who have used LSD for more than 10 times but can even occur after a single use. The drug-induced psychosis is a distortion or disorganization of a person's capacity to recognize reality, think rationally, or communicate with others. LSD-induced psychosis can last for years and can affect people who have no history or other symptoms of psychological disorder. HPPD, more commonly referred to as *flashbacks,* are spontaneous, repeated, and sometimes continuous recurrences of some of the sensory distortions originally produced by LSD. The experience may include hallucinations, but it most commonly consists of such vision disturbances as seeing false motion on the edges of the field of vision, bright or colored flashes, and halos or trails attached to moving objects. Flashbacks can occur for years, normally decreasing in frequency, intensity, and duration over time. There is no established treatment for HPPD although some antidepressant may reduce the symptoms.

INDOLEALKYLAMINES

Indolealkylamines include the two mushroom-derived substances (psilocybin and psilocin), DMT, and bufotenine. Psilocybin and psilocin are obtained from certain mushrooms found in parts of South America, Mexico, and the United States. These substances have the ability to produce muscle relaxation or weakness, dilation of pupils, ataxia, altered perception of time, and an inability to discern fantasy from reality (NIDA, 2009). These substances are normally consumed as dried or brewed mushrooms. The effects are not predictable because they are dependent on the type of mushroom used and the age and preservation of the extract. The mushrooms cause fewer adverse reactions than LSD, although hyperthermia, seizures, and coma have been reported (Parish, 2011). Often these mushrooms are either accidentally or purposely misidentified, with only about one-third of them actually being "magic mushrooms" as they are referred to on the street. Many times the product is simply store-bought mushrooms laced with phencyclidine (PCP).

DMT is a substance found in various plants and seeds and can be produced synthetically. The drug is ineffective when taken orally unless it is taken with another drug to inhibit its metabolism. The usual route of administration for this drug is sniffing, smoking, or snorting. It is a potent psychedelic drug that causes more vision hallucinations and more sympathetic effects than LSD. The experience associated with this drug is very quick (less than 1 hour) and has been nicknamed the "businessman's trip."

Bufotenine is a hallucinogen chemically similar to DMT. It can be found on certain mushrooms and seeds but most notably on the skin glands of Bufo toads. The toads produce venom that has psychoactive properties and are licked or milked for their venom, which may be then ingested or smoked. In general, most naturally occurring bufotenine preparations are extremely toxic and their role as a hallucinogen has to be clearly established. An analogue of the compound 5-MeO-DMT produces the same pharmacologic effects but is less potent than DMT.

PHENYLETHYLAMINES

A third group of hallucinogens includes phenylethylamine derivatives and other hallucinogenic amphetamines. The peyote is a small, spineless cactus and the crown of the plant consists of disc-shaped buttons that are generally chewed or soaked in water to produce an intoxicating liquid. The effects start in about 30 minutes to 2 hours and last for up to 12 hours. Mescaline, a psychogenic amphetamine, occurs naturally in the peyote cactus but can also be synthetically produced. Historically, this substance has been ingested by natives of northern Mexico and the Southwestern United States during religious ceremonies (NIDA, 2009). Today, legal use continues among members of the Native American Church for religious ceremonies (Parish, 2011). The hallucinogenic experience is usually preceded by nausea, vomiting, diaphoresis, and ataxia.

Many of the hallucinogenic amphetamines are synthetically produced analogs of mescaline and amphetamine, otherwise known as "designer drugs." These drugs all have similar psychogenic effects and toxicities and include MDA, MDEA, and MDMA (Ecstasy). The primary reason these substances were produced was to avoid prosecution by the U.S. DEA. The most well-known designer drug is MDMA or Ecstasy, which is found commonly at "raves" or all night dance parties. This substance appears to affect serotonin neurotransmission, causing changes in mood, perception of music, and feelings of intimacy and empathy (Parish, 2011). Some of the common adverse drug effects include hypertension, tachycardia, hyperthermia, physical exhaustion, and dehydration. Tolerance develops quickly with frequent consumption of this substance and increasing doses are required to maintain the desired effect. There is some initial animal research that warns of the potential of permanent neural damage with MDMA use.

In addition, several deaths have been reported with MDMA use related to the serious complication of hyperthermia.

PIPERIDINES

Piperidines include PCP and ketamine, which are dissociative anesthetics that were developed in the 1950s and 1960s. These drugs produce sedative and anesthetic effects. The original purpose for these substances was as anesthesia agents. PCP was approved for veterinary use only; however, ketamine, which was developed after PCP, was approved for both human and veterinary uses. Today, much of the illegal ketamine is diverted from veterinary offices to be used illegally.

PCP is extremely unpredictable and dose dependent. Users may appear wild, calm, disoriented, violent, stuporous, or comatose. Other effects include tachycardia, hypertension, hyperthermia, muscle rigidity, grimacing, and bruxism. The dissociative nature of PCP causes users to be at increased risk for trauma because they perceive little or no harm to their bodies. PCP is associated with a higher risk of death than other hallucinogens due to complications related to severe agitation and hyperthermia.

Ketamine has experienced a resurgence since the 1970s and is a popular drug at all-night dance parties and raves. This drug has a shorter duration than PCP and is much less potent. It is also known as the *date rape drug* and has also been connected with the commission of sexual assaults because it produces a sense of detachment and an amnesia effect.

CANNABINOLS

Marijuana contains the psychoactive substance THC, which is found in the leaf or flower of the plant. This substance is grouped with hallucinogens but rarely causes hallucinations. It is available both naturally and synthetically. The leaves of the plant are smoked and create changes in mood and perception, laughing, increased appetite, conjunctival injection, tachycardia, and minimal central nervous system (CNS) depression. This remains the most commonly abused illegal drug in the United States.

DEXTROMETHORPHAN

Dextromethorphans, such as PCP or ketamine, are N-methyl-D-aspartate (NMDA) antagonists that produce dissociative effects. Dextromethorphan, also known as *DXM* or *robo,* is a cough suppressant found in many over-the-counter (OTC) medications. The most common source of abused dextromethorphan is extra strength cough syrup, which typically contains 3 mg of the drug per ml of syrup. The drug is generally considered safe and effective in therapeutic doses. At doses of about 2 ounces, the user experiences a mild stimulant effect with distorted vision perceptions; at doses of about 10 ounces, the user experiences a sense of complete dissociation from his or her body (NIDA, 2001).

A study by Bryner et al. (2006) identified a tenfold increase in all dextromethorphan abuse cases reported to the California Poison Control System from 1999 to 2004. An increase in these cases has also been reported by the American Association of Poison Control Centers and the Drug Abuse Warning Network. According to the Poison Control Centers, the highest frequency of abuse is being seen among adolescents ages 15 and 16. The reasons contributing to the rise in adolescent abuse are availability, legality, cost, safety issues, and the production of euphoric and hallucinatory effects. Because this is a common over-the-counter drug (OTC), most adolescents fail to recognize the health risks associated with high doses.

A serious concern related to consuming large amounts of OTC cough medications and cold products is the unintended toxicity from pseudoephedrine, acetaminophen, and antihistamies. High doses of acetaminophen can cause liver toxicity and ultimately liver failure. It is important for nurses, primary care providers, pharmacists, educators, counselors, and parents to be aware of this recent trend to help identify potential abuse situations.

SCREENING OF SPECIAL POPULATIONS AND RISK IDENTIFICATION

According to the 2011 National Survey on Drug Use and Health (NSDUH), approximately 36.3 million people in the U.S. ages 12 and older reported trying hallucinogens at least once during their lifetime, representing 14.1% of the population. Additionally 1.6% of the population reported use in the past year and 0.4% reported use in the past month (Substance Abuse and Mental Health Services Administration [SAMHSA], 2012a).

According to the 2012 Monitoring the Future study, past year use of LSD decreased significantly since 2001. For example, in 2001 6.0% of students in grades 8-12 reported past year use of LSD, compared to 3.2% of students in grades 8-12 in 2012 (Johnston, O'Malley, Bachman & Schulenberg, 2013). Additionally, on average, 54% of all three grades of students reported LSD as a "great risk," and in 2004, 12th graders' personal disapproval of trying LSD increased significantly, with little change since.(Johnston, O'Malley, Bachman & Schulenberg, 2012). The survey results indicate that 3.7% of college students and 6.1% of other young adults reported lifetime use of LSD (Johnston et al., 2012).

According to the SAMHSA (2012a), approximately 972,000 people in the U.S. were current (past month) hallucinogen users. Hallucinogenic mushrooms, LSD, and MDMA are popular among junior and senior high school students who use hallucinogens. Teenagers and young adults abuse LSD at raves, nightclubs, and concerts. Presently, the production, distribution, and use of LSD appear to be decreasing and there are currently no indications of resurgence.

RELATED MEDICAL PROBLEMS AND CO-OCCURRING DISORDERS

Acute anxiety and panic reactions are the most common problems related to the use of such hallucinogens as LSD or mescaline. The most common reason for seeking medical care is an acute panic reaction or an accidental ingestion of the drug (Parish, 2011). These drugs are extremely unpredictable and will act differently in the same person on different occasions. Someone with a previous pleasant experience on LSD may have an unpleasant experience or bad trip during a subsequent use. The anxiety and paranoia commonly resolve within 24 hours as the drug is metabolized in the body.

The risk of depression and suicide can last for days after LSD ingestion. A thorough psychiatric examination needs to be conducted with these patients to differentiate among paranoid schizophrenia, LSD psychosis, and other drug-induced psychoses. Toxicology laboratory studies may be helpful but standard toxicology screens detect only a few hallucinogenic agents. Substances readily identified by standard toxicology screens include MDMA (positive for amphetamines), PCP, and marijuana. Generally, the priority of care is to stabilize the patient and then provide supportive treatment.

Long-term effects of hallucinogens include psychoses, depressive reactions, acting out, paranoid states, and flashbacks (Pechnick & Ungerleider, 2005). Flashbacks spontaneously occur weeks to months after the original drug experience and may or may not resemble the original drug experience. The experience involves such perceptual and reality distortion as seeing motion on the edges of the field of vision or bright or colored flashers. The most disturbing or anxiety-producing aspect of this experience is when the person realizes that he or she has no control over it happening (Pechnick & Ungerleider, 2005). Flashbacks have been treated with some selective serotonin reuptake inhibitor antidepressants and psychotherapy. Additionally psychosis can develop after hallucinogen use but it remains unclear whether the drugs caused or had a role in precipitating the illness. Chronic personality changes, such as the shifts in attitudes and the onset of magical thinking, can occur with the use of hallucinogens. Few if any neuropsychological deficits have been attributed to hallucinogens (Pechnick & Ungerleider, 2005).

Complications, such as severe hyperthermia, rhabdomyolysis, myoglobininuric renal failure, and disseminated intravascular coagulation (DIC) have been seen with these drugs (Parish, 2011). PCP has also been associated with memory loss and depression that can persist for years after the drug use has stopped. Hallucinogens, MDMA and PCP have been attributed to several deaths.

PREVENTIVE STRATEGIES AND TREATMENT

High schools and colleges are important targets for prevention strategies because adolescents and young adults are the age-groups most likely to use hallucinogens. Education continues to be the most promising tool for preventing drug abuse. Clear, accurate dissemination of information regarding the effects of these drugs is essential in treating this problem. Peer-led advocacy programs and drug prevention programs are being used in school systems because they incorporate the importance of social context and networks.

Most LSD users voluntarily decrease or stop its use over time because it is not an addictive drug. This, along with the previously discussed trends of decreased LSD use among youth and college students, is an encouraging trend. From 2000 to 2010, the number of admissions for treatment of hallucinogen (such as LSD, mescaline, and peyote) were reported as the primary drugs of abuse decreased from 3,118 to 1,675, representing 0.2% and 0.1% of the total treatment admissions, respectively (SAMHSA, 2012b).

There are no specific treatments for MDMA or Ecstasy abuse. Generally, cognitive behavioral therapies (CBTs) are designed to help modify the abuser's thinking, expectancies, and behaviors and to improve their coping skills (NIDA, 2009). CBT is based on social learning theories and emphasizes modification of the client's thoughts and behaviors. The goal is to encourage abstinence by helping clients learn and master effective coping skills that can help them believe they can resist relapsing to substance abuse. The focus is on the exploration of positive and negative consequences of substance use. This approach is the foundation for relapse prevention because clients are taught the skills needed to prevent a return to substance abuse. Narcotics Anonymous may be effective when combined with behavioral interventions to create periods of long-term drug-free recovery.

Ketamine is a very addictive drug and has no specific treatments. Current behavioral therapies for chemical addictions are recommended. Support groups and recovery networks are helpful in maintaining drug-free periods.

Treatment for acute hallucinogenic intoxication is variable due to the purity of the substance, the dose, the setting, and the individual.

Emergency department visits are often related to a bad trip. The primary goal of treatment is harm prevention for the user and those around him. The treatment space should be quiet, softly lit, and separated from large groups of people. Calm the user by speaking in a reassuring and confident manner. Always address users by name and remind them often of who they are and who you are. If possible, do not leave someone alone when he is experiencing an adverse reaction. In cases where physical restraints are necessary, subdue abusers with at least a team of five people to minimize risks of injury.

Phencyclidine intoxication can produce seizures and severe hypertension, resulting in hypertensive encephalopathy or intracerebral bleeding (NIDA, 2009). The most effective treatment for phencyclidine intoxication is increasing urinary excretion by acidifying the urine with ammonium chloride or ascorbic acid. This treatment can only be used after it has been determined that the patient does not have rhabdomyolysis. If the patient is at low risk for renal or hepatic failure, the urine pH should be monitored and kept around 5.5; a diuretic can be administered to increase drug excretion (Heard & Hoppe, 2012).

There have been no specific treatments identified for use with chronic hallucinogen abusers. Behavioral therapies constitute the bulk of treatment and include CBT, motivational interventions, and contingency management. These therapies are usually initiated after the detoxification period. Behavioral therapies are important strategies that assist the abuser in preventing relapse to substance abuse.

Behavioral treatment can be delivered at an individual or a group level and last for a single session (such as a brief intervention) or longer than 1 year or more. Additional approaches that may complement care include self-help or 12-step groups, family-based treatment, acupuncture, and faith-based groups. No one behavioral therapy appears to be more effective than another.

SUMMARY

Historically, naturally occurring hallucinogens have been used by many different cultures in medicinal, religious, and recreational manners. It has only been since the late 1930s that synthetic hallucinogens were created.

The rise and decline of LSD use can be documented through the cultural revolution of the 1960s. Although LSD is the most potent of the synthetically-produced hallucinogens, its use has been consistently decreasing over the past several years and the DEA does not expect a change in this encouraging pattern.

Areas of concern continue to be the hallucinogen or designer drugs, such as Ecstasy and PCP, because of their availability and use at all-night dances and raves.

EXAM QUESTIONS

CHAPTER 14

Questions 80-84

Note: Choose the one option that BEST answers each question.

80. The hallucinogenic effects of LSD were originally identified in

    a. 1943 when Dr. Albert Hoffman accidentally consumed the substance.
    b. the 1950s when the Central Intelligence Agency tested its use as an interrogation tool.
    c. 1950 when synthesized at a Harvard University Laboratory.
    d. 1962 when Timothy Leary discovered the compound.

81. The most potent hallucinogen is

    a. PCP.
    b. LSD.
    c. mescaline.
    d. MDMA (Ecstasy).

82. Which statement correctly reflects flashbacks as physiological and psychological effects?

    a. They normally occur within 24 hours after ingesting the drug.
    b. They are spontaneous recreations of previous drug experiences with vision and sensory distortions.
    c. They occur only with long-term abuse of the drug.
    d. They are associated with depression.

83. A substantial health risk associated with LSD use is

    a. increased blood pressure.
    b. decreased blood pressure.
    c. increased appetite.
    d. decreased heart rate.

84. Which statement regarding behavioral treatment for hallucinogenic abuse is correct?

    a. Behavioral treatment is most effective when initiated before detoxification.
    b. No one behavioral treatment appears to be more effective than another.
    c. Twelve-step groups are more effective than cognitive behavioral therapies.
    d. Contingency management is the most effective treatment.

REFERENCES

Bryner, J.K., Wang, U.K., Hui, J.W., Bedodo, M., MacDougall, C., & Anderson, I.B. (2006). Dextromethorphan abuse in adolescents: An increasing trend. *Archives of Pediatrics & Adolescent Medicine, 160*(12), 1217-1222.

Drug Enforcement Administration. (n.d.-a). *Hallucinogens.* Retrieved March 15, 2013, from http://www.justice.gov/dea/druginfo/drug_data_sheets/Hallucinogens.pdf

Drug Enforcement Administration. (n.d.-b). *LSD.* Retrieved March 15, 2013, from http://www.justice.gov/dea/druginfo/drug_data_sheets/LSD.pdf

Johnston, L. D., O'Malley, P. M., Bachman, J. G., & Schulenberg, J. E. (2012a). *Monitoring the Future national survey results on drug use, 1975-2011. Volume I: Secondary school students.* Ann Arbor: Institute for Social Research, The University of Michigan.

Johnston, L. D., O'Malley, P. M., Bachman, J. G., & Schulenberg, J. E. (2013). *Monitoring the Future national results on adolescent drug use: Overview of key findings, 2012.* Ann Arbor: Institute for Social Research, The University of Michigan.

Heard, K. & Hoppe, J. (2012). *Phencyclidine (PCP) intoxication in adults.* Retrieved March 15, 2013 from http://www.uptodate.com/contents/phencyclidine-pcp-intoxication-in-adults

McDowell, D. (2005). Marijuana, hallucinogens, and club drugs. In R.J. Frances, S.I. Miller, & A.H. Mack (Eds.), *Clinical textbook of addictive disorders* (3rd ed.). New York: Guilford Press.

National Institute on Drug Abuse. (2001). *Research Report Series: Hallucinogens and Dissociative Drugs Including LSD, PCP, Ketamine, Dextromethorphan.* NIH Publication Number 01-4209. Retrieved March 15, 2013, from http://www.drugabuse.gov/PDF/RRHalluc.pdf

National Institute on Drug Abuse. (2009). *DrugFacts: Hallucinogens – LSD, Peyote, Psilocybin, and PCP.* Retrieved on March 15, 2013, from http://www.drugabuse.gov/publications/drugfacts/hallucinogens-lsd-peyote-psilocybin-pcp

Pechnick, R.N. & Ungerleider, J.T. (2005). Hallucingoens. In J.H. Lodwinson, P. Ruiz, R.B., Millman, & J.G. Langrod (Eds.), *Substance abuse: A comprehensive textbook* (4th ed.). Philadelphia: Lippincott Williams & Wilkins.

Parish, B. (2011). *Hallucinogens.* Retrieved March 15, 2013, from http://emedicine.medscape.com/article/293752-overview

Substance Abuse and Mental Health Services Administration. (2012a). *Results from the 2011 National survey on drug use and health: Summary of national findings* (NSDUH Series H-44, HHS Publication No. (SMA) 12-4713). Rockville, MD. Accessed March 15, 2013 from http://www.samhsa.gov/data/NSDUH/2k11Results/NSDUHresults2011.htm

Substance Abuse and Mental Health Services Administration. (2012b). *Treatment Episode Data Set (TEDS) 2000-2010: National admissions to substance abuse treatment services*. Retrieved March 15, 2013 from http://www.samhsa.gov/data/2k12/TEDS2010N/TEDS2010NWeb.pdf

CHAPTER 15

DESIGNER DRUGS

CHAPTER OBJECTIVE

After completing this chapter, the learner will be able to discuss the characteristics of and issues related to designer drug use.

LEARNING OBJECTIVES

After studying this chapter, the learner will be able to:

1. Identify populations at risk for use of designer drugs.
2. Describe the designer drugs most commonly used.
3. Discuss the health risks related to the use of designer drugs.
4. Identify effective strategies used in designer drug interventions.

OVERVIEW

Designer drugs are synthetic derivatives of federally controlled substances, created by slightly altering the molecular structure of existing drugs. They are produced illegally for illicit use (Hoecker, 2013). Today's most frequently used designer drugs are 3,4-methylenedioxy-N-methamphetamine (MDMA) (Ecstasy), rohypnol, gamma hydroxybutyrate (GHB), ketamine, lysergenic acid diethylamide (LSD), and methamphetamine (National Institute on Drug Abuse [NIDA], 2010). LSD and methamphetamine have been discussed in depth in previous chapters. These drugs are collectively referred to as "designer drugs" because they are used by young adults, who are often part of the nightclub, bar, rave, or trance scenes. Raves and trances are night-long dances that are frequently held in warehouses. Designer drugs are popular with young adults because they are thought to enhance social interactions. The drugs are credited with creating a sense of physical closeness, empathy, and euphoria (Gahlinger, 2004). The low cost and the convenient method of oral administration add to the attractiveness of these substances with young adults. MDMA is particularly popular at raves or all-night dance parties because it allows the user to remain active at these events for up to 3 days and, because it suppresses the need to eat, drink, or sleep, the user can participate in marathon parties (Hess & DeBoer, 2002).

HISTORY

Before the 19th century, psychoactive drugs were only available as plant derivatives. In the late 19th and early 20th centuries, medical chemists began developing methods for producing synthetic chemicals that could alter mood and consciousness, induce pleasure, and decrease unwanted feelings (Morgan, 2005). Their goal was to create improved medications for the treatment of disease. During this growth in medical technology, this knowledge was diverted for the development of illegal chemical substances, which were then marketed for unsanctioned use. The chemical MDMA, known as *Ecstasy,* was first created in 1910 and patented by a pharmaceutical company in 1914. The consumption of illegal synthesized drugs remains low in comparison to such naturally occurring drugs as heroin, cocaine, and cannabis (Morgan, 2005) and, in recent years, only one newly created formula has been identified. Basically, for a synthesized product to enter the market, it must create a desired effect and be economically viable for the producer.

In 1986, the Controlled Substances Act was modified to include the Controlled Substances Analogues Enforcement Act (Morgan, 2005). This modification was necessary to avoid the confusing term of designer drugs. A controlled substance analogue is defined as a chemical substantially similar to an already existing substance classified as a Schedule I or II drug. The courts have had some difficulty clarifying this term but have essentially defined the standard and are relying on the understanding of the jury to determine a controlled-substance analogue.

EPIDEMIOLOGY

General Population

The typical person likely to use designer or "club" drugs is a teenager or young adult who frequently attends bars, clubs, concerts, and parties. According to the 2011 National Survey on Drug Use and Health (NSDUH), nearly 15 million people have tried MDMA, almost 12.0 million have tried methamphetamine, and more than 23.0 million have tried LSD at least once (Substance Abuse and Mental Health Services Administration [SAMHSA], 2012). There are minimal gender differences noted with this type of illicit drug use. Historically, designer drugs are used by the young, White population, but indicators from Chicago and New York suggest an increase in use among Black adults in their 20s and 30s and in other non-White communities (NIDA, 2006). An increase in MDMA use has also been reported in urban gay males. NIDA has reported the emergence of these drugs into more mainstream settings during the past few years (NIDA, 2006). There have been an increasing number of reports of such designer drugs as rohypnol, being used to perpetrate sexual crimes because it incapacitates the user and causes amnesia.

Adolescents and Young Adults

According to 2012 data from Monitoring the Future (MTF) study, declines have continued in use of LSD/GHB, methamphetamine and rohypnol use. Additionally, after a few years of increases, the rate of MDMA and ketamine use has decreased as well (Johnston, O'Malley, Bachman, & Schulenberg, 2013).

Questions regarding the use of MDMA were added to the survey in 1989 for college students and adults, but not for secondary school students until 1996.

The MTF study results showed MDMA use beginning to rise above trace levels in 1995 and continuing to rise through 2001 for young adults. Through 2001, MDMA use rose sharply for grades 8, 10, and 12. Data showed a significant decrease in MDMA use in 2002 (20%) and again in 2003 (40%). The trend of decreasing MDMA use continued through 2004 (through 2009 for eighth graders), but increased for tenth and twelfth graders. Use then increased significantly in the lower grades from 2009 to 2010 (1.3% to 2.4% in 8th grade, and 3.7% to 4.7% in 10th), but then declined in 2011 in both grades. Use among 12th graders increased in 2011, and then declined significantly in all three grades in 2012 (Johnson et al., 2013).

From 2004 to 2011, a troubling drop in perceived risk for all three grades was noted, corresponding to the increase in use in the upper two grades and then in all three grades. In 2012 only 8th grade showed much further decline. This ongoing decline in perceived risk does not explain the recent decline in use (Johnston et al., 2013). Figure 15-1 provides graphic representation of "use" and "risk" data as reported in the 2012 MTF study.

BIOCHEMISTRY

The exact chemical composition of designer or club drugs is not clear. These illegal drugs are manufactured with uncertain drug sources or pharmacological agents and uncertain contaminants, resulting in uncertain toxicity profiles (NIDA, 2004). The varied nature of these compounds makes reporting the effects, symptoms, consequences, and toxicities more difficult. Most of these emerging abused substances do not yield positive results with traditional drug screens (Haroz & Greenberg, 2005). Lastly, these drugs are often used with alcohol and together make a dangerous combination.

MDMA (Ecstasy)

MDMA or Ecstasy is a synthetically-produced illegal drug that acts as a stimulant and psychedelic. It is taken orally, usually in the form of a tablet or a capsule. The average reported dose is one to two tablets and the effects usually last for about 3 to 6 hours. Users of the drug will often take a second dose of the drug as the effects begin to subside. MDMA is rapidly absorbed into the bloodstream and the drug's metabolites interfere with the body's ability to break down the drug. This can potentially result in dangerously high levels of the drug with repeated short interval dosing. It causes

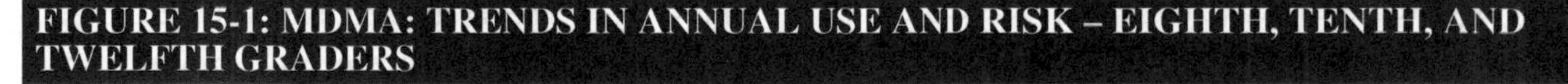
FIGURE 15-1: MDMA: TRENDS IN ANNUAL USE AND RISK – EIGHTH, TENTH, AND TWELFTH GRADERS

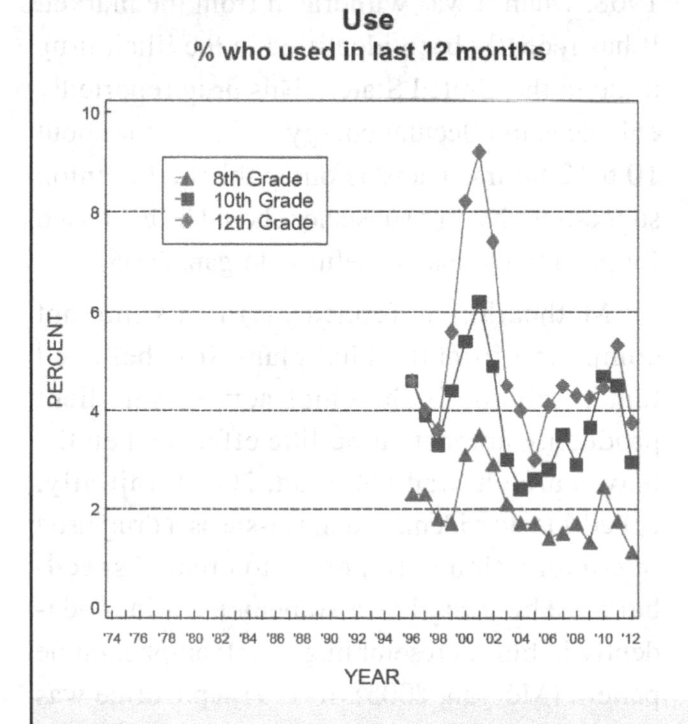

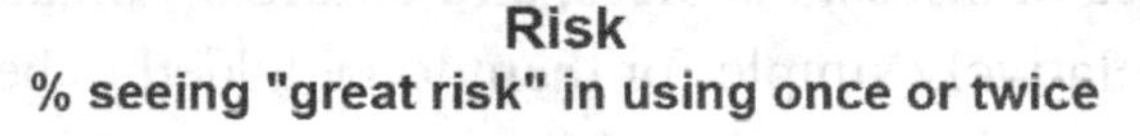

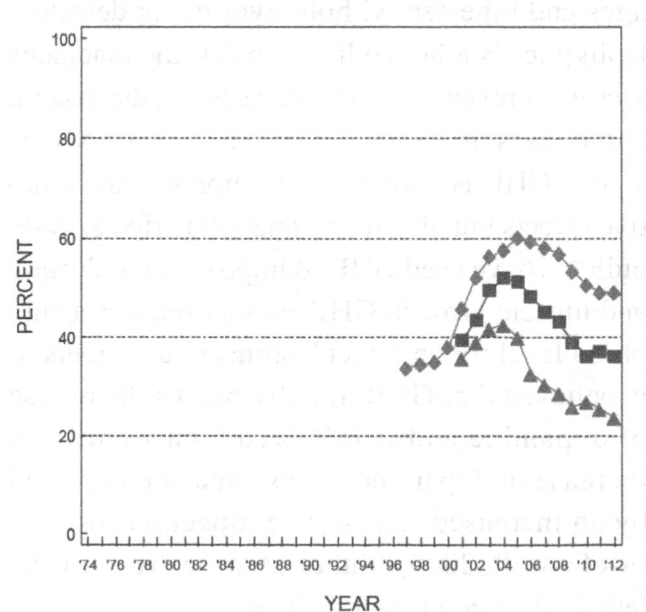

Note. From *The Monitoring the Future National Results On Drug Use: 2012 Overview Key Findings on Adolescent Drug Use* by L.D. Johnston, P.M. O'Malley, J.G. Bachman, & J.E. Schulenberg, 2012, Ann Arbor, MI: University of Michigan News Service.

an energizing effect and distortions of time and perception and enhances enjoyment from tactile stimulation.

The effects of MDMA are caused by altering the activity of many neurotransmitter systems in the brain, primarily affecting serotonin. The drug causes the release of serotonin stores, blocks the reuptake of serotonin, and inhibits the synthesis of new serotonin causing a depletion of this neurotransmitter over time (McDowell, 2005). Though not yet demonstrated in humans, in a study of nonhuman primates, exposure to MDMA for only 4 days caused damage to serotonin nerve terminals that remained evident 6 to 7 years later (NIDA, 2010).

Rohypnol and Gamma Hydroxybutyrate

Rohypnol and GHB are both predominantly central nervous system (CNS) depressants. These drugs have been associated with date rape. They are ingested orally and effects remain constant for about 8 to 10 hours. The drugs are odorless, tasteless, and colorless, making it relatively simple for them to be added to beverages and ingested without ever being detected. Rohypnol is a benzodiazepine; it incapacitates victims, prevents them from resisting the assault, and causes amnesia of the experience (NIDA, 2010). GHB is known for its euphoric and sedative effects but also for its anabolic effects. Body builders have used GHB to improve fat reduction and muscle growth. GHB rapidly reaches a high blood level for an effect lasting about 3 hours. It is believed that GHB initially blocks the release of dopamine and is followed by a significant increase in dopamine release and accompanied by an increased release in endogenous opioids (McDowell, 2005). Either of these drugs can be lethal when combined with alcohol.

Ketamine

Ketamine is an anesthetic that has been approved for both human and animal use. It is commercially available in the form of a liquid. About 90% of illegally used ketamine has been redirected from veterinary use (McDowell, 2005). This drug causes dreamlike states and hallucinations. It is commonly evaporated and the resultant powder either snorted or dabbed on the tongue. Ketamine functions similarly to PCP; it works globally, affecting numerous neurotransmitter systems and causing an increase in dopamine release.

Other Drugs

4-Methylaminorex (4MAM or U4Euh) was the first controlled substance analogue stimulant created in the 1960s. It was originally researched as an anorectic medication. There is minimal evidence of widespread use and its clinical importance is currently unassessed (Morgan, 2005). This drug was never marketed in the United States but was marketed in Europe as Aminorex until 1968, when it was withdrawn from the market. It has recently been identified in the illicit drug trade in the United States. This drug reportedly enhances intellectual energy and lasts for about 10 to12 hours. There is one published opinion suggesting that this substance should be evaluated for potential human benefits (Morgan, 2005).

Methcathinine (ephedrine) is a stimulant compound from the khat plant. It is believed that cathinone is the chief active ingredient producing amphetamine-like effects when the leaves are chewed (Morgan, 2005). Initially, ephedrine was identified in Russia as a drug used in combination with heroin to create "speedballs." This drug has also been used independently in binges resembling a methamphetamine pattern (Morgan, 2005). In 1991, ephedrine was identified in rural Michigan, being manufactured in local clandestine laboratories. In 1992, it was added as a Schedule I of the Controlled Substances Act (Morgan, 2005). In the United States, users usually ingest the drug through the intranasal route. Users report a sense of increased energy, feelings of toughness and invincibility, and increased sexual drive. Magnified effects are seen with subsequent uses, creating increased vision effects (hallucinations), headaches, abdominal cramps, sweating, and tachycardia. It appears that the use of this drug has spread from Michigan to other Midwestern states (Morgan, 2005).

HEALTH EFFECTS

Table 15-1 provides a list of designer drugs and their most common street names. The growing popularity of these drugs is thought to be related to their relatively low cost and their intoxicating high.

MDMA (Ecstasy)

MDMA or Ecstasy has become a popular designer drug due to the perceived positive effects that a person experiences after ingestion. Most users experience feelings of mental stimulation, emotional warmth, empathy toward others, decreased anxiety, and a general sense of well-being. A hallmark of MDMA is the enhanced sensory perceptions. The stimulant effect of this drug allows the users to dance for extended periods, which is associated with the potentially fatal adverse effect of severe increases in body temperature. Some additional adverse effects include nausea, chills, sweating, involuntary teeth clenching, muscle cramping, and blurred vision. Overdose symptoms of MDMA include high blood pressure, faintness, panic attacks, loss of consciousness and seizures. Table 15-2 provides a complete list of the adverse effects of using MDMA (Ecstasy). Ecstasy markedly decreases the user's ability to process information making it dangerous for users to perform complex or skilled tasks. This drug is very addictive in some users and has been shown to be similar to cocaine in that users prefer it to other pleasurable stimuli. About 59% of MDMA users met the criteria for dependence by continued use of the drug, despite knowledge of physical or psychological harm, withdrawal effects, and tolerance; an additional 15% met the criteria for drug abuse. Withdrawal symptoms, including fatigue, loss of appetite, depressed feelings, and trouble concentrating, were reported in about 68% of the users (Cottler, Leung, & Abdaliah, 2009).

Rohypnol

Rohypnol is not manufactured or approved for any medical use in the United States, but it is manufactured in Europe and Latin America, thus remaining the number one sleep medica-

TABLE 15-1: DESIGNER DRUGS – COMMON STREET NAMES

MDMA (3,4-methylenedioxy-N-methamphetamine)	GHB (gamma hydroxybutyrate)	Rohypnol (flunitrazepam)	Ketamine
XTC	Liquid Ecstasy	Roofies	Special K
X	Soap	Rophies	Vitamin K
Ecstasy	Easy lay	Roach	Cat valium
Adam	Vit-G	Roche	Super K
Clarity	Georgia home boy	Forget-me pill	
Hug drug	Grievous bodily harm	Rope	
Love drug			
Lover's speed			
Beans			

TABLE 15-2: EFFECTS OF MDMA (ECSTASY)

Reported Undesirable Effects
(up to 1 week post-MDMA use, or longer)
- Anxiety
- Restlessness
- Irritability
- Sadness
- Impulsiveness
- Aggression
- Sleep disturbances
- Lack of appetite
- Thirst
- Reduced interest in and pleasure from sex
- Significant reductions in mental abilities

Potential Adverse Health Effects
- Nausea
- Sweating
- Involuntary jaw clenchng and teeth grinding
- Muscle cramping
- Blurred vision
- Marked rise in body temperature (hyperthermia)
- Dehydration
- High blood pressure
- Heart failure
- Kidney failure
- Arrhythmia

Symptoms of MDMA Overdose
- High blood pressure
- Faintness
- Panic attacks
- Loss of consciousness
- Seizures

Note. From *Research report series: MDMA (Ecstasy) abuse,* NIH Publication Number 06-4728 by National Institute on Drug Abuse, 2006. Retrieved March 15, 2013, from http://www.drug abuse.gov/PDF/RRmdma.pdf

tion in the world. This drug belongs to the pharmacological class of benzodiazepines and has been associated with date rape because it can be given without the victim's knowledge. The drug is colorless, odorless, and tasteless and is usually added to a victim's beverage without his or her knowledge. It causes the victim to be incapacitated, preventing him or her from resisting a sexual assault, and then usually causes amnesia.

Rohypnol can be fatal when taken with alcohol or other depressants (NIDA, 2010). Neurological effects include sedation, dizziness, memory impairment, decreased coordination, muscle relaxation, decreased blood pressure, slurred speech, impaired judgment, amnesia, loss of inhibitions, loss of consciousness, vision disturbances, and nausea.

Gamma Hydroxybutyrate

GHB is a CNS depressant that is tasteless, colorless, and odorless and usually added to other substances (NIDA, 2010). In the 1950s, it was legally used as an anesthetic but due to such adverse effects as nausea, vomiting, and seizures, its popularity diminished (Klein & Kramer, 2004). The main effects of this drug include euphoria, sedation, and anabolic effects. During the 1980s to 1990s, GHB was legally available in health food stores and was used by body builders for fat reduction and muscle building. Multiple Web sites offer recipes for producing GHB with such simple household items as baking soda and floor stripper (Klein & Kramer, 2004). Withdrawal symptoms related to GHB include insomnia, anxiety, tremors, and sweating. Toxic levels of GHB can cause loss of consciousness, memory impairment, confusion, loss of inhibition, seizures, dizziness, extreme drowsiness, stupor, coma, agitation, nausea, and vision disturbances (Klein & Kramer, 2004).

Ketamine

Ketamine is an anesthetic that is currently used in veterinary and human medicine. About 90% of the drugs used for illegal purposes are diverted from veterinary sources. This drug causes dream-like states and hallucinations often described as out-of-body experiences. Ketamine has been associated with date rape due to the dissociative effect of the drug. Some of the more common adverse effects include delirium, amnesia, depression, high blood pressure, impaired motor function, long-term memory and cognition problems, and potentially fatal respiratory problems (Klein & Kramer, 2004).

SCREENING OF SPECIAL POPULATIONS AND RISK IDENTIFICATION

Adolescents and Young Adults

Populations most likely to use designer or club drugs are adolescents and young adults. The environments in which these substances are found include popular dance clubs, raves, and all-night dance parties. Raves are usually held in more remote settings, such as barns, open fields, and warehouses. Reports indicate that the use of designer drugs is spreading beyond the predominantly White youth to include a wider range of ethnic groups. The use of designer drugs is becoming more common in non-White segments of the community across the country. It should also be noted that gay and bisexual men use MDMA and other designer drugs causing concern related to high-risk sexual behaviors and risks of acquiring human immunodeficiency syndrome (HIV) or sexually transmitted infections (STIs) (NIDA, 2006).

Pregnant and Breast-feeding Women

Because most MDMA users are young and in their childbearing years, the potential for unintentional prenatal drug exposure is significant. Most of these drugs cross the placenta and can cause effects on the fetus (Drug Info Clearinghouse, 2013). It is unclear what effects are attributable solely to a specific drug because many of these abusers are polydrug users. Additionally, there are pregnancy-related concerns due to lifestyle, such as the effects of extreme exercise and dehydration on the viability of the fetus. Although there is no clear evidence to support the harmful effects of MDMA on the fetus, it is advisable that women abstain from this drug (as well as all non-prescribed drugs) during pregnancy.

Behavioral studies in animals have found significant adverse effects on learning and memory tests from exposure to MDMA during a developmental period equivalent to the third trimester in humans; however, more research is needed to determine the effects of MDMA on the developing human fetus (NIDA, 2006). Nursing mothers using MDMA are likely to transmit the drug to the infant through the breast milk (Drug Info Clearinghouse, 2013). Nursing mothers should be particularly cautioned against using MDMA while breastfeeding due to its potential adverse effects on the infant. Specific data related to the effects of other designer drugs on pregnancy could not be found.

Mental Disorders

MDMA is associated with increased risk of the coexistence of other mental disorders. Researchers in Germany reported that 51% of MDMA users had either a current or past diagnosis of panic disorders (Leib, Schuetz, Pfister, vonSydow & Wittchen, 2002). In comparison to non-drug users, the odds of having a mental disorder were three times higher among MDMA users than among non-users, and two times as high as users of other illicit drugs (Leib et al., 2002) Specific data related to the effects of other designer drugs on mental disorders could not be found.

PREVENTIVE STRATEGIES AND TREATMENT

High schools and colleges are important focuses for prevention strategies because adolescents and young adults are most likely to take designer drugs. Education continues to be the most promising tool for preventing drug abuse. Clear, accurate dissemination of information regarding the effects of these drugs is essential to improve this problem. Peer-led advocacy programs and drug prevention programs are promising because they incorporate the importance of social context and networks (NIDA, 2006).

Emergency Care

Designer drugs are illicit substances that have usually been adulterated or substituted and should be considered unknown substances during initial treatment. It is important to remember that many of these drug users are polysubstance abusers. The initial primary goal of treatment is to maintain the cardiorespiratory system.

No standard treatment has been developed for the overdose of designer drugs. The basic management should include cardiac monitoring, pulse oximetry, urinalysis, and a comprehensive chemistry panel to check for electrolyte imbalance, renal toxicity, and possible underlying disorders (Gahlinger, 2004). It is always important to institute seizure precautions.

When a person arrives in the emergency department, it is important to attempt to identify the illicit substance consumed and, if possible, obtain a sample of the substance used. If the substance has been consumed within the previous 60 minutes, then gastric lavage with activated charcoal and a cathartic can be considered. However, this procedure is generally reserved for massive drug doses because it is considered ineffective for small doses and causes increased psychological distress. Initial care includes maintaining adequate cardiorespiratory system function, evaluating basic laboratory values, taking seizure precautions, and minimizing risk of self injury. If rohypnol has been identified as the ingested substance, then the antidote flumazenil can be administered (Gahlinger, 2004). There are no antidotes available for other designer drugs; only supportive care is available. Anxiety and agitation are generally managed with diazepam, lorazepam, or midazolam. The hypertension and tachycardia are usually resolved with managing anxiety and agitation. Hyperthermia can be treated with tepid water baths and fanning. Alkalization of urine is usually accomplished with I.V. fluids and assists with preventing rhabdomyolysis. Administering chlorpromazine and cyproheptadine is useful in treating serotonin syndrome.

After the initial phase of treatment, a psychiatric consult should be obtained. Additionally, it is essential that education be provided to the patient and the family.

Behavioral Therapy

Only behavioral therapy has proven helpful in MDMA abuse. Generally, cognitive behavioral therapies (CBTs) are designed to help modify the abuser's thinking, expectancies, and behaviors, and to improve their coping skills (NIDA, 2006). Behavioral therapies constitute the bulk of treatment and include CBTs, motivational interventions, and contingency management. No one behavioral therapy appears to be more effective than another. Although not typically initiated during the detoxification period, if this time is extended, behavioral therapy can and should be initiated.

Behavioral treatment can be delivered at an individual or a group level and last for a single session, such as a brief intervention, or for more than 1 year. Historically, Narcotics Anonymous has been effective when combined with behavioral interventions to create periods of long-term drug-free recovery.

Rohypnol and GHB are also treated with CBTs. GHB can cause a physiological dependence that appears similar to alcohol withdrawal. The abuser will experience anxiety, tremor, insomnia, and feelings of doom. These symptoms usually resolve within a few weeks. Benzodiazepines can be used with caution to control some of the symptoms (McDowell, 2005).

Ketamine is a very addictive drug and has no specific treatments. Current behavioral therapies for chemical addictions are recommended for treating ketamine abuse. Support groups and recovery networks are helpful in maintaining drug-free periods.

SUMMARY

The dangers and risks associated with the use of designer drugs have been clearly identified. During recent years, some of the nation's best monitoring mechanisms have noted an increase in the popularity of these drugs. The most recent data from the MTF survey indicates a decrease or stabilization in the use of many of these illegal drugs (Johnston et al., 2013), but one concern that should influence our prevention strategies is a significant decrease in the number of high school students who identify a great risk in using MDMA occasionally.

Clearly, designer drugs are a significant health risk in this country. These drugs are commonly used in combination with alcohol, creating an even more dangerous scenario for the user. The development of prevention and treatment strategies targeting these at-risk populations needs to continue to be a priority.

EXAM QUESTIONS

CHAPTER 15

Questions 85-89

Note: Choose the one option that BEST answers each question.

85. Traditionally, the population(s) at highest risk for using designer or club drugs include

    a. Hispanic males older than age 30.
    b. teenagers and young adults.
    c. gay and bisexual males.
    d. Black males.

86. The designer drug that has been associated with such sexual crimes as date rape is

    a. MDMA (Ecstasy).
    b. lysergenic acid diethylamide (LSD).
    c. methamphetamine.
    d. rohypnol.

87. Most designer drugs are consumed by

    a. intravenous injection.
    b. oral ingestion.
    c. snorting.
    d. topical administration.

88. The stimulant effect of MDMA (Ecstasy) allows users to dance for extended periods of time. A potentially fatal adverse effect associated with this behavior is

    a. an increase in body temperature.
    b. muscle cramping.
    c. damage to the liver.
    d. diminished sensory perception.

89. The most promising tool for the prevention of designer drug abuse among high school and college students is

    a. increased criminal penalties for first time offenses.
    b. informational material for parents.
    c. training sessions for teachers.
    d. education and peer led advocacy for students.

REFERENCES

Cottler L.B., Leung K.S., & Abdallah, A.B. (2009). Test-re-test reliability of *DSM-IV* adopted criteria for 3, 4-methylenedioxy-methamphetamine (MDMA) abuse and dependence: a cross-national study. (Abstract) *Addiction,* August 4, 2009. Retrieved March 15, 2013, from http://www.ncbi.nlm.nih.gov/pubmed/19681802

Drug Info Clearinghouse. (2013). *Ecstasy.* Retrieved March 15, 2013, from http://wwwdruginfo.adf.org.au/druginfo/drugs/drugfacts/ecstasy.html

Gahlinger, P. (2004). Club drugs: MDMA, gamma-hydroxybutrate (GHB), rohypnol, and ketamine. *American Family Physican, 69*(11), 2629-26.

Haroz, R. & Greenberg, M.I. (2005). Emerging drugs of abuse. *The Medical Clinics of North America, 89*(6), 1259-1276.

Hess, D. & DeBoer, S. (2002). Ecstasy. *American Journal of Nursing, 102*(4), 45-47.

Hoecker, C. (2013). *Designer drugs of abuse.* Retrieved March 15, 2013, from http://www.uptodate.com/patients/content/topic.do?topicKey=~llv70Ez9tNZ6D&source=HISTORY

Johnston, L. D., O'Malley, P. M., Bachman, J. G., & Schulenberg, J. E. (2013). *Monitoring the Future national results on adolescent drug use: Overview of key findings, 2012.* Ann Arbor: Institute for Social Research, The University of Michigan.

Klein, M. & Kramer, F. (2004). Rave drugs: Pharmacological considerations. *American Association of Nurse Anesthetists, 72*(1), 61-67.

Leib, R., Schuetz, C., Pfister, H., von Sydow, K., & Wittchen, H. (2002). Mental disorders in Ecstasy users: A prospective-longitudinal investigation. *Drug and Alcohol Dependence, 68*(2), 195-207.

McDowell, D. (2005). Marijuana, hallucinogens, and club drugs. In R.J. Frances, S.I. Miller, & A.H. Mack (Eds.), *Clinical textbook of addictive disorders* (3rd ed.). New York: Guilford Press.

Morgan, J. (2005). Designer drugs. In J.H. Lowinson, P. Ruiz, R.B. Millman, & J.G. Langrod (Eds.), *Substance abuse: A comprehensive textbook* (4th ed.). Philadelphia: Lippincott Williams & Wilkins.

National Institute on Drug Abuse. (2004). *NIDA community drug alert bulletin: Club drugs.* Retrieved March 15, 2013, from http://www.drugabuse.gov/ClubAlert/ClubDrugAlert.html

National Institute on Drug Abuse. (2006). *Research report series: MDMA (Ecstasy) abuse.* NIH Publication Number 06-4728. Retrieved March 15, 2013, from http://www.drugabuse.gov/PDF/RRmdma.pdf

National Institute on Drug Abuse. (2010). *DrugFacts: Club Drugs (GHB, Ketamine and Rohypnol).* Retrieved March 15, 2013, from http://www.nida.nih.gov/infofacts/clubdrugs.html

Substance Abuse and Mental Health Services Administration. (2012a). *Results from the 2011 National survey on drug use and health: Summary of national findings* (NSDUH Series H-44, HHS Publication No. (SMA) 12-4713). Rockville, MD. Accessed March 15, 2013 from http://www.samhsa.gov/data/NSDUH/2k11Results/NSDUHresults2011.htm

CHAPTER 16

ANABOLIC STEROIDS

CHAPTER OBJECTIVE

After completing this chapter, the learner will be able to discuss the characteristics of and issues related to anabolic steroid use.

LEARNING OBJECTIVES

After studying this chapter, the learner will be able to:

1. Identify steroids most commonly abused and the methods of abuse.
2. Describe populations at risk for steroid abuse.
3. Distinguish among the presenting signs and symptoms of anabolic steroid abuse for males and females.
4. Select appropriate strategies used in anabolic steroid abuse interventions.

OVERVIEW

The formal scientific term for this class of drugs is *anabolic-androgenic steroids.* These drugs are synthetic substances that are similar to the male hormone testosterone. The scientific term, anabolic-androgenic, can be better understood by reviewing the individual words *anabolic,* meaning muscle building, and *androgenic,* meaning to increase male characteristics (National Institute on Drug Abuse [NIDA], 2009). The most common reason these drugs are used is to promote physical strength, athletic endurance, and muscle size.

HISTORY

The first documented use of anabolic steroids as performance enhancers in the United States was with Bob Hoffman, a World War I veteran, who invented the barbell in 1923. Later, anabolic steroids were used during World War II to help increase the muscle size and strength of German soldiers. After World War II, anabolic steroids were used to promote weight gain in concentration camp survivors (McDuff & Barron, 2005). A Maryland physician, John Zeigler, studied the effects of anabolic steroids on weightlifting athletes and, as a result, in 1958, methandrostenalone was the first mass-produced anabolic steroid. In 1960, U.S. weightlifters started using anabolic steroids and by 1968, the use of steroids in the Olympics had become so common that routine urine testing became necessary.

During the 1970s and 1980s, the use of steroids continued to grow. In 1991, the Anabolic Steroid Control Act was passed making anabolic steroids a Schedule III drug requiring a prescription (Drug Enforcement Administration [DEA], n.d.). The Dietary Supplement Health and Education Act of 1994 was responsible for promoting the use of legal nutritional supplements as opposed to illegal anabolic steroids. Today, anabolic steroid use remains a significant health problem in the United States due to the steroids being smuggled from other countries, obtained from the internet, or diverted illegally from U.S. pharmacies (NIDA, 2000).

MEDICAL INDICATIONS

There are many different types of anabolic steroids available by prescription in the United States. There are various therapeutic indications for these medications used by many different fields of medicine. Anabolic steroids are appropriate treatment for people who do not produce testosterone naturally, for some cancers, for some anemias, for burn victims, and for wasting diseases such as human immunodeficiency syndrome (HIV) or tuberculosis (Brown, 2005).

STEROID ADMINISTRATION AND USE

Steroids can be administered orally, intramuscularly, or topically. Two of the more common street names for these drugs are *roids* or *juice*. Table 16-1 includes a list of common steroid street names. The most common steroids used today include anadrol, oxandrin, dianabol, winstrol, deca-durabolin, and equipoise (NIDA, 2006). Table 16-2 identifies the mode of use, generic name, and brand name for these commonly abused steroids.

Steroid abusers use extremely high doses of these medications, often 20 to 200 times higher than the prescribed doses (Eisenberg & Galloway, 2005). Steroid abusers have specific regimens for using the drugs such as cycling, stacking, and pyramiding. *Cycling* is a technique of alternating between use and non-use of steroids. By *cycling,* the user is attempting to minimize the unwanted adverse drug effects. Cycling usually involves administering the specific steroids every 4 to 18 weeks, followed by a drug-free period of 1 month to 1 year. A second technique is called *stacking;* a common practice where the users use multiple different steroids to maximize the effect on muscle size. A third dosing technique is *pyramiding,* initially administering a low dose of the steroid, gradually increasing the dose to the middle of the cycle, and then tapering the dose to

TABLE 16-1: COMMON STREET NAMES FOR STEROIDS

Street Names
Arnolds
Gym candy
Juice
Product
Pumpers
Roids
Sauce
Slop
Stackers
Vitamins
Weight trainers

TABLE 16-2: COMMONLY ABUSED STEROIDS

Form	Generic Name	Brand Name
Oral	Oxymetholone	Adroyd Anadrol-50 Anapolon Oxitosona Plenastril
	Oxandrolone	Lonavar Oxandrin (U.S.)
	Methandrosenolone	Metaboline Dianabol
	Stanozolol	Stromba
Injectable	Methandrosenolone	Winstrol
	Boldenone undecylenate	Equipoise
	Nortestosterone	Deca-Durabolin (U.S.) Androlone-D

complete the cycle. A final dosing alternative is known as *stacking the pyramid* that combines the dosing techniques. Abusers are often extremely exacting in the dosing and timing of their steroid regimens. It should be noted that the perceived benefits of these techniques has not been scientifically documented (Eisenberg & Galloway, 2005).

EPIDEMIOLOGY

The spread of anabolic steroid use has been significant in the United States yet it has gone relatively unnoticed. In 2004, amendments to the Controlled Substances Act caused many forms of anabolic steroids, including the steroid precursors previously available in health food stores, in gyms and health clubs, and over the internet to become illegal (Anabolic Steroid Control Act of 2004, 2004). There is limited data available to quantify the extent of anabolic steroid abuse in the general adult population, due primarily to the hesitance to report the use of illegal substances (Brown, 2005), but scientific evidence indicates that anabolic steroid abuse among athletes may range between one and six percent (NIDA, 2006).

In 2011, 1.2% of 19-30 year olds reported having used steroids in their lifetime. The highest rate of annual use is among 12th graders at 1.2%. Annual and 30-day rates for steroid use were very low for college students and young adults at 0.2%. Steroid use remains higher in males then females (Johnston, O'Malley, Bachman, & Schulenberg, 2012). Of the high school students surveyed, 1.2% of eighth graders, 1.4% of tenth graders and 1.8% of twelfth graders indicated they have used steroids in their lifetime (Johnston et al., 2012).

The incidence of anabolic steroid abuse is especially high among athletes, particularly competitive bodybuilders and weight lifters. Steroid abuse is also related to a behavioral syndrome called *muscle dysmorphia,* where the person has a distorted body image. Some people use steroids to increase their muscle size after experiencing either sexual or physical abuse. Generally speaking, most people who initiate steroid use are psychologically normal when they begin but develop abnormal personality traits and disturbances that can be attributed to steroid use (Eisenberg & Galloway, 2005).

BIOCHEMISTRY

Anabolic steroids are synthetic derivatives of the male sex hormone *testosterone*. Testosterone is a steroid hormone produced in male testes; however, it is also present in females in smaller amounts, produced by the adrenal glands and the ovaries. In females, the testosterone is acted upon in adipose tissue and converted into estrogen. Males maintain plasma concentration levels of 300 to 1000 ng/dL, whereas females maintain levels between 15 and 65 ng/dL. Testosterone is metabolized extensively in the liver (Brown, 2005). This hormone promotes the growth of skeletal muscle, and the development of male sex characteristics (Volkow, 2005a).

Some steroid supplements can be found over the counter (OTC) in most health food stores and are advertised as dietary supplements. These items are popular with athletes because they advertise their ability to increase muscle mass. The concern is that when these substances are consumed in high doses, there is a significant rise in the body's testosterone level similar to that of prescription anabolic steroids. Currently, research has not been conducted to identify the adverse effects of these substances. However, it is thought that they will produce the same types of adverse effects as seen with anabolic steroids (NIDA, 2006).

SCREENING OF SPECIAL POPULATIONS AND RISK IDENTIFICATION

Middle and high school-age children – particularly athletes – are at significant risk for steroid abuse. The three most significant warning signs for abuse include prominent acne, gynecomastia, and cutaneous striae. Parents should also pay particular attention to teenagers who increase their time at the gym and have a preoccupation with weight training. Athletes who experience a large increase in muscle mass (greater than 20 lb of muscle) in a relatively short amount of time may be abusing steroids.

Steroids commonly cause dramatic changes in personality, such as moodiness, aggression, and extreme irritability. Users may also experience paranoid jealousy, delusions, and feelings of invincibility resulting in impaired judgment. Males will have an increase in breast tissue called *gynecomastia* and a decrease in testicular size (NIDA, 2013). Both males and females may notice stretch marks called *cutaneous striae* around the breast area. An increased amount of acne on the face, back, and chest is also common. Additionally, the face may appear puffy due to fluid retention. Users may also have an elevated blood pressure and increased heart rate. Parents who identify at least three of these signs in their child should consult their primary care provider to consider steroid abuse. Testicular atrophy is a hallmark of steroid abuse and should always be evaluated by the primary care provider.

Other groups at high risk for steroid abuse include competitive athletes and body builders (NIDA, 2006). Laboratory drug testing is commonly required for professional athletes during competitive events to ensure fairness. Urine drug testing is very reliable when done by a qualified laboratory, but not all laboratories test for all steroids and there are new steroids on the market all the time. Therefore, a negative laboratory test does not rule out abuse, particularly in cases where body composition indicates otherwise. Many athletes have learned how to avoid a positive test by stopping use for an appropriate amount of time to allow for the drugs to leave their system. Some athletes use combinations of drugs, such as probenecid and diuretics, to decrease the urinary concentrations of steroids and avoid potential positive tests (Eisenberg & Galloway, 2005). Additionally, the detection of testosterone is complicated because it is a naturally occurring hormone and testing must rely on ratios of testosterone to epitestosterone. Some athletes have also been found to self-administer epitestosterone in an attempt to nullify the laboratory tests.

In general, the amount of time steroids remain detectable in a person's system is dependent on the length of use, the doses used, and the individual's ability to clear the drug. Most intramuscular steroids are detectable for 3 to 4 months after ceasing use and oral steroids are detectable for 1 to 4 weeks after the last use (Eisenberg & Galloway, 2005).

RELATED MEDICAL PROBLEMS AND CO-OCCURRING DISORDERS

General

Anabolic steroid abuse has been associated with various adverse effects that range in severity from abnormal changes in appearance to those that are life threatening. Generally, most of these effects are considered reversible after the abuser stops using the drugs, but some are permanent. Most of the data on long-term adverse effects has been compiled through case reports as opposed to formal epidemiological

TABLE 16-3: EFFECTS OF ANABOLIC STEROIDS BY SYSTEM
Cardiovascular
Myocardial infarctions
Thromboyctosis
Lipodystrophy
Hypertension
Cerebral vascular accident (stroke)
Endocrine
Male
Testicular atrophy
Infertility
Gynecomastia
Increase in sex drive
Female
Amenorrhea
Masculinazation (voice deepening, breasts shrinking)
Excessive growth of body hair
Clitoris enlargement
Both genders
Male-pattern Baldness
Infection
Hepatitis B
Hepatitis C
HIV
Bacterial endocarditis
Abcesses
Hepatic
Hepatic tumors
Peliosis
Hepatomegly
Musculoskeletal
Short stature
Ruptured tendons
Avulsions
Dermatologic
Acne
Cutaneous striae
Increased oily scalp
Psychiatric
Increased violence and aggression
Depression
Mania
Delusions
Major mood swings
Restlessness
Hallucinations
Irritability

studies. Medically-related problems have been noted in the endocrine, musculoskeletal, cardiovascular, and integumentary systems, as well as causing liver, psychiatric, and infection problems (NIDA, 2006). A summary of these medical problems is provided in Table 16-3.

Endocrine

The endocrine system is seriously altered by the use of anabolic steroids. A decrease in sperm production and atrophy of the testicles are reversible effects noted in male steroid abusers. Gynecomastia, breast development, and male-pattern baldness are irreversible effects that occur in male steroid abusers more than 50% of the time. It has also been found that male steroid users complain of breast pain and experience a decrease in naturally occurring gonadotropins, which results in variable effects on sexual interest, spontaneous erections, the prostate, and fertility (Eisenberg & Galloway, 2005).

In females, anabolic steroids have been used therapeutically to treat osteoporosis and menopause; to date, the role of these drugs in breast growth and development has not been completely determined. Steroid abuse in females causes masculinization – notably, a decrease in breast size, increase in facial and body hair growth, decrease in scalp hair growth, deepening of the voice, and coarseness of the skin (NIDA, 2000). Females also experience a decrease in body fat, increase in menstrual irregularities, and clitoral enlargement. In contrast to males, female adverse effects are usually irreversible.

Both males and females who use steroids experience an increase in insulin resistance. Currently research is being conducted to explore the supraphysiologic dose of anabolic androgenic steroids on glucose metabolism (Eisenberg & Galloway, 2005). Fortunately, it appears that these symptoms are reversible when the drugs are withdrawn.

Musculoskeletal

The musculoskeletal system responds to rising androgenic steroids by triggering bone growth during puberty and adolescence. In young adults who have not reached this increased state by naturally occurring hormones, but experience the increase of hormones through steroid abuse, stunted height may occur due to the increased levels of steroids signaling the bones to stop growing (Volkow, 2005b). Another issue with steroid abuse is the increase of muscular skeletal injuries as a result of the drugs. The steroids cause the muscle to grossly increase in size resulting in stress on the tendons and ligaments. Tendon rupture (unilaterally and bilaterally) and avulsions can result from bulking due to steroids. Bilateral quadriceps tendon rupture is rare and only seen in athletes abusing steroids (Eisenberg & Galloway, 2005).

Cardiovascular

Some of the more lethal adverse effects have been seen in the cardiovascular system. Myocardial infarctions, sudden cardiac death, and stroke have been diagnosed in athletes younger than age 30 (DEA, n.d.). Many cases of adverse cardiovascular events related to the use of steroids have been documented but researchers have not been able to clearly identify a causal relationship. Coagulation abnormalities, hypertension, cardiomegaly, and serum lipid abnormalities have been identified as potential health issues seen in otherwise previously healthy, young steroid users (Eisenberg & Galloway, 2005).

It is suspected that the relationship between cardiovascular effects and the use of steroids is complicated and multi-faceted. Oral steroids are known to increase the low-density lipoprotein (LDL) cholesterol and decrease the high-density lipoprotein (HDL) cholesterol, which increases the risk of atherosclerosis. Testosterone is known to increase platelet activation in steroid abusers and has caused thrombosis (blood clot) in weightlifters with no evidence of atherosclerosis. Anabolic steroids cause an increase in hemoglobin and hematocrit due to the increased synthesis of erythropoietin, which is beneficial in the treatment of anemia, but contributes to thrombosis (Eisenberg & Galloway, 2005).

Dermatologic

Dermatologic effects of steroids are readily apparent. An increase in sebaceous secretions creates noticeably oily hair and skin. Acne is a common effect of the steroid abuse. Cystic acne and pitting scars are significant findings when screening for steroid use. Steroids have also been associated with linear keloids, striae, hirsutism, seborrheic dermatitis, and secondary infections (Eisenberg & Galloway, 2005).

Hepatic

Chronic anabolic androgenic steroid use has been associated with various serious changes in the liver. Current studies are not adequate to draw causal relationships between steroid use and liver disease due to the limitations in research design, such as no controls for muscle damage, alcohol consumption, other illnesses, or medications. There does seem to be an increase in hepatic tumors in susceptible persons. Such liver diseases as hepatomegaly, enlarged liver, and peliosis (blood-filled cysts that can rupture causing hemorrhage and death) have also been seen in chronic steroid users. Other hepatic disorders, such as biliary stasis, jaundice, and hepatorenal syndrome have been documented with steroid use. Although liver toxicities are expected to occur with supratherapeutic doses of steroids, further research needs to be conducted to clearly define the extent of the disease risks (Eisenberg & Galloway, 2005).

Psychiatric

The psychiatric effects of steroid abuse have not been prospectively studied, but individual case reports and a few small studies show a possible link. Increased irritability and aggressive behavior have been noted in many steroid abusers. There have been criminal reports of previously non-violent steroid abusers fighting, committing armed robbery, or forcibly committing crimes against properties. Anger and explosive outbursts associated with steroid abuse have been identified by the media as "roid rage" (Eisenberg & Galloway, 2005). These events can occur even with very low doses of steroids.

Withdrawal of steroids can cause serious and dangerous symptoms of depression that could lead to suicide. Confusion, forgetfulness, and distractibility are some of the cognitive changes noted with steroid use. Euphoria, behavioral changes, mood swings, increased energy, and increased sexual arousal has also been reported with steroid use (Eisenberg & Galloway, 2005).

Addiction is a problem seen in some steroid abusers; it is identified through continued drug use despite serious physical and behavioral problems. Anabolic steroids are different from other drugs of abuse in that many of their "reinforcing effects" (those effects that keep a person using a drug) are not experienced immediately or rapidly (Volkow, 2005b). The main reason people abuse steroids is to improve their performance in sports or their appearance (to increase their muscle size and/or reduce their body fat). These effects take time to develop, but once developed, they may be strong incentives for continued anabolic steroid abuse (Volkow, 2005a). Symptoms of dependence include loss of control, withdrawal symptoms, and interference with other activities. Acute withdrawal symptoms include drug cravings and depression. Other withdrawal symptoms are anxiety, increased blood pressure and heart rate, chills, piloerection, hot flashes, diaphoresis, nausea, anorexia, vomiting, insomnia, and irritability. The duration of withdrawal seems to be related to the dosage taken and length of drug use. The most severe withdrawal symptom, depression, has been known to resolve within 100 days or persist for more than 1 year (Volkow, 2005a).

Infections

Another health problem related to injected steroids is infections. Injection abusers commonly use nonsterile needles, poor injection techniques, and nonsterile drugs, which can cause serious infection risks. Injection steroid abusers are at risk for such life-threatening infections as HIV, hepatitis B and C, and bacterial endocarditis. Infections at the injection sites due to bacteria could result in serious abscesses (NIDA, 2000).

PREVENTIVE STRATEGIES AND TREATMENT

Prevention research is currently ongoing in this country. Starting in 1993, NIDA funded research at Oregon Health and Science University to develop steroid prevention programs and programs focusing on improving health behaviors in high school students. The results have been positive, and gender-specific peer-led drug prevention and health promotion programs have been effective. These specific programs are Athletes Training and Learning to Avoid Steroids (ATLAS) and Athletes Targeting Healthy Exercise and Nutrition Alternatives (ATHENA) (Volkow, 2005a).

The ATLAS program is a multi-focused approach that promotes nutrition and strength training as alternatives to steroid abuse, drug refusal role play, and an anti-steroid media campaign (Goldberg et al., 1996). This program also includes a parent component designed to inform, support, and encourage parents in communicating with their susceptible teenagers.

Prevention strategies for amateur and professional athletes have been focused on changes in federal laws, rules and regulations of professional sports, and the International Olympic Committee. In 1999, the World Anti-Doping Agency was established to develop standard drug testing protocols, accredit drug testing laboratories, and compile and publish current information on its Web site (http://www.wada-ama.org) (Eisenberg & Galloway, 2005). Other important prevention targets include health clubs and health food stores. In 2004, President Bush addressed the current steroid abuse problem during the State of the Union Address, calling upon coaches, players, and team owners to rectify this broad problem (Eisenberg & Galloway, 2005).

It is estimated that there are approximately 1 million steroid abusers in this country; only a small percentage of these users seek or receive treatment. The initial concern in initiating treatment is the psychiatric status of the client. Some steroid abusers can have serious psychiatric changes and will require inpatient care. It is important to note that assessments of potential steroid abusers should be conducted individually because there is a risk of relationship violence. Treatment must be tailored to individual clients because they may be motivated differently than other drug abusers.

The expected changes, both psychological and physical, should be reviewed with the user. If the abuser is using the drug for its mood-altering effects, then conventional drug treatment would be warranted. If abusers are using the drugs to alter body size or composition, it is important to set realistic goals and develop a balanced diet and exercise program. Previous behaviors must be modified to avoid people and places that trigger use or memories of use. Peer counseling and support groups are excellent methods of reinforcing positive behaviors. Pharmacological therapy is currently limited to the management of serious depression and suicidal thoughts (Eisenberg & Galloway, 2006).

SUMMARY

Anabolic steroid abuse remains a serious health problem in this country. As a society, the message is being sent that physical beauty and athletic accomplishments are valued and worth the physical, psychological, and legal risks to achieve.

President Bush identified the need for us to change our thinking and behavior related to shortcuts in training and performance (Eisenberg & Galloway, 2005). Winning a competition while sacrificing character and fairness should not be acceptable in the United States or other countries.

EXAM QUESTIONS

CHAPTER 16

Questions 90-95

Note: Choose the one option that BEST answers each question.

90. Stacking is a technique used by steroid abusers to
    a. increase the dose of the steroid being administered.
    b. use many different steroids to maximize the desired effects.
    c. vary the dose of steroids being administered.
    d. allow the body to have drug-free periods.

91. Today, the population most at risk for steroid abuse is
    a. military personnel.
    b. burn victims.
    c. athletes.
    d. disaster survivors.

92. Tom, age 16, has been training hard all summer for the school football team. His mother notices that he has significantly increased his muscle mass and she is concerned that he is overtraining. Later, she overhears him talking on the telephone about "roids." Your advice to the mother should be
    a. "Have your son evaluated for possible steroid abuse by your primary care provider."
    b. "Do not worry about the situation; it is perfectly normal."
    c. "Ask your son's friends if he is using steroids."
    d. "Search his room for evidence of drug use."

93. The abuse of steroids can cause serious reversible and irreversible adverse effects. The irreversible adverse effects seen in male abusers include
    a. testicular atrophy.
    b. increased lipid levels.
    c. infertility.
    d. gynecomastia.

94. ATLAS and ATHENA are
    a. prevention programs targeting males and females designed to prevent steroid abuse and promote health behaviors and attitudes.
    b. street names for steroids.
    c. project names for the National Institute on Drug Abuse public service project.
    d. names of steroid abuse screening tools.

95. Violent behavior is commonly associated with steroid abuse and withdrawal from steroids can cause serious symptoms of depression. These depression symptoms
    a. are transient effects that will resolve within 2 to 3 weeks.
    b. are only seen with unusually high doses of steroid abuse.
    c. can lead to suicide and should be closely assessed.
    d. are only seen in specific steroids and do not require further evaluation.

REFERENCES

Anabolic Steroid Control Act of 2004. (2004). Retrieved April 3, 2013, from http://www.qpo.gov/fdsys/plig/BILLS-108s2195enr.pdf

Brown, J. (2005). Anabolic steroids: What should the emergency physician know? *Emergency Medicine Clinics of North America August.* *23*(3), 815-826.

Drug Enforcement Administration. (n.d.). *Steroids.* Retrieved March 15, 2013, from http://www.justice.gov/dea/druginfo/drug_data_sheets/Steroids.pdf

Eisenberg, E. & Galloway, G. (2005). Anabolic-Androgenic steroids. In J.H. Lowinson, P. Ruiz, R.B. Millman & J.G. Langrod (Eds.), *Substance abuse: A comprehensive textbook* (4th ed.). Philadelphia: Lippincott Williams & Wilkins.

Goldberg, L., Elliot, D.L., MacKinnon, D.P., Moe, E., Zoref, L., Green, C., et al. (1996). Effects of a multi-dimensional anabolic steroid prevention intervention: The A.T.L.A.S. (adolescents training and learning to avoid steroids) program. *JAMA, 276,* 1555-1562.

Johnston, L. D., O'Malley, P. M., Bachman, J. G., & Schulenberg, J. E. (2012). *Monitoring the Future national survey results on drug use, 1975-2011. Volume I: Secondary school students*. Ann Arbor: Institute for Social Research, The University of Michigan.

McDuff, D. & Baron, D. (2005). Substance use in athletics: A sports psychiatry perspective. *Clinics in Sports Medicine, 24*(4), 885-89.

National Institute on Drug Abuse. (2000). *NIDA community alert bulletin: Anabolic steroids.* Retrieved March 15, 2013, from http://www.drugabuse.gov/SteroidAlert/SteroidAlert.html

National Institute on Drug Abuse. (2006). *Anabolic steroid abuse.* Research report series (NIH Publication No. 06-3721). Retrieved March 15, 2013, from http://www.nida.nih.gov/ResearchReports/steroids/AnabolicSteroids.html

National Institute on Drug Abuse. (2013). *DrugFacts: Anabolic steroids (anabolic-androgenic).* Retrieved March 15, 2013, from http://www.nida.nih.gov/infofacts/steroids.html

Volkow, N.D. (2005a). *Consequences of the abuse of anabolic steroids – before the Committee on Government Reform – United States House of Representatives.* Statement for the Record. March 17, 2005. Retrieved March 15, 2013, from http://www.drugabuse.gov/Testimony/3-17-05Testimony.html

Volkow, N.D. (2005b). *Message from the Director: Consequences of the abuse of anabolic steroids.* Retrieved March 15, 2013, from http://www.drugabuse.gov/about/welcome/messagesteroids305.html

CHAPTER 17

IMPAIRED PRACTICE IN HEALTHCARE PROFESSIONALS

CHAPTER OBJECTIVE

After completing this chapter, the learner will be able to describe the ethical and legal implications of impaired practice and the role of health care professionals in identifying and reporting impaired practice.

LEARNING OBJECTIVES

After completing this chapter, the learner will be able to:

1. Describe the definition of impaired practice by a health care professional.
2. Identify the prevalence of substance use disorders in health care professionals.
3. Describe the clinical indicators of impaired practice.
4. Explain rationales for reporting a healthcare professional with impaired practice to the appropriate resource for treatment.

OVERVIEW

Substance abuse disorders among healthcare professionals present special challenges to the profession. The prevalence of alcohol and drug abuse in medicine, social work, and nursing is believed to be equal to the general population, about 8.5% (Siebert, 2005). Healthcare professionals commonly view themselves as immune to developing substance use disorders because of their knowledge and position. Often, the opposite is true. It is estimated that one-half of all Americans will develop a mental disorder at some point in their lives (Kessler, Berglund, Demler, Jin, Merikangas, & Walters, 2005; Kessler, Chiu, Demler, Merikangas, & Walters, 2005). In addition, about 26% of individuals older than age 18 report experiencing at least one psychiatric disorder within a 12-month period – most commonly anxiety disorders, mood disorders, impulse control disorders, and substance abuse disorders (Kessler, Berglund, et al., 2005; Kessler, Chiu, et al., 2005).

Healthcare professionals are just as vulnerable to mental health and substance use disorders as the general public. Impaired practice includes not only clinicians with substance use disorders, but any mental health or personal problem and/or distress that interferes with the quality and safety of patient care. For the purposes of this chapter, impairment will be narrowly defined as caused by or related to a substance use disorder. The impact of impairment on the quality and safety of patient care is of great concern to all healthcare professionals; health consumers; boards of nursing, medicine, and social work; and policy makers.

HISTORY

The history of drug and alcohol abuse in health care has been documented since the 1800s. Jane Gibson, a young nurse who accompanied Florence Nightingale to the battlefields of the Crimean war, was fired from her postwar nursing position for coming to work under the influence of alcohol. The press vilified her, implying that she had ruined the image of the "Nightingale Nurses" – an image replete with behaviors described as angelic, pure, caring, and virginal (Monahan, 2003).

Additionally, Dr. William Oster described the addiction of a legendary surgeon, Dr. William Halstad. Oster states, "I saw him in severe chills, and this was the first information I had that he was still taking morphia. Subsequently, I had many talks about it and gained his full confidence. He had never been able to reduce the amount to less than three grains daily; on this, he could do his work comfortably and maintain his excellent physical vigor. I do not think that anyone suspected him" (Noland & Halstad, 1991, p.17).

Dr. Halstad continued in his surgical practice; however, Ms. Gibson's fate was more reflective of the public and professional response to healthcare professionals with impaired practice. Historically, the response was usually overwhelmingly punitive and resulted in devastating personal and professional losses (Monahan, 2003). Since the 1980s, the healthcare professions have worked to develop a more measured response that focuses on protecting the public safety while providing a non-punitive opportunity for treatment and rehabilitation. Each health discipline has developed a Code of Ethics that addresses the issue of an impaired practice associated with a substance use disorder. These Codes of Ethics are developed by such organizations as the American Nurses Association (ANA), the American Medical Association (AMA), and the National Association of Social Workers (NASW). The Codes of Ethics are unique to each organization, but they are consistent in their mandates that require healthcare professionals report all instances of impaired practice of a colleague to the appropriate resource. These resources vary by state law and include administrators, licensing boards, or professional organizations. The Codes of Ethics require that the professional must not only report unsafe or incompetent practices (again, for the purposes of this chapter "incompetent practice" will be defined as "impaired practice associated with substance abuse"), but also all reasonable suspicions of impaired practice.

The Codes of Ethics espoused by professional organizations are considered an ethical mandate. However, licensing boards, specifically the Board of Nursing, Board of Medical Examiners, and Board of Social Work, exist in each state to protect the public and regulate and license the profession. Licensing boards carry the force of law (Reid, 1999). Therefore, it is both an ethical and legal responsibility to report a colleague whose practice is impaired.

Impaired nursing practice may be defined as the inability of a registered nurse to perform her role and responsibilities because of a chemical dependency on drugs and/or alcohol. The ANA Code of Ethics states that a nurse with impaired practice "may have difficulty remaining accountable to herself and others for her own actions or in assessing self-competence" (ANA, 2001, p. 14; Blair, 2002).

Impaired social work practice may be defined as any impairment due to personal problems, psychosocial distress, substance abuse, or mental health difficulties that interferes with practice effectiveness (NASW, 1999). The Association of Social Work Boards states, "a social worker shall not practice while impaired by medication, alcohol, drugs, or other chemicals. A social worker shall not practice under a mental or physical condition that impairs the ability to safely practice" (Association of Social Work Boards, 1997, p. 56).

EPIDEMIOLOGY

The key risk factors for alcohol and drug abuse among healthcare professionals involve personal, genetic, environmental, and occupational risks. As previously noted, healthcare professionals commonly consider themselves to be at low-risk for substance use disorders by virtue of their extensive education and training; however, these professionals are no different from the general population in terms of their risk.

Personal risk factors for a substance abuse disorder include a genetic predisposition to addiction, a family history of substance abuse, a chaotic family history, low self-esteem, a history of victimization, and chronic pain (Coombs, 1997). These risk factors are not unique to healthcare workers but predispose an individual for a substance use disorder.

Occupational and environmental risks factors include work in a stressful and demanding environment that can result in burnout; variable shift work and sleep patterns that can result in sleep deprivation and self-medication with stimulants and sedatives; increased access and familiarity with drugs and controlled substances; the emphasis placed on drugs as a treatment tool; self-medicating behaviors; and, inherent to the helping professions, a focus on the needs of others, not self (Lillibridge, Cox, & Cross, 2002).

Healthcare professionals working in the same specialty area tend to abuse similar substances. This is particularly true with nurses and doctors. Nurses in emergency departments, intensive care units, or operating rooms report easier access to controlled substances and more prescription-type substance abuse than non-critical care nurses (Dunn, 2005; Trinkoff & Storr, 1998). Emergency department nurses are 3.5 times as likely to use marijuana or cocaine as general practice nurses, and oncology and administration nurses are twice as likely to engage in binge drinking than general practice nurses (Trinkoff & Storr, 1998).

Nurses in general are more likely to abuse prescription drugs than other substances. The foundation for alcohol and drug abuse commonly begins in college, with at-risk behaviors and heavy drinking occurring in nursing, medical, or social work school. Research has determined that more than one-half of healthcare professionals who develop impaired practice began abusing drugs before they finished their professional education. Polysubstance abuse, a term used to define abuse of multiple drugs or drugs plus alcohol, was the most common form of abuse (Kenna & Wood, 2004).

CLINICAL FINDINGS

Early identification is critical to the safety and quality of patient care and crucial to the long-term recovery of the professional. The importance of early identification of impairment cannot be overstated. It usually occurs when a professional is suspicious of a colleague's impairment. Recognition of unsafe or incompetent practice protects the safety and quality of care and improves treatment outcomes. Early identification is challenging and usually difficult because job performance is one of the last areas affected in an addicted healthcare professional's life.

The sequence of impairment and negative consequences related to a substance abuse disorder follows a common pattern. First, the substance abuser's family is affected. This is characterized by dysfunctional relationships, conflict, acting out, and co-dependence. Next, the substance abuser's standing and interaction with his or her community is impaired. Financial difficulties follow, along with spiritual and emotional health problems. Next, physical health problems associated with alcohol or drug abuse occur. Often, the root cause of these health problems is not identified and the health problem is treated in isolation. Lastly, job performance is affected and impacted negatively.

As previously stated, early identification is critical to the long-term recovery of the healthcare professional. A pattern of behavior with resulting negative consequences provides cues for early identification (see Table 17-1). Such cues include withdrawal from family activities and family dysfunction. Examples of withdrawal from activities include increasing isolation from family and friends and displaying inappropriate or embarrassing behaviors at community functions. Legal and financial problems include financial difficulties and driving under the influence of the substance. Spiritual and emotional difficulties are exhibited by labile moods, mental health disorders, and rationalization behaviors. Physical indicators include episodes of gastritis or gastrointestinal problems, weight loss, sniffing, sneezing, watery eyes, unexplained bruises, trauma, and frequent visits for healthcare. Occupational indicators include deteriorating performance, excessive use of sick time or tardiness, and poor judgment (Blair, 2002; Dunn, 2005; Kenna & Wood, 2004; Siebert, 2003; Siebert, 2005).

Physical and occupational indicators that are red flags would be the frequent use of mouthwash or mints, tremors, changes in speech patterns, unsteady gait, lethargy, and the smell of alcohol on the breath. Other indicators include requests for the night shift or for positions with less supervision; frequent trips to the bathroom or the "locked door" syndrome; and poor boundaries in asking colleagues for prescriptions or patient medications (Dunn, 2005; Ponech, 2000; Talbot & Wilson, 2004).

TABLE 17-1: CUES FOR EARLY IDENTIFICATION	
Family	• Withdrawal from family activities • Marital conflict • Acting out by children • Sexual problems
Community	• Withdrawal from community activities • Embarrassing behaviors at community functions
Financial and Legal Difficulities	• Legal problems • Driving under the influence • Financial difficulities
Spiritual and Emotional Difficulties	• Changes in emotional health • Mood swings • Anger • Denial and rationalization • Depression, anxiety, and panic disorders • Forgetfullness
Physical Problems	• Poor personal hygiene • Weight loss • Sniffing, sneezing, watery eyes • Cough • Unexplained bruises • Frequent visits for health care • Multiple prescriptions • Chronic pain
Job Performance	• Deteriorating job performance • Excessive use of sick time • Calling in sick on Fridays and/or Mondays • Poor judgment • Disorganization • Withdrawal from co-workers

TREATMENT

The ANA Code of Ethics states, "In a situation where a nurse suspects another's practice may be impaired, the nurse's duty is to take action designed both to protect patients and to assure that the impaired individual receives assistance in regaining optimal function" (ANA, 2001, p. 7). The Code further states, "if impaired practice poses a threat or danger to self or others, regardless of whether the individual has sought help, the nurse must take action to report the individual to persons authorized to address the problem" (ANA, 2001, p. 7). See Table 17-2. It is clear and unequivocal that patient safety is paramount and that it is the responsibility of the nurse to report questionable practice. The Code is also quite clear that compassion, treatment, and rehabilitation are the goals of care for the impaired healthcare professional.

The NASW has a similar Code of Ethics that states, "social workers should not allow their own personal problems, psychosocial distress, legal problems, substance abuse, or mental health difficulties to interfere with their professional judgment and performance or to jeopardize the best interests of people for whom they have a professional responsibility" (NASW, 1999, p. 14). Further, "social workers whose personal problems, psychosocial distress, legal problems, substance abuse, or mental health difficulties interfere with their professional judgment and performance should immediately seek consultation and take appropriate remedial action by seeking professional help, making adjustments in workload, terminating practice, or taking any other steps necessary to protect clients and others" (NASW, 1999, p. 14). The Code clearly articulates the ethical responsibility of a professional to report an impaired social worker to the appropriate resource that is authorized to address the problem. See Table 17-3. Again, patient safety is paramount.

It is not uncommon for the colleagues of the professional with a substance use disorder to be suspicious and recognize the subtle signs of drug and/or alcohol abuse. However, many choose not to document or communicate these suspicions, allowing the impaired practice to continue. The literature suggests that healthcare professionals

TABLE 17-2: AMERICAN NURSES ASSOCIATION CODE OF ETHICS: ADDRESSING IMPAIRED PRACTICE

3.6 Addressing impaired practice

Nurses must be vigilant to protect the patient, the public, and the profession from potential harm when a colleague's practice, in any setting, appears to be impaired. The nurse extends compassion and caring to colleagues who are in recovery from illness or when illness interferes with job performance. In a situation where a nurse suspects another's practice may be impaired, the nurse's duty is to take action designed both to protect patients and to assure that the impaired individual receives assistance in regaining optimal function. Such action should usually begin with consulting supervisory personnel and may also include confronting the individual in a supportive manner and with the assistance of others or helping the individual to access appropriate resources. Nurses are encouraged to follow guidelines outlined by the profession and policies of the employing organization to assist colleagues whose job performance may be adversely affected by mental or physical illness or by personal circumstances. Nurses in all roles should advocate for colleagues whose job performance may be impaired to ensure that they receive appropriate assistance, treatment, and access to fair institutional and legal processes. This includes supporting the return to practice of the individual who has sought assistance and is ready to resume professional duties.

If impaired practice poses a threat or danger to self or others, regardless of whether the individual has sought help, the nurse must take action to report the individual to persons authorized to address the problem. Nurses who report others whose job performance creates a risk for harm should be protected from negative consequences.

Advocacy may be a difficult process and the nurse is advised to follow workplace policies. If workplace policies do not exist or are inappropriate, that is, they deny the nurse in question access to due legal process or demand resignation, the reporting nurse may obtain guidance from the professional association, state peer assistance programs, employee assistance program, or a similar resource.

Note. From *Code of Ethics for Nurses* by American Nurses Association, 2001, Washington, DC. Accessed on March 15, 2013, from http://www.nursingworld.org/MainMenuCategories/ThePracticeofProfessionalNursing/EthicsStandards/CodeofEthics.aspx

TABLE 17-3: NATIONAL ASSOCIATION OF SOCIAL WORKERS CODE OF ETHICS

Social Workers' Ethical Responsibilities to Colleagues

2.09 Impairment of Colleagues

(a) Social workers who have direct knowledge of a social work colleague's impairment that is due to personal problems, psychosocial distress, substance abuse, or mental health difficulties and that interferes with practice effectiveness should consult with that colleague when feasible and assist the colleague in taking remedial action.

(b) Social workers who believe that a social work colleague's impairment interferes with practice effectiveness and that the colleague has not taken adequate steps to address the impairment should take action through appropriate channels established by employers, agencies, NASW, licensing and regulatory bodies, and other professional organizations.

Social Workers' Ethical Responsibilities as Professionals

4.05 Impairment

(a) Social workers should not allow their own personal problems, psychosocial distress, legal problems, substance abuse, or mental health difficulties to interfere with their professional judgment and performance or to jeopardize the best interests of people for whom they have a professional responsibility.

(b) Social workers whose personal problems, psychosocial distress, legal problems, substance abuse, or mental health difficulties interfere with their professional judgment and performance should immediately seek consultation and take appropriate remedial action by seeking professional help, making adjustments in workload, terminating practice, or taking any other steps necessary to protect clients and others.

Note. From *Code of Ethics* by National Association of Social Workers, 1999. Accessed March 15, 2013, from http://www.socialworkers.org/pubs/code/code.asp

address their impaired colleagues in one of three manners: choose to take no action; enable the behavior; or report suspected impairment (Blair, 2002; Dunn, 2005). The professional may choose to take no action because of fear about repercussions, lack of awareness of a policy that addresses the process of reporting impairment, or concerns about personal liability. The healthcare professional may choose to perform the duties or cover the mistakes of an impaired colleague in an attempt to protect the colleague's job or to act as a counselor. These professionals enable the continued impaired practice of their colleague. In either instance, a professional who is aware of a colleague with a substance use disorder and willfully does not report this colleague is jeopardizing patient safety and could face disciplinary action.

"Good-faith reporting of unsafe or incompetent practice is a matter of both law and ethics; it must not be avoided and should not be considered unfair or disloyal" (Reid, 1999, p. 291). If a healthcare professional has a reasonable suspicion of impairment, is concerned about patient safety, is reporting this suspicion in good faith, and has documented his or her concerns, successful litigation by the professional with impaired practice is highly unlikely. This is true even in the event that the professional may benefit personally from reporting the individual (Reid, 1999).

If a healthcare professional subverts the reporting process and chooses to cover the mistakes or duties of their colleague or, worse yet, treats the colleague with a substance use disorder, he or she is jeopardizing his or her license. "Treating a fellow clinician without reporting a patient-threatening condition may seem humane, but is usually a real mistake" (Reid, 1999, p. 293). A healthcare professional who chooses this approach is legally and ethically in jeopardy.

A healthcare professional who chooses to report the suspected impaired practice should document his or her concerns and address these concerns in terms of facts to the appropriate resource. This resource is defined by state law and may be an administrator, a licensing board, or a professional organization. The healthcare professional should carefully consider the ramifications of confronting his or her colleague with his or her suspicions. If he or she chooses to discuss his or her suspicions of impaired practice with this colleague, it is important to address the facts, the effect on patient safety, and the opportunity for treatment. This should not be a punitive discussion, but a discussion that is both factual and hopeful. An approach similar to motivational interviewing may be employed. State concerns; provide facts that describe reasons for concerns (it helps to focus on patient safety); and remind the colleague that compassion, treatment, and rehabilitation are the goals of care for the healthcare professional and that treatment is available. Remember: minimization, denial, and rationalizations are the hallmarks of a substance use disorder. The professional must not accept a colleague's promise to report him- or herself for treatment. If the colleague agrees to treatment, the professional may offer to accompany the colleague when he or she reports him- or herself (either in person or by telephone while you listen in on an extension). If the colleague is unwilling to seek care and denies impaired practice, the professional must report his or her concerns to the appropriate resource.

Patient safety and treatment are the goals of the intervention; this is done best with assistance of a supervisor and appropriate employee assistance program (EAP) personnel. The information and the intervention are considered confidential. Currently, 37 states offer non-disciplinary, confidential, and voluntary programs for healthcare professionals with substance use disorders that do not result in loss of licensure (Blair, 2002). The success of these treatment programs rely on defined reporting and intervention processes; support groups such as Narcotic Anonymous or a Alcoholics Anonymous; random drug/alcohol screening; and return-to-work contracts. These contracts include the recovering professional, the EAP, and the treatment program (ANA, n.d.). The recovering healthcare professional typically participates in these programs for at least 2 to 3 years or longer.

After the recovering professional returns to work, safeguards are put in place to protect the individual and the institution. The recovering professional should be assigned to areas with limited drug availability and should not be dispensing opioids or holding the keys that will access opioids. He or she should not be floating or working in relatively unstructured clinical areas and should be on a predictable schedule allowing for the opportunity to participate in meetings and rehabilitation (Blair, 2002; Dunn, 2005).

SUMMARY

In summary, the importance of early identification of an impaired colleague with timely reporting to an appropriate administrator is critical to the rehabilitation of the professional and the protection of the patient. Table 17-4 provides a list of internet resources that focus on identifying treatment of healthcare professionals with impaired practice.

TABLE 17-4: INTERNET RESOURCES FOR IMPAIRED PRACTICE IN THE HEALTHCARE PROFESSIONS
American Society of Addiction Medicine, www.asam.org
Association of Social Work Boards, http://www.aswb.org
Exceptional Nurse, www.exceptionalnurse.com
Hazelden Foundation, www.hazelden.org
International Nurses Society on Addictions, www.intnsa.org
National Association of Social Workers, www.socialworkers.org
National Institute on Alcohol Abuse and Alcoholism, www.niaaa.nih.gov
National Organization of Alternative Programs, www.alternativeprograms.org

EXAM QUESTIONS

CHAPTER 17

Questions 96-100

Note: Choose the one option that BEST answers each question.

96. Impaired practice by a healthcare professional is best defined as

    a. impaired clinical practice due to a substance use disorder that jeopardizes the quality and safety of patient care.
    b. direct clinical practice that occurs under the influence of drugs or alcohol.
    c. clinical practice that involves direct and indirect patient care, which occurs under the influence of drugs or alcohol.
    d. a trend of persistently impaired clinical practice that occurs under the influence of illegal substances.

97. The prevalence of impaired practice in health care workers is

    a. significantly lower than the general public – approximately 3.0%.
    b. the same as the general public – approximately 8.5%.
    c. significantly higher than the general public – approximately 12%.
    d. unknown; the risks of disclosing substance abuse are too great.

98. The last clinical indicator of the progression of a substance use disorder in an addicted healthcare professional's life is usually problems with

    a. family.
    b. community.
    c. finances.
    d. job performance.

99. The healthcare professional who chooses to perform the tasks of his or her impaired colleague while personally offering treatment is

    a. providing a humane approach to the problem.
    b. legally and ethically in jeopardy.
    c. protecting the colleague's career while the colleague seeks help.
    d. making the best of a very difficult situation.

100. The importance of early reporting of an impaired healthcare professional is initiation of a referral to an employee assistance program. This referral and subsequent treatment is most likely to result in the clinician's

     a. loss of licensure for a 2- to 3-year period.
     b. return to work with safeguards to protect him or her and the institution.
     c. disclosure of his or her impairment to his or her colleagues and asking for forgiveness.
     d. inability to work in a health care institution for at least 2 years.

This concludes the final examination.
Please answer the evaluation questions found on page v of the accompanying instruction booklet.

REFERENCES

American Nurses Association. (n.d.). *Impaired nurses resource center.* Accessed March 15, 2013, from http://www.nursingworld.org/MainMenuCategories/WorkplaceSafety/Healthy-Work-Environment/Work-Environment/ImpairedNurse

American Nurses Association. (2001). *Code of ethics for nurses.* American Nurses Publishing: Washington, D.C. Accessed March 15, 2013, from http://www.nursingworld.org/MainMenuCategories/ThePracticeofProfessionalNursing/EthicsStandards/CodeofEthics.aspx

Association of Social Work Boards. *Model social work practice act.* Accessed March 15, 2013, from http://www.aswb.org/pdfs/Model_law.pdf

Blair, P.D. (2002). Report impaired practice-stat. *Nursing Management, 33*(1), 24-5, 51.

Coombs, R.H.(1997). *Drug-impaired professionals.* Boston: Harvard University Press.

Dunn, D. (2005). Substance use among nurses – Defining the issues. *AORN Journal, 82*(4), 573-82, 585-8, 592-96.

Kenna, G.A. & Wood, M.D. (2004). Substance use by pharmacy and nursing practitioners and students in a northeastern state. *American Journal of Health-System Pharmacists, 61*(9), 921-930.

Kessler R.C., Berglund P., Demler O., Jin R., Merikangas K.R., & Walters E.E. (2005). Lifetime prevalence and age-of-onset distributions of *DSM-IV* disorders in the National Comorbidity Survey Replication. *Archives of General Psychiatry, 62*(6), 593-602.

Kessler, R.C., Chiu W.T., Demler, O., Merikangas, K.R., & Walters, E.E. (2005). Prevalence, severity, and comorbidity of 12-month DSM-IV disorders in the National Comorbidity Survey Replication. *Archives of General Psychiatry, 62*(6), 617-27.

Lillibridge, J., Cox, M., & Cross, W. (2002). Uncovering the secret: Giving voice to the experiences of nurses who misuse substances. *Journal of Advanced Nursing, 39*(3), 219-229.

Monahan, G. (2003). Drug use/misuse among health professionals. *Substance Use & Misuse, 38*(11-13), 1877-1881.

National Association of Social Workers. (2008). *Code of ethics.* NASW Press. Accessed March 15, 2013, from http://www.socialworkers.org/pubs/code/code.asp

Noland, S. & Halstad, W.S. (1991) Idiosyncrasies of a surgical legend. *Harvard Medical Alumni Bulletin, 65,* 17-23.

Ponech, S. (2000). Telltale signs. *Nursing Management, 31*(5), 32-38.

Reid, W. (1999). Law and psychiatry-impaired colleagues. *Journal of Practical Psychiatry and Behavioral Health, 9,* 291-293.

Siebert, D.C. (2003). Denial of AOD use: An issue for social workers and the profession. *Health & Social Work, 28*(2), 89-97.

Siebert, D.C. (2005). Help seeking for AOD misuse among social workers: Patterns, barriers and implications. *Social Work, 50*(1), 65-75.

Talbott, G. & Wilson, C. (2004). In J.H. Lowinson, P. Ruiz, R.B. Millman, & J.G. Langrod (Eds.), *Substance abuse: A comprehensive textbook* (4th ed.). Philadelphia: Lippincott Williams & Wilkins.

Trinkoff, A.M. & Storr, C.L. (1998). Substance use among nurses: Differences between specialties. *American Journal of Public Health, 88*(4), 581-585.

RESOURCES

INTERNET RESOURCES

Alcoholics Anonymous (AA)
http://www.aa.org

American Nurses Association
http://www.nursingworld.org

American Society of Addiction Medicine
http://www.asam.org

Association of Social Work Boards
http://www.aswb.org

Center for Substance Abuse Treatment
http://www.samhsa.gov/about/csat.aspx

Centers for Disease Control and Prevention
http://www.cdc.gov

Department of Health and Human Services. Tobacco: Quick Reference Guide for Clinicians – Treating Tobacco Use and Dependence
http://health.state.tn.us/Downloads/TQL_Quick%20Reference.pdf

Department of Health and Human Services, Agency for Health Care Research and Quality
http://www.ahrq.gov

Drugs of Abuse
http://www.justice.gov/dea/docs/drugs_of_abuse_2011.pdf

KCI: The Anti-Meth Site
http://www.kci.org

National Association of Social Workers
http://www.socialworkers.org

National Clearinghouse for Alcohol and Drug Information
http://store.samhsa.gov/home

National Institute on Alcohol Abuse and Alcoholism (NIAAA)
http://www.niaaa.nih.gov

National Institute on Drug Abuse (NIDA)
http://www.nida.nih.gov

National Institute on Drug Abuse: Preventing drug abuse among children and adolescents
http://www.drugabuse.gov/Prevention/risk.html

Smoking and Nicotine Abuse Prevention Resources
http://www.cdc.gov/tobacco/stateandcommunity/index.htm

Society for Research on Nicotine and Tobacco
http://srnt.org/

Substance Abuse and Mental Health Administration
http://www.samhsa.gov

Substance Abuse Treatment Facility Locator
http://dasis3.samhsa.gov

The Caffeine Awareness Alliance
http://www.caffeineawareness.org

U. S. Public Health Service
http://www.surgeongeneral.gov

Why Quit News
http://whyquit.com

World Health Organization
http://www.who.int/en

TEXTS

Frances, R.J., Miller, S.I., & Mack, A.H. (Eds.). Clinical textbook of addictive disorders (3rd ed.). New York: Guilford Press, 2005.

International Nurses Society on Addictions. (2006). *The core curriculum of addiction nursing* (2nd ed.). United States.

Ruiz, P. & Strain, E. (Eds.). *Lowinson and Ruiz's Substance abuse: A comprehensive textbook* (5th ed.). Philadelphia: Lippincott Williams, & Wilkins, 2011.

GLOSSARY

abstinence: Refraining from use of a drug an individual was addicted to.

abstinence syndrome: A constellation of symptoms occurring as a result of sudden withdrawal from a particular substance.

abuse: A maladaptive pattern of substance use leading to clinically significant impairment or distress.

addiction: Compulsive physical or psychological need for a substance.

agonist: A substance that binds to and activates its receptor.

antagonist: A substance that binds to but does not activate its receptor.

applied epidemiology: The application or practice of epidemiology to address public health issues.

cannabinoids: Chemicals that help control mental and physical processes when produced naturally by the body and that produce intoxication and other effects when absorbed from marijuana.

carbohydrate deficient transferring: A laboratory marker for chronic alcohol use.

cocaethylene: A product produced by the body when cocaine and alcohol are consumed simultaneously.

cycling: Technique of alternating between use and non-use of steroids to decrease unwanted adverse effects.

depressant: Drugs that dampen function of the central nervous system.

detoxification: Withdrawing clients from substances safely and effectively.

dopamine: A brain chemical classified as a neurotransmitter that is found in regions of the brain that regulate movement, emotion, motivation, and pleasure.

dysphoria: An emotional state characterized by irritability, anxiety, and depression.

epidemiology: A discipline basic to all fields of public health that may be defined as the study of the distribution and dynamics of disease in human populations. Its purpose is to identify factors relative to people and their environment to determine the occurrence of disease and to provide a basis for programs in preventive medicine and public health. Epidemiologic methods are used to assess the variance, severity, and magnitude of disease and related risks and resource needs; to evaluate the efficacy of new preventive and therapeutic treatments; and to evaluate the impact of new organizational patterns of health care delivery.

gamma glutamyl transpeptidase: A hepatic enzyme reflecting liver cell damage.

hippocampus: An area of the brain crucial for learning and memory.

hydrocarbon: Any chemical compound containing only hydrogen and carbon.

incidence rate: A measure of the frequency with which an event, such as a new case of illness, occurs in a population over time. The denominator is the population at risk; the numerator is the number of new cases occurring during a given period.

indicated prevention: A strategy designed for persons who are identified as having minimal but detectable signs or symptoms or precursors of some illness or condition, but whose condition is below the threshold of a formal diagnosis of the condition.

inhalants: Volatile solvents and substances that produce chemical vapors that are inhaled for purposes of producing a mind-altering effect.

norepinephrine: A neurotransmitter of the brain that affects regulation of arousal.

physical dependence: Occurrence of an abstinence syndrome after abrutpt total withdrawal or substantial reduction from the offending drug.

prevalence rate: The proportion of persons in a population who have a particular disease or attribute at a specified point in time or over a specified period.

prevention: The public health model of prevention includes primary, secondary, and tertiary prevention. An Institute of Medicine committee (1994) set forth another definition in which prevention refers to those interventions that take place before the onset of a disorder.

protective factors: Factors that include individual resilience and other circumstances that reduce the likelihood to substance use.

pseudoaddiction: Drug behaviors seen as a result of inadequate pain management.

psychedelic: 1960s term for the class of drugs that produces visionary effects.

psychoactive: Having a specific effect on the mind.

psychological dependence: Craving a drug or its effects.

resilience: The ability to quickly recover from problems or setbacks.

risk factors: Factors that increase a vulnerability to the initiation, continuation, or escalation of substance use.

selective prevention: Strategy designed for individuals who are members of population subgroups whose risk of developing an imminent or lifetime disease or disability is significantly above average.

serotonin: A neurotransmitter of the brain that affects regulation of hunger.

solvents: Industrial or household solvents or solvent-containing products, including paint thinners or solvents, degreasers (dry-cleaning fluids), gasoline, glues, art or office supply solvents, correction fluids, felt-tip marker fluid, and electronic contact cleaners.

stimulant: Classification of drugs that produces wakefulness and a sense of energy.

THC: Delta-9-tetrahydrocannabinol; the main active ingredient in marijuana that acts on the brain to produce its effects.

tolerance: When increasing amounts of drugs are needed to obtain the same level of effect.

universal prevention: Prevention designed for everyone in the eligible population, both the general public and all members of specific eligible groups.

volatile solvents: Liquids that vaporize at room temperature.

withdrawal: Symptoms that occur after use of a drug is reduced or stopped.

INDEX

T